Periodontal Re
Second E

MW01132220

Library of Congress Cataloging-in-Publication Data

Names: Termeie, Deborah, author.
Title: Periodontal review Q&A / Deborah A. Termeie.
Other titles: Periodontal review
Description: Second edition. | Batavia, IL : Quintessence Publishing Co,
    Inc, [2020] | Preceded by Periodontal review / Deborah A. Termeie.
    c2013. | Includes bibliographical references and index. | Summary:
    "Study guide review of periodontal literature on topics such as
    periodontal anatomy, diagnosis and treatment planning, nonsurgical and
    surgical therapy, regeneration, and implants, presented in a question
    and answer format"-- Provided by publisher.
Identifiers: LCCN 2019055802 (print) | LCCN 2019055803 (ebook) | ISBN
    9780867158298 (paperback) | ISBN 9781647240110 (ebook)
Subjects: MESH: Periodontal Diseases | Periodontics | Periodontium |
    Examination Question
Classification: LCC RK450.P4 (print) | LCC RK450.P4 (ebook) | NLM WU 18.2
    | DDC 617.6/32--dc23
LC record available at https://lccn.loc.gov/2019055802
LC ebook record available at https://lccn.loc.gov/2019055803

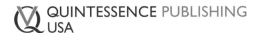
QUINTESSENCE PUBLISHING
USA

© 2020 Quintessence Publishing Co, Inc
Quintessence Publishing Co, Inc
411 N Raddant Road
Batavia, IL 60510
www.quintpub.com

5 4 3 2 1

Editor: Zachary Kocanda
Design: Sue Zubek
Production: Sarah Minor

Printed in the United States

Periodontal Review Q&A

Second Edition

Deborah A. Termeie, DDS
Clinical Instructor
Department of Periodontics
School of Dentistry
University of California, Los Angeles
Los Angeles, California

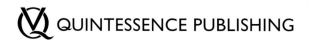 QUINTESSENCE PUBLISHING

Berlin | Chicago | Tokyo
Barcelona | London | Milan | Mexico City | Moscow | Paris | Prague | Seoul | Warsaw
Beijing | Istanbul | Sao Paulo | Zagreb

About the Author

Deborah A. Termeie, DDS, is a clinical instructor in the Department of Periodontics at the University of California, Los Angeles. She is a diplomate of the American Board of Periodontology (ABP), and it was her experience preparing for the ABP qualifying exams that inspired her to write this book. Dr Termeie is also an editor and author of *Avoiding and Treating Dental Complications: Best Practices in Dentistry* (John Wiley & Sons, 2016) and has published on the topics of evidence-based dentistry and implantology. She is the recipient of several awards, including the Excellence in Implantology Research award from the California Society of Periodontics, and has been invited to participate in the American Academy of Periodontics Leadership, Engagement, Action, and Development (LEAD) Program. She maintains a private practice in Beverly Hills, California.

Contents

Preface

The first edition of *Periodontal Review Q&A* was very well received, and I am grateful for the opportunity to author this second edition. The new edition contains many new figures, tables, and treatment planning cases as well as a comprehensive review of new classifications. I wrote this book because despite a plethora of study materials and information, there is no comprehensive single source study guide to help students prepare for their examinations. *Periodontal Review Q&A* was specifically written to address this void.

The material in this book is presented in a question and answer format for ease of study. The classic literature is cited as well as more recent and practical literature on topics such as diagnosis, nonsurgical therapy, surgical therapy, regeneration, and implants. Literature evidence for opposing viewpoints is also presented throughout the book. Additionally, each chapter contains clear and relevant tables, illustrations, and pictures. This comprehensive and yet concise approach to periodontics is aimed at preparing the candidate for periodontal examinations and clinical practice.

Periodontal Review Q&A is a useful resource for residents, practicing periodontists preparing for board certification, dental students, and dental hygiene students seeking a broader appreciation and in-depth understanding of periodontics. Topics chosen are those emphasized in periodontal residency graduation examinations as well as the oral examination of the American Board of Periodontology. Readers are urged to study all literature preceding their examination, including literature that may be made available subsequent to this textbook's publication.

Acknowledgments

I would like to acknowledge my mentors, Drs Philip R. Melnick, Thomas N. Sims, Paulo M. Camargo, Thomas Han, Henry H. Takei, and Perry R. Klokkevold, for their advice and guidance. Thank you to all the reviewers, Drs Dennis P. Tarnow, Russell Christensen, Jack G. Caton, Michael P. Rethman, Mary E. Neill, and Sejal R. Thacker.

I would like to thank my loving husband, David; my children, Gabriella and Elliot; and my parents. Without their love and support this book would not have been possible.

I appreciate Quintessence and the editorial staff, especially Zachary Kocanda and Bryn Grisham, whose knowledge and dedicated care to every word and idea made this book what it is.

Evidence-Based Dentistry

1

Background

Q: What is the evidence-based approach?

Evidence-based dentistry is the merging of clinically pertinent scientific evidence to the patient's oral and medical condition and history as well as the dentist's experience (Fig 1-1). The dentist uses the evidence to make sound decisions about diagnosis, prognosis, and treatment. Evidence-based decision making consists of formulating patient-centered questions (Population-Intervention-Comparison-Outcome [PICO]); examining and critically evaluating the evidence; and relating the evidence to practice.[1]

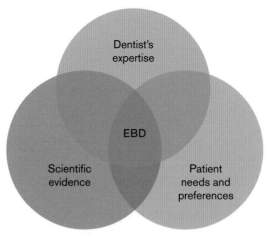

Dentist's expertise

EBD

Scientific evidence

Patient needs and preferences

Fig 1-1 Three parts of the decision-making process. (Redrawn from the American Dental Association[1] with permission.)

Q: What is the PICO question?

The *PICO question* is a question that includes a *p*opulation to be examined, the nature of the *i*ntervention to be inspected, a *c*omparison statement, and the type of *o*utcome to be evaluated. It should be problem-focused and concise.

Example: In patients with horizontal alveolar ridge deficiencies (population), what is the effect of horizontal bone augmentation procedures (intervention) compared with controls (comparison) on peri-implant health (outcome)?

Q: What is the step-by-step process for making an evidence-based decision in a dental practice?

The steps involved in evidence-based decision making in a dental practice are shown in Fig 1-2.

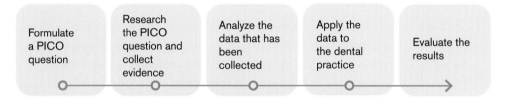

Fig 1-2 Evidence-based decision making. (Based on data in Chiappelli et al.[2])

Studies

Q: What are the different study types (ranked from highest level of evidence to lowest)?

The different types of studies are shown, ranked in order of highest to lowest level of evidence, in Fig 1-3.

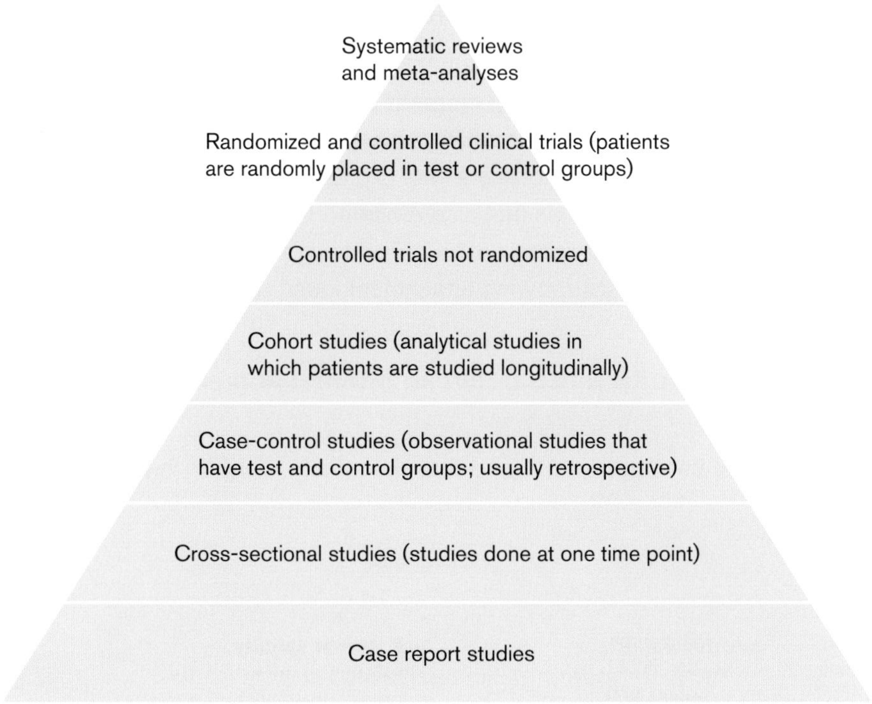

Systematic reviews
and meta-analyses

Randomized and controlled clinical trials (patients
are randomly placed in test or control groups)

Controlled trials not randomized

Cohort studies (analytical studies in
which patients are studied longitudinally)

Case-control studies (observational studies that
have test and control groups; usually retrospective)

Cross-sectional studies (studies done at one time point)

Case report studies

Fig 1-3 Different studies ranked from highest level of evidence to lowest. (Based on Nocini et al.[3])

Q: Describe the difference between a cross-sectional study and a longitudinal study.

A cross-sectional study is done at one time point, whereas a longitudinal study ranges over a period, allowing temporal relationships to be investigated.

Q: What is the P value?

The P value is the probability of obtaining a test statistic at least as extreme as the one observed, assuming that the null hypothesis is true. The smaller the P value, the less likely the effect was due to chance. A P value less than or equal to .05 usually indicates statistical significance.

Q: What is the difference between sensitivity and specificity?

Sensitivity is the ability of a test to correctly identify diseased individuals. *Specificity* is the ability of a test to correctly identify a healthy individual.

For instance, the diagnostic sensitivity of a clinical parameter (suppuration, gingival plaque) in predicting disease was expressed as the proportion of sites showing attachment loss that also exhibited the given parameter. Diagnostic specificity was expressed as the proportion of sites not exhibiting the clinical parameter and not showing attachment loss.[4]

Q: What is the difference between internal and external validity?

The difference between internal and external validity is shown in Fig 1-4.

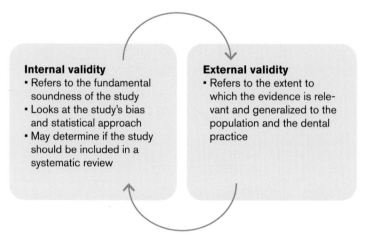

Internal validity
- Refers to the fundamental soundness of the study
- Looks at the study's bias and statistical approach
- May determine if the study should be included in a systematic review

External validity
- Refers to the extent to which the evidence is relevant and generalized to the population and the dental practice

Fig 1-4 Internal and external validity.

Q: Why practice evidence-based dentistry?[5]

1. There are thousands of articles published monthly in dental magazines. It would take hundreds of hours to read the dental literature. Using evidence-based review databases eases the necessary time spent evaluating dental literature.
2. Practicing evidence-based dentistry keeps dentists current on recent evidence and practice standards.
3. A thorough and analytical literature review should be carried out before proceeding in clinical research.

References

1. American Dental Association. About EBD. https://ebd.ada.org/en/about. Accessed 10 October 2019.
2. Chiappelli F, Brant XMC, Oluwadara OO, Neagos N, Ramchandani MH. Introduction: Research synthesis in evidence-based clinical decision-making. In: Chiappelli F, Brant XMC, Neagos N, Oluwadara OO, Ramchandani MH (eds). Evidence-Based Practice: Toward Optimizing Clinical Outcomes. London: Springer, 2010:5.
3. Nocini PF, Verlato G, De Santis D, et al. Strengths and limitations of the evidence-based movement aimed to improve clinical outcomes in dentistry and oral surgery. In: Chiappelli F, Brant XMC, Neagos N, Oluwadara OO, Ramchandani MH (eds). Evidence-Based Practice: Toward Optimizing Clinical Outcomes. London: Springer, 2010:151.
4. Haffajee AD, Socransky SS, Goodson JM. Clinical parameters as predictors of destructive periodontal disease activity. J Clin Periodontol 1983;10:257–265.
5. Boston University Alumni Medical Library website. Why practice EBM? www.bumc.bu.edu/medlib/resources/tutorials/introduction-to-evidence-based-medicine/ebm-intro-p10/. Accessed 12 Nov 2019.

Periodontal Anatomy

2

Anatomy

Q: Identify the anatomical structures of the periodontium shown below.

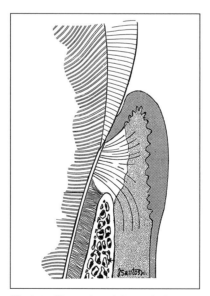

Fig 2-1a Illustration of the periodontium. (Reprinted from Fan and Berry[1] with permission.)

The answers are shown on the next page in Fig 2-1b.

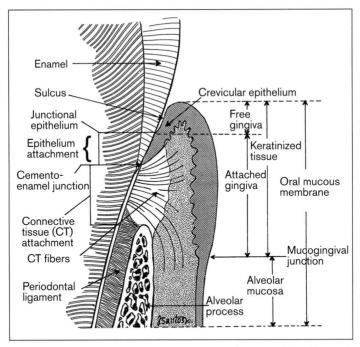

Fig 2-1b Labeled anatomy of the periodontium. (Reprinted from Fan and Berry[1] with permission.)

Q: Where does the vascular supply of the periodontium originate?

The external carotid artery and its main branches, which include the lingual, facial, and maxillary arteries, are the vascular supply for the periodontium. Locally, the blood supply comes from the supraperiosteal vessels and vessels from the periodontal ligament (PDL) and bone.[2]

Q: What is the main innervation for the periodontium?

The trigeminal nerve and its branches provide the main innervation for the periodontium.

Definitions

Q: What is attached gingiva?

The *attached gingiva* is the area from the base of the sulcus to the mucogingival junction. It prevents the free gingiva from being separated from the tooth. Its height is determined by subtracting the sulcus probing depth from the total width of the keratinized tissue. It consists of thick lamina propria and deep rete pegs. Goaslind et al[3] reported that the attached gingival thickness is 1.25 ± 0.42 mm.

Q: What is keratinized attached gingiva?

The *keratinized attached gingiva* is that found from the gingival margin to the mucogingival junction.

Q: What is alveolar mucosa?

Alveolar mucosa is the covering of the alveolar process that is nonkeratinized, unstippled, and movable. It extends from the mucogingival junction to the floor of the mouth and vestibular epithelium.

Q: What is clinical attachment loss (CAL)?

If the marginal gingiva is below the cementoenamel junction (CEJ):

CAL = pocket depth + [CEJ to marginal gingiva]

If the marginal gingiva is above the CEJ:

CAL = [marginal gingiva to CEJ] − [marginal gingiva to bottom of pocket]

Q: What is Ante's law?

Ante's law states that the root surface area of the abutment teeth must be equal to or greater than that of teeth being replaced with pontics. This helps determine the number of abutments needed for a fixed partial denture.

Gingival Epithelium

Q: What are the characteristics of healthy gingiva?

Healthy gingiva is coral pink, firm, follows the CEJ of the teeth, and may be stippled. The color of the gingiva is associated with the pigmentation of the patient. In dark-haired individuals, the gingiva can be darker than that in blond patients.

Q: What are the five types of gingival fibers?

There are five types of gingival fibers:

1. Dentogingival group: There are three types of fibers within this group.
   - Fibers extending coronally toward the gingival crest
   - Fibers extending laterally to the facial gingival surface
   - Fibers extending horizontally beyond the alveolar crest height and then apically along the alveolar bone cortex
2. Alveologingival group: Fibers in this group run coronally into the lamina propria from the periosteum at the alveolar crest.
3. Dentoperiosteal fibers: These fibers insert into the periosteum of the alveolar crest and fan out to the adjacent cementum.
4. Circular group: These are the only fibers that are confined to the gingiva and do not attach to the teeth.
5. Transseptal group: These fibers bridge the interproximal tissue between adjacent teeth and insert into the cementum.

Q: What is the composition of the oral mucosa (the tissue lining the oral cavity)?

The oral mucosa is composed of masticatory, lining, and specialized tissues (Fig 2-2).

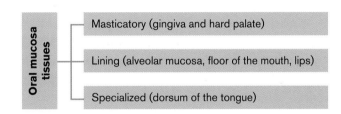

Fig 2-2 Composition of the oral mucosa. (Based on Avery.[4])

Oral mucosa tissues
- Masticatory (gingiva and hard palate)
- Lining (alveolar mucosa, floor of the mouth, lips)
- Specialized (dorsum of the tongue)

Q: What is the composition of the gingival epithelium?

The gingival epithelium consists of oral (masticatory), oral sulcular, and junctional epithelia (average width < 1 mm) (Fig 2-3).

Oral (masticatory) epithelium	Oral sulcular epithelium	Junctional epithelium
• Orthokeratinized, stratified squamous • Surface cells lose their nuclei and contain keratin • Made of the following: free gingiva (base of the sulcus to the free gingival margin, ie, the most coronal part of the gingiva), attached gingiva, and palatal tissue	• Epithelium that lines the sulcus • No rete pegs in healthy tissue	• Attaches to the tooth via a hemidesmosomal layer and a basal lamina • Nonkeratinized and has a fast turnover • Permeable • Most apical part lies at the CEJ in healthy tissue

Fig 2-3 Composition of the gingival epithelium. (Based on Clerehugh et al.[5])

Q: What are the four layers of cells that comprise the masticatory epithelium?

There are four layers of cells that comprise the masticatory epithelium[2]:

1. Stratum basale: Cuboidal cells found at the basement membrane; epithelial cell replication takes place in this location. This layer contains melanocytes and Merkel cells.
2. Stratum spinosum: The "spines" are desmosomes allowing intracellular contacts. It is the thickest layer and contains Langerhans cells, which are derived from bone marrow and take part in immune surveillance.
3. Stratum granulosum: Cells in this layer appear flat. Keratinocytes migrating from the underlying stratum spinosum become known as *granular cells* in this layer. These cells contain keratohyalin granules, protein structures that promote hydration and cross-linking of keratin. $\rightarrow$

4. Stratum corneum: Outermost layer containing dead cells and consisting of ortho- and parakeratinization. It is composed of compactly packed tonofilaments.

Q: Where are the widest and narrowest zones of gingiva?

The average thickness of the gingiva is 1.25 mm.[3] The widest zone of gingiva is in the maxillary anterior region; the narrowest zone is at the facial aspect of the mandibular first premolar.[2]

Connective Tissue

Q: What is the composition of connective tissue?

Connective tissue (average width slightly greater than 1 mm) is fibrous, consisting of mostly type I collagen, ground substances, and mucopolysaccharides. It also contains white blood cells, blood vessels, lymphatics, and nerves.[2]

Q: What determines whether epithelium is keratinized or nonkeratinized?

The underlying connective tissue determines whether the epithelium is keratinized.[6]

Q: What is periosteum? What is its function?

The *periosteum* is a highly vascular connective tissue sheath covering the external surface of all bones except areas of articulation and muscle attachment. It consists of an inner cambium layer (contains osteoblasts and osteoprogenitor cells) and an outer fibrous layer.[7]

The periosteum is involved in bone healing and bone regeneration.[8] It also serves as protection as well as a channel for the blood supply and nutrients for bone tissue.

Periodontal Ligament (PDL)

Q: Where is the average width of the PDL greatest and where is it narrowest?

The width of the PDL is greatest at the apex and narrowest in the middle. Older individuals have thicker fiber bundles in the PDL than younger individuals. The average width of the PDL is 0.2 mm.

Q: What provides the blood supply to the PDL?

Superior and inferior alveolar arteries provide the blood supply to the PDL, which is a vascular tissue.

Q: What are the functions of the PDL?

- Protect vessels and nerves
- Transmit occlusal forces
- Attach the tooth to bone
- Perform formative and remodeling functions

Q: What are the fibers of the PDL?

The fibers of the PDL include the alveolar crest, horizontal, oblique (most numerous), interradicular, and apical fibers.

Q: Describe and define ankylosis.

Ankylosis is the fusion of the cementum and alveolar bone with obliteration of the PDL. It develops after chronic periapical inflammation, tooth reimplantation, and occlusal trauma.

Alveolar Bone

Q: What is the composition of alveolar bone?

Alveolar bone consists of[2]:

- Cortical bone
- Cancellous trabeculae (more prevalent in the maxilla)
- Alveolar bone proper (lines the tooth socket)

Q: What are the functions of the alveolar bone?

The alveolar bone has three functions[2]:

1. Protection
2. Support
3. Calcium metabolism

Cementum

Q: Where are acellular cementum and cellular cementum located?

- Acellular cementum is located on the enamel at the CEJ. It does not contain cementocytes and forms slowly.
- Cellular cementum is located at the apical third of the root. It is more irregular and forms rapidly. With age, there is an increase in width of the cellular cementum.

Q: What percentage of the cementum and enamel overlap?

- 60% of the cementum and enamel overlap.
- 30% of the cementum and enamel form a butt joint.
- 10% of the cementum and enamel are separated by a gap.

Q: What is the difference between extrinsic and intrinsic cementum?

Extrinsic fibers are made of Sharpey fibers from the PDL, whereas intrinsic fibers are cementum fibers produced by cementoblasts (Fig 2-4).

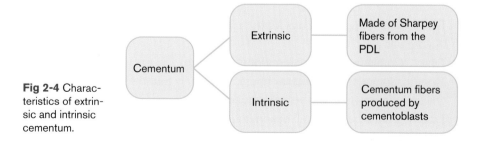

Fig 2-4 Characteristics of extrinsic and intrinsic cementum.

Cementum
- Extrinsic — Made of Sharpey fibers from the PDL
- Intrinsic — Cementum fibers produced by cementoblasts

Q: How does the junctional epithelium attach to the cementum?

The junctional epithelium attaches to the cementum via hemidesmosomes and replicates every 5 days.

Temporomandibular Joint (TMJ)

Q: What is the composition of the TMJ disc (meniscus)?

The TMJ disc is composed of dense connective tissue.

Q: Describe the movement of the TMJ.

The meniscus divides the joint into two compartments. The upper compartment has translational movement, and the lower compartment has rotational movement.

Q: What is meniscal derangement with and without reduction?

- With reduction: The disc as well as the posterior band of the meniscus is anteriorly displaced in front of the condyle upon opening. This causes a popping or clicking sound.
- Without reduction: In some patients, the meniscus remains anteriorly displaced at full opening. This is a much more serious condition.

Collagen

Q: Describe the four different types of collagen.

- Type I: Skin, tendon, vascular ligature, organs, bone (main component of the organic part of bone)
- Type II: Cartilage (main component of cartilage)
- Type III: Comprised of reticular fibers, commonly found alongside type I collagen, found mostly in smooth muscle
- Type IV: Forms basis of cell basement membrane

Supracrestal Tissue Attachment (Previously Biologic Width)

Q: What is supracrestal tissue attachment?

The *supracrestal tissue attachment* is defined as the physiologic dimension of the junctional epithelium and connective tissue attachment. It is measured from the most coronal part of the junctional epithelium to the crest of the alveolar bone. In studies on cadavers, Gargiulo[9] found a connective tissue attachment of 1.07 mm and a junctional epithelium attachment of 0.97 mm. Therefore, the supracrestal tissue attachment is about 2 mm. He also found the sulcus, which is not part of the supracrestal tissue attachment, to be 0.69 mm.

Q: What results from violation of the supracrestal tissue attachment?

If subgingival restorations violate the supracrestal tissue attachment, periodontal bone loss and inflammation may occur. The body will try to make room between the margin of the restoration and the alveolar bone to allow for reestablishment of the supracrestal tissue attachment.

Günay[10] did a study comparing crowns with interproximal margins placed at different distances from the alveolar bone. The three groups were ≤ 1 mm (I), 1 to 2 mm (II), and ≥ 2 mm (III) between crown margin and alveolar crest. It was observed that probing depth and papillary bleeding index was greater for group I (which had an encroachment of its crown margins within the supracrestal tissue attachment).

Miscellaneous

Q: What is the most common area of recurrent pockets?

The mesial aspect of the maxillary first premolars and first molars are the most common areas of recurrent pockets.

Q: What is the relationship between tooth support and root morphology?[11]

1. Root curvatures and concavities increase periodontal support because they increase the surface area and allow for multidirectional fiber orientation, which makes the tooth more stable.
2. Multirooted teeth have increased support and resistance to applied forces (the more coronal the furcation, the more stability).
3. Divergent roots increase stability and allow for more bone support.
4. Conical roots have less attachment area and are not as stable.
5. Enamel pearls can weaken periodontal attachment.
6. Root fractures can lead to periodontal destruction.

Many other factors can influence tooth stability, such as inflammation, occlusion, and the density and structure of bone.

Q: Which muscles elevate and depress the mandible?

- Elevate: Temporalis, medial pterygoid, and masseter
- Depress: Lateral pterygoid, digastric, and mylohyoid

References

1. Fan PP, Berry TG. Cast-gold restorations. In: Summitt JB, Robbins JW, Hilton TJ, Schwartz RS (eds). Fundamentals of Operative Dentistry: A Contemporary Approach, ed 3. Chicago: Quintessence, 2006:543.
2. Serio FG, Hawley C. Manual of Clinical Periodontics. Hudson, OH: Lexi-Comp, 2002.
3. Goaslind GD, Robertson PB, Mahan CJ, Morrison WW, Olson JV. Thickness of facial gingiva. J Periodontol 1977;48:768–771.
4. Avery J. Oral Development and Histology, ed 3. Stuttgart, Germany: Thieme Medical, 2002:250.
5. Clerehugh V, Tugnait A, Genco R.J. Periodontology at a Glance. Oxford: Wiley-Blackwell, 2009:3.
6. Karring T, Lang NP, Löe H. The role of gingival connective tissue in determining epithelial differentiation. J Periodontal Res 1975;10:1–11.
7. Mahajan A. Periosteum: A highly underrated tool in dentistry. Int J Dent. 2012;2012:717816.
8. Lin Z, Fateh A, Salem DM, Intini G. Periosteum: Biology and applications in craniofacial bone regeneration. J Dent Res 2014;93:109–116.
9. Gargiulo AW. Dimensions and relations of the dentogingival junction in humans. J Periodontol 1961;32:261–267.
10. Günay H, Seeger A, Tschernitschek H, Geurtsen W. Placement of the preparation line and periodontal health—A prospective 2-year clinical study. Int J Periodontics Restorative Dent 2000;20:171–181.
11. Scheid RC, Weiss G. Woelfel's Dental Anatomy, ed 8. Philadelphia: Wolters Kluwer, 2012:220.

Furcations

3

Background

Q: Define furcation lesion.

A *furcation lesion* has been defined as "the pathologic resorption of bone in the anatomic area of a multi-rooted tooth where the roots diverge."[1]

Q: What is the prevalence of furcation involvement?

In a study on periodontal patients, Svärdström and Wennström[2] found a greater prevalence of furcation involvement in maxillary molars than in mandibular molars. The narrowest furcation entrance was found on the buccal aspect of maxillary and mandibular molars, and the highest frequency of involvement was the distal aspect of the maxillary first molar. The mesial aspect of the second molar had the least frequency of furcation involvement.

Q: What is a furcation fornix?

The *furcation fornix* is the roof of the furcation.

Q: Is the Nabers probe a valid and efficient tool for detecting furcation invasion?

Eickholz and Kim[3] found that the Nabers probe, marked in 3-mm increments, is a valid method of diagnosing furcation lesions.

Classification

Q: Describe the Hamp classification.

The classification by Hamp et al[4] involves a horizontal measurement:

- F0: No furcation involvement.
- F1: The probe can penetrate the furcation less than 3 mm.
- F2: The furcation can be probed greater than 3 mm, but it is not a through and through furcation involvement.
- F3: Through and through furcation involvement.

Q: Describe the Glickman classification.

The Glickman[5] classification is presented in Fig 3-1.

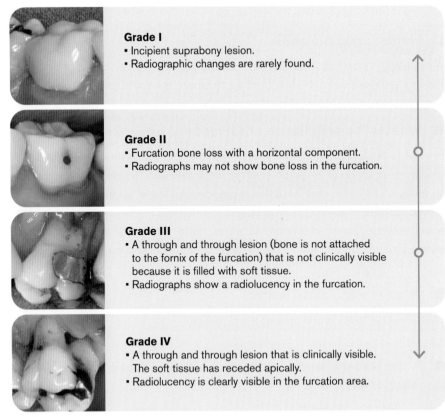

Grade I
- Incipient suprabony lesion.
- Radiographic changes are rarely found.

Grade II
- Furcation bone loss with a horizontal component.
- Radiographs may not show bone loss in the furcation.

Grade III
- A through and through lesion (bone is not attached to the fornix of the furcation) that is not clinically visible because it is filled with soft tissue.
- Radiographs show a radiolucency in the furcation.

Grade IV
- A through and through lesion that is clinically visible. The soft tissue has receded apically.
- Radiolucency is clearly visible in the furcation area.

Fig 3-1 Glickman classification.

Q: Describe the Tarnow classification.

The classification by Tarnow and Fletcher[6] is a subclassification of the Glickman furcation classification that measures the vertical probing depth from the roof of the furca:

- A: 0 to 3 mm
- B: 4 to 6 mm
- C: Greater than 7 mm

Treatment Options

Q: What are the treatment options for furcation defects?

- Nonsurgical debridement
- Surgical debridement
- Surgical exposure of the furcation
- Regeneration (guided tissue regeneration [GTR] and enamel matrix derivative [EMD])
- Extraction
- Root resection
- Tunnel preparation

Q: Is open/closed flap scaling and root planing effective in furcation lesions?

A review by Cobb[7] demonstrated a less favorable response to scaling and root planing by molars with furcation involvement compared with those without furcation lesions and single-rooted teeth. He surmised that this was related to the inability to remove all pathogenic microbial flora due to the furcal anatomy restricting access for mechanical therapy.

Bower[8] found that 81% of the time the furcation entrance is 1 mm or less. The study also found that 58% of the time the furcation entrance is 0.7 mm or less. The blade width of commonly used periodontal curettes is 0.75 mm. The ultrasonic (smaller) tip would fit better than the tip of a Gracey curette in a grade II or III furcation.

Wylam et al[9] found no significant difference between open and closed flap root planing. The study further concluded that root planing is inefficient in the debridement of furcation lesions and does not allow for periodontal regeneration.

Q: **What are guidelines for root resection?**[10]

Situations favorable for root resection:

- The candidate tooth is of critical importance to the overall dental treatment plan (abutments, important to a prosthesis).
- The tooth has enough attachment present to function.
- No other cost-effective therapy is available.
- Patient has good oral hygiene.

How to determine which root to remove:

- Remove the root that eliminates the furcation.
- Remove the root that has the greatest amount of bone and attachment loss.
- Remove the root that eliminates periodontal bone loss on adjacent teeth.
- Remove the root with the most anatomical problems.
- Remove the root that would complicate future treatment the least.
- The most common root resected is the distobuccal root of the maxillary first molar.

See chapter 10 for more information—eg, indications, contraindications—on root resections.

Q: **Would you have endodontic therapy done before a root resection and why?**

Endodontic therapy should be done prior to root resection for the following reasons:

- Little/no pain.
- It would be prudent to do the root canal therapy so that if a perforation, fracture, or other adverse outcome occurs, the patient does not have to have the resection done.[10]

Q: **Describe the technique for root resection.**[10]

1. Facial and lingual flaps are elevated.
2. Debridement and exposure of the furcation of the root to be resected.
3. Removal of a small amount of buccal or palatal bone to allow access for elevation and root removal.
4. An oblique cut is made with the high-speed handpiece using a carbide bur (surgical length) through the tooth.
5. The root is elevated from the socket, and if necessary odontoplasty and/or periodontal surgery are done on adjacent teeth. →

6. Sutures should be placed.
7. Occlusion may have to be adjusted because of removal of the root.

Q: **Can a grade I, II, III, IV furcation be treated successfully? Which treatment is the most effective?**

According to the 2015 consensus report from the American Academy of Periodontology[11] (Table 3-1):

Table 3-1	Most effective treatments
Hamp classification	**Most effective treatment**
F1	Regenerative therapy may be helpful, although generally F1 furcation defects may be treated successfully with non-regenerative therapies.
F2	Regenerative periodontal therapy should be considered before resective therapy or extraction. A combined therapeutic approach (membrane, bone graft with or without biologics) appears more beneficial over monotherapeutic algorithms.
F3	Proof of histologic periodontal regeneration in mandibular F3 defects is limited to one case report. Favorable outcomes after regenerative therapy for maxillary F3 furcation defects are limited to clinical case reports.

According to a systematic review by Huynh-Ba et al,[12] treatment for the maintenance of teeth with furcation defects (ie, open flap debridement [OFD], tunneling, root amputation, hemisection, and regeneration) are associated with high survival rate ranges, with GTR being the highest one with a survival rate range of 83.3% to 100% after 5 to 12 years. These survival rates are pretty close to implant survival rates in periodontal patients for the same time period (see implant chapter).

Huynh-Ba et al[12] also found the most recurrent complications after resective treatment were not related to periodontal disease but were related to endodontic failures and vertical root fractures. It is important to note that full furcation closure was not predictably attained following GTR or the application of EMD in maxillary and mandibular molars. →

Kinaia et al[13] did a meta-analysis and discovered, "guided tissue regeneration with the use of resorbable membranes was superior to non-resorbable membranes in vertical bone fill. Both types of membranes were more effective than open flap debridement in reducing vertical probing depths and gaining vertical attachment levels and in gaining vertical and horizontal bone."

Chen et al[14] did a meta-analysis and found that the GTR and GTR with osseous grafting (OG) groups obtained greater vertical/horizontal bone fill, furcation closure rate, and vertical/horizontal attachment level gain than the OFD group in mandibular molars. The GTR group obtained greater vertical attachment level gain and vertical/horizontal bone fill than the OFD group in maxillary molars. The GTR with OG group achieved better clinical outcomes than the GTR group did in all the studies comparing outcomes in mandibular molar.

Similarly, Murphy and Gunsolley[15] performed a systematic review and discovered that GTR is more effective than OFD in the treatment of furcation defects. The study also found that in furcation lesions vertical probing depth, vertical probing attachment levels, and horizontal open probing attachment levels—but no intrabony outcomes—were improved by augmentation with a particulate graft in conjunction with the GTR barrier.

Evans et al[16] reviewed 50 papers that studied 1,016 grade II furcations. The teeth had received various treatments such as bone grafts, OFD, and GTR. The study found complete closure of the furcation in 20% of the grade II furcations and an improvement of a grade II to a grade I furcation in 33% of the cases. In general, there was a 50% improvement for grade II furcations. The most effective treatment was a bone graft with GTR, and the least effective treatment was OFD (2% of the grade II furcations had complete closure).

Bowers et al,[17] who treated his patients with a combination therapy using an expanded polytetrafluoroethylene (ePTFE) membrane and demineralized freeze-dried bone allograft (DFDBA), discovered complete closure of grade II mandibular furcations in 50% of patients. There was a 68% improvement of a grade II to a grade I furcation.

Q: What factors influence the success of treatment?

Bowers et al[17] found poorer results in the treatment of furcation lesions in smokers. Smokers had a 62.5% chance of having a grade II residual defect compared with nonsmokers, who had a 14.3% chance. Furcation fill decreases at an increased horizontal and vertical presurgical probing attachment level (greater than 5 mm). The following were found to reduce the frequency of clinical closure: →

- Increased distance between the roof of the furcation and the crest of bone
- Increased distance between the roof of the furcation and the base of the defect
- The depth of the horizontal defect
- Increased divergence of roots at the crest of bone

Q: Are teeth that undergo the tunnel preparation in the furcation area prone to caries?

Hellden et al[18] studied 156 teeth with advanced periodontal furcation defects that were treated by tunnel preparations. The study found that 25% of the teeth developed caries.

A retrospective study by Feres et al[19] demonstrated that a history of root caries was the only factor with a positive association with caries incidence in tunnels.

Q: Are biologic mediators effective in furcation lesions?

Enamel matrix derivative (EMD)

Because grade II or III furcation defects are noncontained defects, the use of biologic materials has the significant limitation that, because of their fluid or gel-like quality, any space-making effect is prevented, and therefore the regenerative possibility of such tools may be inadequate in furcation lesions.[1]

A study by Araújo and Lindhe[20] used EMD and a barrier in the test defects and just a barrier in control defects. The test defect was found to have acellular cementum in the apical portion, while in the coronal portion a thick cellular cementum, similar to the cementum found in the control group, was detected. Both the test and control group furcation defects were found to be clinically closed and to contain bone and periodontal ligament tissue that appeared structurally similar to newly formed root cementum.

A randomized clinical trial by Jepsen et el[21] comparing membrane placement and EMD treatment of buccal grade II furcation involvement in mandibular molars found a significantly greater reduction in horizontal furcation depth and a comparatively lower incidence of postoperative swelling/pain following EMD compared to membrane therapy.

Although enamel matrix protein therapy has exhibited clinical improvements in the treatment of buccal grade II furcation defects in mandibular molars, complete closure of the furcation lesion is attained only in a minority of cases.[1]

$\rightarrow$

Recombinant human osteogenic protein-1 (OP-1)

Giannobile et al[22] found distinct stimulation of osteogenesis, regenerative cementum, and new attachment formation in sites treated with three different concentrations of OP-1.

Platelet-rich plasma (PRP)

Pradeep et al[23] reported that although the grade II status of the studied furcation defects was unchanged, sites treated with PRP showed a statistically significant difference in all clinical and radiographic parameters compared with those receiving OFD.

Anatomical Factors

Q: What anatomical factors are associated with furcation lesions?

The anatomical factors associated with furcation lesions are shown in Fig 3-2.

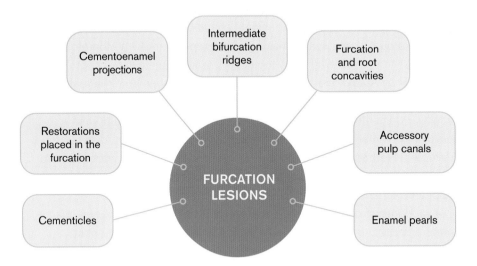

Fig 3-2 Anatomical factors associated with furcation lesions.

Q: **What percentage of molars have accessory canals in the furcation?**

Gutmann[24] studied 102 molars and found that 28.4% (29.4% of mandibular molars and 27.4% of maxillary molars) have accessory canals in the furcation.

Q: **What is the classification for cervical enamel projections?**

Masters and Hoskins[25] classified cervical enamel projections as follows:

- Grade 1: Extends from the CEJ to the furcation
- Grade 2: Approaches the furcation
- Grade 3: Extends into the furcation horizontally

Q: **What is the frequency of cervical enamel projections?**

Swan and Hurt[26] discovered that mandibular second molars had the highest incidence of cervical enamel projections (51.0%), while the lowest incidence was found in the maxillary first molars (13.6%). The most frequently encountered enamel projections in the study were grade 1, and the buccal surfaces were the most common location of cervical enamel projections.

Roussa[27] observed 60 teeth and discovered cervical enamel projections in 30% of the teeth examined.

Q: **Is there a relationship between cervical enamel projections and furcations?**

It is believed that the existence of cervical enamel projections inhibits connective tissue attachment and makes management of the furcation difficult.

Swan and Hurt[26] showed a positive correlation between grade 2 and grade 3 cervical enamel projections and periodontally involved furcations. However, the study did not find a relationship between grade 1 projections and furcation involvements.

A review by Lima and Hebling[28] found an association between cervical enamel projection, inflammatory periodontal disease, and molar furcation involvement.

Q: Describe how root concavities can affect prognosis of a tooth. Where are the concavities located on the first molars?

It is much more difficult to perform scaling and root planing on teeth with concavities, and as a result they can have a deleterious effect on the prognosis of a tooth. It is also challenging for the patient to maintain oral hygiene.

The root concavities for the first molars, as described by Bower,[29] are presented in Fig 3-3.

They are present in all two-rooted maxillary premolars.

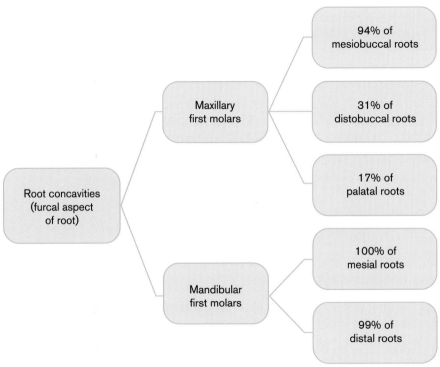

Fig 3-3 Anatomy of root concavities.

Q: How do different furcations compare in regard to entrance width?

The differences in furcation entrance width are as follows[29]:

- Mandibular molars: Buccal furcation entrance width is greater than lingual furcation entrance width. Further, the buccal furcation entrance in the mandibular first molar is positioned close to the cementoenamel junction (CEJ), whereas it is more apically located in the mandibular second molars.[1]

$\rightarrow$

▪ Maxillary molars: Mesial entrance width is greater than distal entrance width, which is greater than buccal entrance width. The mesial–palatal furcation entrance of the maxillary first molar is located close to the palatal third of the tooth, whereas the distal–palatal furcation is in the middle portion of the tooth.[1]

Q: Where are enamel pearls (see Fig 3-4) found most often? How can they contribute to furcation lesions?

According to Moskow and Canut,[30] enamel pearls (spherical in shape) have a tendency to originate in the furcation areas of molars, especially the maxillary second and third molars. The study found an incidence of 1.1% to 9.7%.

As with cervical enamel projections, the existence of enamel pearls inhibits connective tissue attachment and makes management of the furcation difficult.

Fig 3-4 Cone beam image of enamel pearl in the furcation of the mandibular left second molar.

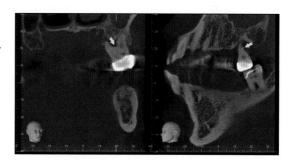

Q: How much attachment loss occurs for a furcation entrance to be observed in a maxillary molar?

According to Gher and Dunlap,[31] the mean distances from the CEJ to the mesial, facial, and distal furcation entrances are 3.6, 4.2, and 4.8 mm, respectively. Attachment loss of 6 mm is associated with a grade III furcation.

Q: How much surface area does each of the maxillary roots comprise?

According to Hermann et al,[32] the roots comprise the following surface areas:

▪ Mesiobuccal: 36%
▪ Palatal: 35%
▪ Distobuccal: 28%

Q: What is an intermediate bifurcation ridge? How can it contribute to a furcation lesion?

Everett et al[33] first described the ridges. He studied 328 mandibular teeth and found that 73% had an intermediate bifurcation ridge, which is cementum extending from the mesial to the distal of a furcation opening on a mandibular molar. Its existence can hamper effective plaque control by the patient and the dentist.

Q: Describe cementicles and their contribution to furcation lesions.

Cementicles are calcified masses adherent to or separated from the tooth's root. Similar to intermediate bifurcation ridges, they compromise effective scaling and root planing by the dentist and oral hygiene by the patient.

Restorations

Q: Do restored molars have a higher percentage of furcation lesions than teeth without restorations?

Wang et al[34] demonstrated a higher percentage of furcation involvement but no greater mobility in molars with a crown or proximal restoration when compared with nonrestored molars. Restored molars also showed a greater mean probing periodontal attachment loss than nonrestored molars, but the difference was only marginally significant.

References

1. Sanz M, Jepsen K, Eickholz P, Jepsen S. Clinical concepts for regenerative therapy in furcations. Periodontol 2000 2015;68:308–332.
2. Svärdström G, Wennström JL. Prevalence of furcation involvements in patients referred for periodontal treatment. J Clin Periodontol 1996;23:1093–1099.
3. Eickholz P, Kim TS. Reproducibility and validity of the assessment of clinical furcation parameters as related to different probes. J Periodontol 1998;69:328–336.
4. Hamp SE, Nyman S, Lindhe J. Periodontal treatment of multirooted teeth. Results after 5 years. J Clin Periodontol 1975;2:126–135.
5. Glickman I. Clinical Periodontology: The Periodontium in Health and Disease; Recognition, Diagnosis and Treatment of Periodontal Disease in the Practice of General Dentistry. Philadelphia: Saunders, 1953.
6. Tarnow D, Fletcher P. Classification of the vertical component of furcation involvement. J Periodontol 1984;55:283–284.

7. Cobb CM. Non-surgical pocket therapy: Mechanical. Ann Periodontol 1996;1:443–490.

8. Bower RC. Furcation morphology relative to periodontal treatment. Furcation entrance architecture. J Periodontol 1979;50:23–27.

9. Wylam JM, Mealey BL, Mills MP, Waldrop TC, Moskowicz DC. The clinical effectiveness of open versus closed scaling and root planing on multi-rooted teeth. J Periodontol 1993;64:1023–1028.

10. Ammons WF, Harrington GW. Furcation: Involvement and treatment. In: Newman MG, Takei HH, Klokkevold PR, Carranza FA. Carranza's Clinical Periodontology, ed 10. St Louis: Saunders, 2006:997.

11. Reddy MS, Aichelmann-Reidy ME, Avila-Ortiz G, et al. Periodontal regeneration—Furcation defects: A consensus report from the AAP Regeneration Workshop. J Periodontol 2015;86(2 suppl):S131–S133.

12. Huynh-Ba G, Kuonen P, Hofer D, Schmid J, Lang NP, Salvi GE. The effect of periodontal therapy on the survival rate and incidence of complications of multirooted teeth with furcation involvement after an observation period of at least 5 years: A systematic review. J Clin Periodontol 2009;36:164–176.

13. Kinaia BM, Steiger J, Neely AL, Shah M, Bhola M. Treatment of Class II molar furcation involvement: Meta-analyses of reentry results. J Periodontol 2011;82:413–428.

14. Chen TH, Tu YK, Yen CC, Lu HK. A systematic review and meta-analysis of guided tissue regeneration/osseous grafting for the treatment of Class II furcation defects. J Dent Sci 2013;8:209–224.

15. Murphy KG, Gunsolley JC. Guided tissue regeneration for the treatment of periodontal intrabony and furcation defects. A systematic review. Ann Periodontol 2003;8:266–302.

16. Evans GH, Yukna RA, Gardiner DL, Cambre KM. Frequency of furcation closure with regenerative periodontal therapy. J West Soc Periodontol Periodontal Abstr 1996;44(4):101–109.

17. Bowers GM, Schallhorn RG, McClain PK, Morrison GM, Morgan R, Reynolds MA. Factors influencing the outcome of regenerative therapy in mandibular Class II furcations: Part I. J Periodontol 2003;74:1255–1268.

18. Hellden LB, Elliot A, Steffensen B, Steffensen JE. The prognosis of tunnel preparations in treatment of class III furcations. A follow-up study. J Periodontol 1989;60:182–187.

19. Feres M, Araujo MW, Figueiredo LC, Oppermann RV. Clinical evaluation of tunneled molars: A retrospective study. J Int Acad Periodontol 2006;8(3):96–103.

20. Araújo MG, Lindhe J. GTR treatment of degree III furcation defects following application of enamel matrix proteins. An experimental study in dogs. J Clin Periodontol 1998;25:524–530.

21. Jepsen S, Heinz B, Jepsen K, et al. A randomized clinical trial comparing enamel matrix derivative and membrane treatment of buccal Class II furcation involvement in mandibular molars. Part I: Study design and results for primary outcomes. J Periodontol 2004;75:1150–1160.

22. Giannobile WV, Ryan S, Shih MS, Su DL, Kaplan PL, Chan TC. Recombinant human osteogenic protein-1 (OP-1) stimulates periodontal wound healing in class III furcation defects. J Periodontol 1998;69:129–137.

23. Pradeep AR, Pai S, Garg G, Devi P, Shetty SK. A randomized clinical trial of autologous platelet-rich plasma in the treatment of mandibular degree II furcation defects. J Clin Periodontol 2009;36:581–588.

24. Gutmann JL. Prevalence, location, and patency of accessory canals in the furcation region of permanent molars. J Periodontol 1978;49:21–26.

25. Masters DH, Hoskins SW. Projection of cervical enamel into molar furcations. J Periodontol 1964;35:49–53.

26. Swan RH, Hurt WC. Cervical enamel projections as an etiologic factor in furcation involvement. J Am Dent Assoc 1976;93:342–345.

27. Roussa E. Anatomic characteristics of the furcation and root surfaces of molar teeth and their significance in the clinical management of marginal periodontitis. Clin Anat 1998;11:177–186.

28. Lima AF, Hebling E. Cervical enamel projection related to furcation involvement. Braz Dent J 1994;5:121–127.

29. Bower RC. Furcation morphology relative to periodontal treatment. Furcation root surface anatomy. J Periodontol 1979;50:366–374.

30. Moskow BS, Canut PM. Studies on root enamel (2). Enamel pearls. A review of their morphology, localization, nomenclature, occurrence, classification, histogenesis and incidence. J Clin Periodontol 1990;17:275–281.

31. Gher MW Jr, Dunlap RW. Linear variation of the root surface area of the maxillary first molar. J Periodontol 1985;56:39–43.

32. Hermann DW, Gher ME Jr, Dunlap RM, Pelleu GB Jr. The potential attachment area of the maxillary first molar. J Periodontol 1983;54:431–434.

33. Everett FG, Jump EB, Holder TD, Williams GC. The intermediate bifurcational ridge: A study of the morphology of the bifurcation of the lower first molar. J Dent Res 1958;37:162–169.

34. Wang HL, Burgett FG, Shyr Y. The relationship between restoration and furcation involvement on molar teeth. J Periodontol 1993;64:302–305.

Epidemiology and Etiology

4

Risk Factors and Risk Indicators

Q: What is the difference between a risk factor and a risk indicator?

A *risk factor* is a characteristic that places an individual at increased risk of contracting a disease. A *risk indicator* is a probable or putative risk factor that has been identified in cross-sectional correlation studies but not confirmed through longitudinal studies.

Q: What are the risk factors for gingivitis and periodontitis?

Poor oral hygiene

- Listgarten[1] suggested increased plaque mass or reduced host defense may precipitate episodes of periodontal destruction.
- Löe et al[2] observed 480 tea plantation workers that were not exposed to preventive care for 15 years. They found that 8% of the population had rapid progression to periodontal disease, 11% had no progression, and 81% had moderate progression.

Dental plaque biofilm retention factors

- Certain tooth anatomical factors that facilitate plaque accumulation at and apical to the gingival margin (eg, enamel pearl).
- Subgingival restoration margins may be detrimental to gingival and periodontal health.[3] Another study found that when plaque control →

and periodontal maintenance measures are described, and the patient complies, subgingival margins do not act as a plaque retentive factor that causes gingivitis.[4]

- A direct or indirect restoration with overhanging margins can be associated with localized gingivitis, increase in pocket depth, and interproximal bone loss.[4]
- Tooth position (eg, crossbite, malalignment, and crowding).[4]

Oral dryness

- Reduced cleansing, which can lead to increased dental plaque and enhanced gingival inflammation.

Smoking

- Strongest modifiable risk factor and predictor of future disease.
- According to Grossi,[5] smokers are 2.7 times more likely to have periodontal disease than nonsmokers.
- Smokers have 18 times more periodontal pathogens compared with nonsmokers.

Diabetes

- Three times more bone loss and attachment loss has been found in patients with diabetes.
- After treatment of periodontal disease, there is a 10% drop in sugar levels.[6]

Genetics

- In a study by Kornman et al,[7] 86.0% of the severe periodontitis patients were either smokers or had the interleukin-1 genotype.
- According to Michalowicz et al,[8] 50% of enhanced risk for periodontitis can be accounted for by genetics alone.

Q: What are the risk indicators for periodontitis?

Following are the risk indicators for periodontitis:

- Age: Increased age is associated with increased extent and severity of chronic periodontitis.
- Sex: Male patients have poorer hygiene than female patients.
- Socioeconomic status: Those with lower socioeconomic status have less education and limited access to care. →

- Race: There is a greater incidence of periodontitis in black and Hispanic populations. Blacks were found to be at much greater risk of aggressive periodontitis than whites.[9]
- Obesity: Adipose tissue can produce cytokines, which can lead to a hyperinflamed state. Gorman et al[10] found that overall obesity and central adiposity are associated with an increased hazard of periodontal disease progression in men.
- Alcohol: Shepherd[11] found evidence suggesting that alcohol consumption is a risk indicator for periodontitis. Gay et al[12] found alcohol consumption was associated with an increase in the likelihood of having periodontitis, especially severe periodontitis.
- Stress: Genco et al[13] found that financial stress and the coping mechanism of the patient were related to periodontal disease. They found that the effects of stress on periodontal disease can be moderated by adequate coping behaviors.
- Contraceptives: There is a possible association between injectable progesterone contraceptives and poor periodontal health, as indicated by a study that found an increased likelihood of indicators of poor periodontal health, including gingivitis and periodontitis, in women who had taken or were currently taking depot medroxyprogesterone acetate (DMPA) injectable contraceptives.[14]
- Recreational cannabis: Researchers have discovered that recurrent recreational cannabis use—which includes marijuana, hashish, and hash oil—may be linked with elevated risk of periodontal disease. When compared to study participants who used cannabis less regularly, those who had taken it at least once a month for a year showed increased indicators of mild, moderate, and severe periodontal disease. The National Health and Nutrition Examination Survey 2011 to 2012[15] found frequent recreational cannabis is associated with deeper pocket depths, more clinical attachment loss, and higher odds of having severe periodontitis.

Epidemiology Terminology

Q: What is an odds ratio?

An *odds ratio* is the probability that a person with an adverse outcome was exposed to risk. An odds ratio that is greater than 1 has a positive association.

Q: What is the difference between sensitivity and specificity?

Sensitivity is the proportion of subjects with a disease who test positive, and *specificity* is the proportion of subjects without the disease who test negative. (See chapter 1.)

Q: What is the difference between prevalence and incidence?

Prevalence is defined as the total number of cases (or cases of the risk factor) in the population at a given time, divided by the number of individuals in the population. *Incidence* is a measure of the risk of developing a new condition within a specified period of time.

Prevalence is a good measure for generalized chronic periodontitis since it develops slowly over time. Incidence is a better tool for toothache since it usually has a rapid onset; however, a specified period of time measurement might miss a lot of cases.

Indices

Q: What is gingival crevicular fluid?

The volume of gingival crevicular fluid (GCF) has been adopted in clinical trials to measure the severity of gingival inflammation.[16] There is a strong relationship between GCF volume and other clinical parameters of gingival inflammation. Measuring GCF is a very reliable quantitative method to assess plaque-induced inflammation in a research setting; however, in clinical practice, measurement of GCF is challenging, time consuming, and costly.

Q: What is the Gingival Index?

The Gingival Index (GI; Löe[17]) incorporates bleeding on probing (BOP) and color change:

- 0: Normal gingiva
- 1: Mild inflammation, slight color change, slight edema, and no BOP
- 2: Moderate inflammation, redness, edema, glazing, and BOP
- 3: Severe inflammation, marked redness, edema, ulceration, and spontaneous bleeding →

BOP sites (GI = 2) have a higher chance of attachment loss compared to non-bleeding sites (GI = 0 or 1).[18]

The average GI in a representative American adult population that approximates a recent US Census is 1.055, with 93.9% of subjects having a GI ≥ 0.50 and 55.7% ≥ 1.00.[19]

Q: How is BOP assessed?

A BOP score is assessed as the proportion of bleeding sites (no/yes evaluation) when a standardized probe with a 25-g force is placed at the bottom of the sulcus at six sites (distobuccal, buccal, mesiobuccal, distolingual, lingual, and mesiolingual) on all present teeth.[16,20]

Q: What factors can increase BOP? Decrease BOP?

See Fig 4-1 below.

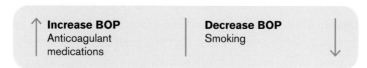

Fig 4-1 Factors that increase and decrease BOP.

Q: What is the modified Gingival Index?

Following is the modified Gingival Index:

- 0: Absence of inflammation
- 1: Mild inflammation, slight color change, and slight edema but not involving the entire marginal or papillary unit and no BOP
- 2: Mild inflammation, slight color change, and slight edema involving the entire marginal or papillary unit and no BOP
- 3: Moderate inflammation, redness, edema, glazing, BOP, and hypertrophy of the entire marginal unit
- 4: Severe inflammation: Marked redness and edema, ulceration with spontaneous bleeding

Q: How early can BOP occur?

BOP can occur as early as 2 days after gingivitis begins.

Q: Describe the Periodontal Index.

In the Periodontal Index (Russell[21]), the supporting tissues around the tooth are scored. Periodontal probing is not recommended.

- 0: Negative
- 1: Mild inflammation
- 2: Gingivitis
- 6: Gingivitis with pocket formation
- 8: Advanced destruction with loss of masticatory function

Q: What is the Periodontal Disease Index? What teeth are used in the index?

The teeth used in the Periodontal Disease Index (Ramfjord[22]) are the maxillary right first molar, left central incisor, and first premolar as well as the mandibular left first molar, right central incisor, and first premolar. The cementoenamel junction is used as the fixed landmark to measure periodontal attachment loss.

- G0: Absence of disease
- G1: Mild to moderate inflammation not extending around the tooth
- G2: Mild to moderate inflammation extending around the tooth
- G3: Severe gingivitis and redness

Q: What is the Plaque Index?

The Plaque Index (Löe[17]) is based on the thickness of soft deposits found around a tooth by running a probe along the gingival crevice.

- 0: No plaque
- 1: Film of plaque
- 2: Moderate accumulation of plaque within the gingival pocket or on the tooth and gingival margin that can be seen with the naked eye
- 3: Abundance of plaque within the gingival pocket or on the tooth and gingival margin

Prevalence of Gingivitis, Periodontitis, and Gingival Recession

Q: What is the prevalence of gingivitis?

Albandar and Kingman[23] found a prevalence of 32.3% (limited, 21.8%; extensive, 10.5%).

Mild localized clinical inflammation is found in 95% of the population.[24]

Q: What percentage of tooth extractions are caused by periodontitis?

According to Brown et al,[25] less than 20% of all missing teeth were recorded as missing as a result of periodontal disease.

Overall, in the general population, including people with and without periodontitis, mean annual attachment loss was 0.1 mm per year, and mean annual tooth loss was 0.2 teeth per year. Attachment loss per year for periodontitis patients is 0.6 mm.[26]

Q: What percentage of the population has aggressive, chronic, and severe periodontitis?

- Severe periodontitis is the sixth most prevalent disease of mankind, and it affects 11% of the world population with the prevalence increasing with age. The peak global incidence is at age 38.[27]
- Localized aggressive periodontitis: 0.53% (greater prevalence in blacks[9]; many studies have proposed that there may be a defect in neutrophil function)
- Generalized aggressive periodontitis: 0.13%

The 2009–2014 National Health and Nutrition Examination Survey[28] found the following data on the prevalence of periodontitis among adults in the United States:

- 42.2% of dentate adults 30 years or older had periodontitis: 7.8% with severe periodontitis and 34.4% with nonsevere (ie, mild to moderate) periodontitis.
- 3.3% of all periodontally probed sites or 9.1% of all teeth had probing depth of 4 mm or greater. →

- 19% of sites or 37.1% of teeth had clinical attachment loss of 3 mm or greater.
- Severe periodontitis was most prevalent among Mexican Americans, non-Hispanic blacks, smokers, and adults 65 years or older.
- Periodontitis significantly co-occurred with diabetes and increasing number of missing teeth but not obesity.

Q: What percentage of adults have gingival recession?

Cross-sectional epidemiologic studies have shown that 88% of people 65 years of age and older and 50% of people 18 to 64 years of age have one or more sites with recession.[29]

Association of Periodontitis with Other Conditions

Q: Is there a relationship between periodontitis and preterm births and low birth weight?

A *preterm birth* is defined as one that occurs before 37 weeks gestation; low birth weight is less than 2,500 grams. According to Offenbacher et al,[30] the incidence of preterm birth was 11.2% among women with no periodontal disease and 28.6% in women with moderate to severe periodontitis. Michalowicz et al[31] found treatment of periodontitis in pregnant women was safe and improved periodontitis, but it did not alter rates of preterm birth. Furthermore, nonsurgical periodontal therapy, ie, scaling and root planing, does not improve birth outcomes in pregnant women with periodontitis.[32]

López et al found: "The results of epidemiological, molecular, microbiological and animal-model studies support a positive association between maternal periodontal disease and preterm birth. However, the results of intervention studies carried out to determine the result of periodontal treatment on reducing the risk of preterm birth are controversial."[33]

Figure 4-2[34] presents the current theory of the relationship between periodontitis and preterm birth.

Ide and Papapanou[35] found preeclampsia is significantly associated with maternal periodontitis. →

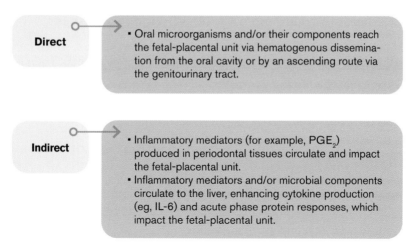

Direct → • Oral microorganisms and/or their components reach the fetal-placental unit via hematogenous dissemination from the oral cavity or by an ascending route via the genitourinary tract.

Indirect → • Inflammatory mediators (for example, PGE$_2$) produced in periodontal tissues circulate and impact the fetal-placental unit.
• Inflammatory mediators and/or microbial components circulate to the liver, enhancing cytokine production (eg, IL-6) and acute phase protein responses, which impact the fetal-placental unit.

Fig 4-2 Current theory of the relationship between periodontitis and preterm birth. PGE$_2$, prostaglandin E$_2$; IL, interleukin.

Q: Does food impaction contribute to periodontal pathosis?

Open contacts are correlated with food impaction, and food impaction is correlated with increased probing depth. However, there is no direct relationship between open contacts and increased pocket depth.[36]

Jernberg et al[37] found less plaque but increased probing depth and attachment loss at open contacts.

Q: Do overhanging dental margins contribute to periodontal pathosis?

Overhanging dental margins can be a nidus of periodontal pathogens due to their bulk and roughness and make dental hygiene challenging for the patient and the provider. Pack et al[38] studied 100 patients and found that the percentage of pockets greater than 3 mm was 64.3% among those adjacent to overhanging margins but only 49.2% in pockets neighboring restored surfaces in the absence of overhanging margins and 23.1% in those next to unrestored surfaces.

Brunsvold and Lane[39] found an increase in bleeding, gingivitis, and bone loss in tissues next to overhanging dental margins. They also reported that removal of the overhanging margins improved the effectiveness of hygiene procedures.

Q: Does mouth breathing affect the periodontal tissues?

Mouth breathing can cause dehydration of the gingival tissues, which can result in greater gingivitis in the anterior region. Gulati et al[40] found that in study participants with an incompetent lip seal, GI was higher in those who breathed through the mouth compared with those who breathed normally.

Q: Is there an association between malalignment of the teeth and periodontal disease?

With controls for social group and sex, periodontal disease was found more commonly in the maxilla in connection with overjet, crowding, and crossbite. No association was found in the mandible.[41]

Another study found significant periodontal disease progression associated with certain incisor malalignment qualities (ie, maxillary incisor crowding, maxillary incisor spacing, mandibular incisor mild crowding, mandibular incisor moderate-to-severe crowding, mandibular incisor moderate irregularity, and mandibular incisor severe irregularity).[42]

Smoking and Periodontal Disease

Q: What oral disorders is smoking associated with?

Smoking is associated with increased risk of root caries, impaired oral wound healing, oral pain, and a wide range of other oral soft tissue changes (eg, oral leukoplakia, nicotine stomatitis, acute necrotizing ulcerative gingivitis, halitosis, staining, dental plaque, and calculus).[43]

Q: How does smoking affect periodontitis?

Figure 4-3 presents the relationship of smoking and periodontitis. Smoking increases expression of the cytokines involved in periodontal destruction. Furthermore, the acrolein and acetaldehyde in smoke inhibit human gingival fibroblasts. Lastly, it can cause negative effects on polymorphonuclear leukocytes (PMNs), causing abnormal phagocytosis.

- Grossi et al[44] found that heavy smokers have six to seven times more alveolar bone loss.
- It has also been shown that 90% of persons with refractory periodontitis are smokers.[45] $\rightarrow$

- Haffajee and Socransky[46] found that smokers have increased bacteria subgingivally.
- An association has been shown between the prevalence of moderate to severe periodontal disease and the number of cigarettes smoked and years that the patient has smoked. Attachment loss severity was increased by 0.5% by smoking one cigarette per day, while smoking up to 10 and 20 cigarettes a day increased attachment loss by 5% and 10%, respectively.[47]

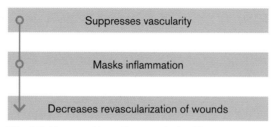

Suppresses vascularity

Masks inflammation

Decreases revascularization of wounds

Fig 4-3 How smoking affects periodontitis.

Q: How does smoking affect healing after surgery?

- There are differing conclusions on smoking's effect on the success of subepithelial connective tissue grafts.[48,49] Martins et al[50] found a correlation between failure to cover the root and heavy smoking.
- Root coverage following a free gingival graft is diminished by heavy cigarette smoking. A 100% correlation between failure to obtain root coverage and heavy smoking (ie, greater than 10 cigarettes a day) was reported.[51]
- Clinical attachment improvements are also less in smokers as compared to nonsmokers after regenerative procedures.[52,53]
- Smoking is a factor that has the potential to negatively affect the outcome of implant treatment and healing.[54] Studies have shown that implant success rates are reduced in smokers.[55]

Q: How should a dentist manage a patient who smokes?

The dental professional should follow the five As for managing patients who smoke[43,56]: $\longrightarrow$

1. Ask about smoking at each appointment (eg, "Do you ever smoke or use any type of tobacco?").
2. Advise and educate the patient on the benefits of quitting. In a strong, clear, nonjudgmental, and personalized manner, urge every tobacco user to quit (eg, "It is important you know that quitting smoking can protect your current and future health.").
3. Assess the patient's willingness to quit (eg, "Would you be willing to try to quit in the next couple of months? If so, the office can help.").
4. Assist the patient with developing a plan to quit.
5. Arrange for follow-up visits. Ask the patient again at the next visit.

Q: Does smoking cessation affect periodontal therapy?

Kaldahl et al[57] found that a history of smoking did not adversely affect the outcome of therapy: Both past smokers and nonsmokers responded more favorably to therapy compared with heavy and light smokers. Hyman and Reid[58] found the adjusted odds ratios for mean loss of attachment were greatest for current smokers and decreased for former smokers as the number of years since quitting smoking increased.

Hujoel et al[59] estimated that severe periodontitis incidence decreased 31% from 1955 to 2000, attributable to a decrease in the number of smokers in the United States population.

Q: Is there a difference between smoking a pipe or cigars versus cigarettes?

In a study on 690 dentate men, Krall et al[60] found an increased risk for tooth loss in men who smoked cigars or pipes and for alveolar bone loss in cigar smokers similar to that observed in cigarette smokers. As a result, the authors recommended that smoking prevention and cessation programs should be targeted to users of all tobacco products.

Tverdal and Bjartreit[61] found that pipe smoking is not safer than cigarette smoking.

Q. How does vaping affect the periodontal tissues?

Sundar et al[62] observed that e-cigarettes with flavorings produce increased oxidative/carbonyl stress and inflammatory cytokine release in human peri-odontal ligament fibroblasts. →

Wadia et al[63] found that replacement of smoking with vaping was associated with a statistically significant increase in gingival BOP.

Biofilms and Plaque

Q: What are some characteristics of biofilms?

Biofilms are dynamic and optimally organized to make use of nutrients. They have greater stability, more cohesiveness, and greater antibiotic resistance compared with their free-living counterparts.

Q: What are plaque and calculus?

Plaque is an organized mass consisting mainly of microorganisms that adhere to the teeth. It consists of bacterial byproducts such as enzymes, food debris, calcium, and phosphate. The organic composition is polysaccharides and proteins, and the inorganic composition is calcium and phosphorus. *Calculus* is made of calcium phosphate salts.

Q: What are the specific and nonspecific plaque hypotheses (Loesche and Giordano[64])?

- Specific plaque hypothesis: Only certain microorganisms cause disease.
- Nonspecific plaque hypothesis: Periodontitis and caries are the result of noxious agents from the entire bacterial population.

Bacteria

Q: Describe the bacteria present in periodontitis.

Table 4-1 presents the properties of bacteria found in periodontitis.[65,66] →

Table 4-1	Bacteria in periodontitis				
Bacteria	**Oxygen requirement**	**Motility**	**Properties**		**Virulence factors**
Aggregatibacter actinomycetem-comitans	Facultative anaerobe	Nonmotile	• Short, gram-negative rod • Fibroblast inhibiting factor • Lymphocyte suppressing factor • Associated with localized aggressive periodontitis		• Leukotoxin: Kills PMNs and macrophages • Lipopolysaccharide (LPS): Produces collagenase and can induce bone resorption • Hemolytic
Porphyromonas gingivalis	Obligate anaerobe	Nonmotile	• Gram-negative, non–spore forming • Contains porphyrin pigments and fimbriae • *Bacteroides* genus • Associated with advanced periodontal disease		• Gingipains cleave the host proteins between arginine and lysine • Significant hemolytic activity • LPS: Produces collagenase and can induce bone resorption • Inhibits interleukin 8
Prevotella intermedia	Anaerobe	Nonmotile	• Gram-negative, black pigmented • Contain fimbriae • Common in pregnancy because of increased steroid uptake • Common in patients with necrotizing ulcerative gingivitis		• High hemolytic activity • Matrix metalloproteinases destroy the connective tissue • Involved in actin polymerization of the cytoskeleton

Table 4-1 (cont)	Bacteria in periodontitis			
Bacteria	**Oxygen requirement**	**Motility**	**Properties**	**Virulence factors**
Fusobacterium nucleatum	Anaerobe (can grow in 6% oxygen)	Nonmotile	• Gram-negative, non–spore forming, spindle shaped • Principal and frequent bacterial species associated with gingivitis and periodontitis	• Butyric acid: Inhibits fibroblasts and decreases wound healing • Can act as a bridge between other-wise noncoagulating pairs of species • PMN apoptosis • Supports growth of *P gingivalis* in oxygenated or carbon dioxide–depleted environments • LPS: Produces collagenase and can induce bone resorption
Tannerella forsythia	Anaerobe	Nonmotile	• Gram-negative, filament shaped • Found in refractory and advanced periodontitis • Associated with early implant failure	• Contains a surface layer that is believed to delay the host immune response[65] • Trypsin-like protease • Hemolytic activity • Sialidase involved in tissue destruction • Bacterial surface protein A is involved in binding and induces an antibody reaction in periodontal disease[66]
Treponema denticola	Anaerobe	Highly motile	• Spiral shaped • Difficult to study because it is hard to cultivate and slow growing • Found in necrotizing gingivitis	• Spore-forming surface protein • Acylated protease complex • Mediates adherence, proteolytic activity, and cytotoxic effects

Q: Describe the red, yellow, orange, and green bacterial complexes first described by Socransky et al[67] in 1998.

Figure 4-4 presents the bacterial complexes. The red complex bacteria increase in prevalence and numbers with increasing pocket depth. Similarly, all species in the orange complex show a significant association with increasing pocket depth as exemplified by *P intermedia* and *F nucleatum*. The remaining complexes showed no statistically significant relationship with pocket depth.

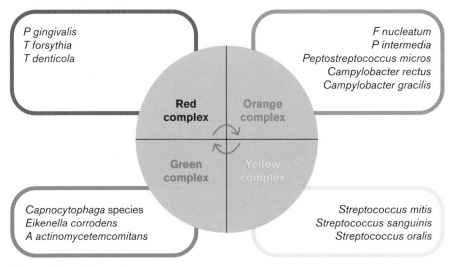

Fig 4-4 Bacterial complexes.

Q: What bacterial changes occur in the transition from health to disease?

Figure 4-5 presents bacterial properties in periodontal health and disease.

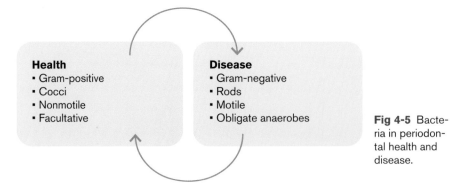

Fig 4-5 Bacteria in periodontal health and disease.

Q: **What percentages of gram-positive and gram-negative bacteria are harbored in gingivitis?**

The bacteria in gingivitis are about 50% gram-positive and 50% gram-negative.

Q: **Which bacteria are associated with health? Gingivitis? Localized aggressive periodontitis (molar/incisor pattern)? Chronic periodontitis (using old classification)?**

- Health: Bacteria associated with health include *Streptococcus sanguis*, *Streptococcus mitis*, *Actinomyces viscosus*, and *Actinomyces naeslundii*.
- Gingivitis: Lie et al[68] found *Prevotella nigrescens* at the start of gingivitis and after 14 days of experimental gingivitis. Tanner et al[69] studied 56 individuals and found that the predominant species in gingivitis were *A naeslundii*, *Campylobacter gracilis*, and *T forsythia*.
- Aggressive periodontitis (molar/incisor pattern): *A actinomycetemcomitans* is associated with localized aggressive periodontitis.
- Chronic periodontitis: *P gingivalis*, *T forsythia*, *F nucleatum*, and *P intermedia* are strongly associated with chronic periodontitis.

Q: **Which bacteria are associated with refractory periodontal disease? HIV/AIDS? Necrotizing periodontal diseases?**

The bacteria associated with refractory periodontitis, HIV/AIDS, and necrotizing periodontal diseases are shown in Fig 4-6.

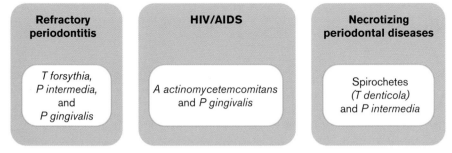

Refractory periodontitis	HIV/AIDS	Necrotizing periodontal diseases
T forsythia, *P intermedia*, and *P gingivalis*	*A actinomycetemcomitans* and *P gingivalis*	Spirochetes (*T denticola*) and *P intermedia*

Fig 4-6 Bacteria associated with refractory periodontitis, HIV/AIDS, and necrotizing periodontal diseases.

Q: Which bacteria are associated with implant failure? Diabetes? Preterm birth?

- Implant failure: *T forsythia*, spirochetes, and *P gingivalis*
- Diabetes: *Capnocytophaga* species, *P gingivalis*, and *P intermedia*
- Preterm birth and low birth weight: *A actinomycetemcomitans*, *P gingivalis*, *T forsythia*, and *T denticola*

Q: Can bacteria associated with periodontal disease be transmitted from one individual to another?

Offenbacher et al[70] examined 14 married couples to determine the degree of similarity of periodontal flora. They found three times greater odds of observing medium spirochetes and 30% greater odds of the presence of filaments in a patient if the spouse carried the same morphotype. They further stated that, according to their analysis, the presence of these morphotypes in the spouse conferred risk but was not required for the presence of the morphotype in an individual. Asikainen et al[71] found parent-child transmission of *A actinomycetemcomitans* in 6 of 19 (32%) families. *P gingivalis* was not transmitted from parent to child in any of the families.

Q: How have bacterial species been detected from oral clinical samples?

Many studies have utilized polymerase chain reaction–based methods to detect specific species directly from oral clinical samples.[72]

Viruses

Q: Do viruses play any role in periodontal disease?

According to Slots et al,[73] active cytomegalovirus and Epstein-Barr infections have been implicated in the etiopathogenesis of apical periodontitis. In addition, the release of tissue-destructive cytokines, the overgrowth of pathogenic bacteria, and the initiation of cytotoxic or immunopathologic events in periapical pathosis may be caused by herpesviruses.

References

1. Listgarten MA. Pathogenesis of periodontitis. J Clin Periodontol 1986;13:418–430.
2. Löe H, Anerud A, Boysen H, Morrison E. Natural history of periodontal disease in man. Rapid, moderate and no loss of attachment in Sri Lankan laborers 14 to 46 years of age. J Clin Periodontol 1986;13:431–445.
3. Schätzle M, Land NP, Anerud A, Boysen H, Bürgin W, Löe H. The influence of margins of restorations of the periodontal tissues over 26 years. J Clin Periodontol 2001;28:57–64.
4. Ercoli C, Caton JG. Dental prostheses and tooth-related factors. J Periodontol 2018;89(suppl 1):S223–S236.
5. Grossi S. Smoking and stress: Common denominators for periodontal disease, heart disease, and diabetes mellitus. Compend Contin Educ Dent Suppl 2000;(30):31–39.
6. Grossi SG, Skrepcinski FB, DeCaro T, et al. Treatment of periodontal disease in diabetics reduces glycated hemoglobin. J Periodontol 1997;68:713–719.
7. Kornman KS, Crane A, Wang HY, et al. The interleukin-1 genotype as a severity factor in adult periodontal disease. J Clin Periodontol 1997;24:72–77.
8. Michalowicz BS, Aeppli D, Virag JG, et al. Periodontal findings in adult twins. J Periodontol 1991;62:293–299.
9. Löe H, Brown LJ. Early onset periodontitis in the United States of America. J Periodontol 1991;62:608–616.
10. Gorman A, Kaye EK, Apovian C, Fung TT, Nunn M, Garcia RI. Overweight and obesity predict time to periodontal disease progression in men. J Clin Periodontol 2012;39:107–114.
11. Shepherd S. Alcohol consumption a risk factor for periodontal disease. Evid Based Dent 2011;12(3):76.
12. Gay IC, Tran DT, Paquette DW. Alcohol intake and periodontitis in adults aged ≥ 30 years: NHANES 2009–2012. J Periodontol 2018;89:625–634.
13. Genco RJ, Ho AW, Grossi SG, Dunford RG, Tedesco LA. Relationship of stress, distress and inadequate coping behaviors to periodontal disease. J Periodontol 1999;70:711–723.
14. American Academy of Periodontology. Media Alert: Injectable Progesterone Contraceptives May Be Associated with Poor Periodontal Health. https://www.perio.org/consumer/contraceptives. Accessed 16 September 2012.
15. Shariff JA, Ahluwalia KP, Papapanou PN. Relationship between frequent recreational cannabis (marijuana and hashish) use and periodontitis in adults in the United States: National Health and Nutrition Examination Survey 2011 to 2012. J Periodontol 2017;88:273–280.
16. Trombelli L, Farina R, Silva CO, Tatakis DN. Plaque-induced gingivitis: Case definition and diagnostic considerations. J Clin Periodontol 2018;89(suppl 1):S46–S73.
17. Löe H. The Gingival Index, the Plaque Index and the Retention Index Systems. J Periodontol 1967;38(6 suppl):610–616.
18. Schätzle M, Löe H, Bürgin W, Anerud A, Boysen H, Lang NP. Clinical course of chronic periodontitis. I. Role of gingivitis. J Clin Periodontol 2003;30:887–901.
19. Li Y, Lee S, Hujoel P, et al. Prevalence and severity of gingivitis in American adults. Am J Dent 2010;23:9–13.
20. Ainamo J, Bay I. Problems and proposals for recording gingivitis and plaque. Int Dent J 1975;25:229–235.
21. Russell AL. A system of classification and scoring for prevalence surveys of periodontal disease. J Dent Res 1956;35:350–359.
22. Ramfjord SP. The Periodontal Disease Index (PDI). J Periodontol 1967;38(6 suppl):602–610.
23. Albandar JM, Kingman A. Gingival recession, gingival bleeding, and dental calculus in adults 30 years of age and older in the United States, 1988–1994. J Periodontol 1999;70:30–43.

24. Chapple ILC, Mealey BL, Van Dyke TE, et al. Periodontal health and gingival diseases and conditions on an intact and a reduced periodontium: Consensus report of workgroup 1 of the 2017 World Workshop on the Classification of Periodontal and Peri-Implant Diseases and Conditions. J Periodontol 2018;89(suppl 1):S74–S84.

25. Brown LJ, Oliver RC, Löe H. Periodontal diseases in the U.S. in 1981: Prevalence, severity, extent, and role in tooth mortality. J Periodontol 1989;60:363–370.

26. Needleman I, Garcia R, Gkranias N, et al. Mean annual attachment, bone level, and tooth loss: A systematic review. J Periodontol 2018;89(suppl 1):S120–S139.

27. Kassebaum NJ, Bernabé E, Dahiya M, Bhandari B, Murray CJ, Marcenes W. Global burden of severe periodontitis in 1990–2010: A systematic review and meta-regression. J Dent Res 2014;93:1045–1053.

28. Eke PI, Thornton-Evans GO, Wei L, Borgnakke WS, Dye BA, Genco RJ. Periodontitis in US Adults: National Health and Nutrition Examination Survey 2009–2014. J Am Dent Assoc 2018;149:576–588.e6.

29. Offenbacher S, Boggess KA, Murtha AP, et al. Progressive periodontal disease and risk of very preterm delivery. Obstet Gynecol 2006;107:29–36.

30. Kassab MM, Cohen RE. The etiology and prevalence of gingival recession. J Am Dent Assoc 2003;134:220–225.

31. Michalowicz BS, Gustafsson A, Thumbigere-Math V, Buhlin K. The effects of periodontal treatment on pregnancy outcomes. J Periodontol 2013;84(4 suppl):S195–S208.

32. Michalowicz BS, Hodges JS, DiAngelis AJ, et al. Treatment of periodontal disease and the risk of preterm birth. N Engl J Med 2006;355:1885–1894.

33. López NJ, Uribe S, Martinez B. Effect of periodontal treatment on preterm birth rate: A systematic review of meta-analyses. Periodontol 2000 2015;67:87–130.

34. Sanz M, Kornman K; Working group 3 of joint EFP/AAP workshop. Periodontitis and adverse pregnancy outcomes: Consensus report of the Joint EFP/AAP Workshop on Periodontitis and Systemic Diseases. J Clin Periodontol 2013;40(suppl 14):S164–S169.

35. Ide M, Papapanou PN. Epidemiology of association between maternal periodontal disease and adverse pregnancy outcomes—Systematic review. J Clin Periodontol 2013;40(suppl 14):S181–S194.

36. Hancock EB, Mayo CV, Schwab RR, Wirthlin MR. Influence of interdental contacts on periodontal status. J Periodontol 1980;51:445–449.

37. Jernberg GR, Bakdash MB, Keenan KM. Relationship between proximal tooth open contacts and periodontal disease. J Periodontol 1983;54:529–533.

38. Pack AR, Coxhead LJ, McDonald BW. The prevalence of overhanging margins in posterior amalgam restorations and periodontal consequences. J Clin Periodontol 1990;17:145–152.

39. Brunsvold MA, Lane JJ. The prevalence of overhanging dental restorations and their relationship to periodontal disease. J Clin Periodontol 1990;17:67–72.

40. Gulati MS, Grewal N, Kaur A. A comparative study of effects of mouth breathing and normal breathing on gingival health in children. J Indian Soc Pedod Prev Dent 1998;16(3):72–83.

41. Helm S, Petersen PE. Causal relation between malocclusion and periodontal health. Acta Odontol Scand 1989;47:223–228.

42. Alsulaiman AA, Kaye E, Jones J, et al. Incisor malalignment and the risk of periodontal disease progression. Am J Orthod Dentofacial Orthop 2018;153:512–522.

43. Walsh MM, Ellison JA. Treatment of tobacco use and dependence: The role of the dental professional. J Dent Educ 2005;69:521–537.

44. Grossi SG, Genco RJ, Machtei EE, et al. Assessment of risk for periodontal disease. II. Risk indicators for alveolar bone loss. J Periodontol 1995;66:23–29.

45. Johnson GK, Slach NA. Impact of tobacco use on periodontal status. J Dent Educ 2001;65:313–321.

46. Haffajee AD, Socransky SS. Relationship of cigarette smoking to the subgingival microbiota. J Clin Periodontol 2001;28:377–388.

47. Research, Science, and Therapy Committee of the American Academy of Periodontology. Position paper: Tobacco use and the periodontal patient. J Periodontol 1999;70:1419–1427.

48. Harris RJ. The connective tissue with partial thickness double pedicle graft: The results of 100 consecutively-treated defects. J Periodontol 1994;65:448–461.

49. Zucchelli G, Clauser C, De Sanctis M, Calandriello M. Mucogingival versus guided tissue regeneration procedures in the treatment of deep recession type defects. J Periodontol 1998;69:138–145.

50. Martins AG, Andia DC, Sallum AW, Sallum EA, Casati MZ, Nociti Júnior FH. Smoking may affect root coverage outcome: A prospective clinical study in humans. J Periodontol 2004;75:586–591.

51. Miller PD Jr. Root coverage with the free gingival graft. Factors associated with incomplete coverage. J Periodontol 1987;58:674–681.

52. Rosen PS, Marks MH, Reynolds MA. Influence of smoking on long-term clinical results of intrabony defects treated with regenerative therapy. J Periodontol 1996;67:1159–1163.

53. Trombelli L, Kim CK, Zimmerman GJ, Wikesjö UM. Retrospective analysis of factors related to clinical outcome of guided tissue regeneration procedures in intrabony defects. J Clin Periodontol 1997;24:366–371.

54. Chrcanovic BR, Albrektsson T, Wennerberg A. Smoking and dental implants: A systematic review and meta-analysis. J Dent 2015;43:487–498.

55. Baig MR, Rajan M. Effects of smoking on the outcome of implant treatment: A literature review. Indian J Dent Res 2007;18:190–195.

56. Clerehugh V, Tugnait A, Genco RJ. Periodontology at a Glance. West Sussex, UK: Wiley-Blackwell, 2009:72.

57. Kaldahl WB, Johnson GK, Patil KD, Kalkwarf KL. Levels of cigarette consumption and response to periodontal therapy. J Periodontol 1996;67:675–681.

58. Hyman JJ, Reid BC. Epidemiologic risk factors for periodontal attachment loss among adults in the United States. J Clin Periodontol 2003;30:230–237.

59. Hujoel PP, del Aguila MA, DeRouen TA, Bergström J. A hidden periodontitis epidemic during the 20th century? Community Dent Oral Epidemiol 2003;31:1–6.

60. Krall EA, Garvey AJ, Garcia RI. Alveolar bone loss and tooth loss in male cigar and pipe smokers. J Am Dent Assoc 1999;130:57–64.

61. Tverdal A, Bjartveit K. Health consequences of pipe versus cigarette smoking. Tob Control 2011;20:123–130.

62. Sundar IK, Javed F, Romanos GE, Rahman I. E-cigarettes and flavorings induce inflammatory and pro-senescence responses in oral epithelial cells and periodontal fibroblasts. Oncotarget 2016;7: 77196–77204.

63. Wadia R, Booth V, Yap HF, Moyes DL. A pilot study of the gingival response when smokers switch from smoking to vaping. Br Dent J 2016;221:722–726.

64. Loesche WJ, Giordano JR. Treatment paradigms in periodontal disease. Compend Contin Educ Dent 1997;18:221–226,228–230,232.

65. Sekot G, Posch G, Messner P, et al. Potential of the *Tannerella forsythia* S-layer to delay the immune response. J Dent Res 2011;90:109–114.

66. Hall LM, Dunford RG, Genco RJ, Sharma A. Levels of serum immunoglobulin G specific to bacterial surface protein A of *Tannerella forsythia* are related to periodontal status. J Periodontol 2012;83:228–234.

67. Socransky SS, Haffajee AD, Cugini MA, Smith C, Kent RL Jr. Microbial complexes in subgingival plaque. J Clin Periodontol 1998;25:134–144.

68. Lie MA, van der Weijden GA, Timmerman MF, Loos BG, van Steenbergen TJ, van der Velden U. Occurrence of *Prevotella intermedia* and *Prevotella nigrescens* in relation to gingivitis and gingival health. J Clin Periodontol 2001;28:189–193.

69. Tanner A, Maiden MF, Macuch PJ, Murray LL, Kent RL Jr. Microbiota of health, gingivitis, and initial periodontitis. J Clin Periodontol 1998;25:85–98.

70. Offenbacher S, Olsvik B, Tonder A. The similarity of periodontal microorganisms between husband and wife cohabitants. Association or transmission? J Periodontol 1985;56:317–323.

71. Asikainen S, Chen C, Slots J. Likelihood of transmitting *Actinobacillus actinomycetemcomitans* and *Porphyromonas gingivalis* in families with periodontitis. Oral Microbiol Immunol 1996;11:387–394.
72. Paster BJ, Dewhirst FE. Molecular microbial diagnosis. Periodontol 2000 2009;51:38–44.
73. Slots J, Sabeti M, Simon JH. Herpesviruses in periapical pathosis: An etiopathogenic relationship? Oral Surg Oral Med Oral Pathol Oral Radiol Endod 2003;96:327–331.

Pharmacology

Background

Q: **What are the United States Food and Drug Administration pharmaceutical pregnancy categories?**[1]

- A: Adequate and well-controlled studies in pregnant women have failed to demonstrate a risk to the fetus in the first trimester of pregnancy (and there is no evidence of risk in later trimesters).
- B: Animal reproduction studies have failed to demonstrate a risk to the fetus, but there are no adequate and well-controlled studies in pregnant women.
- C: Animal reproduction studies have shown an adverse effect on the fetus. There are no adequate and well-controlled studies in humans, but the benefits from the use of the drug in pregnant women may be acceptable despite its potential risks.
- D: There is positive evidence of human fetal risk based on adverse reaction data from investigational or marketing experience or studies in humans, but the potential benefits from the use of the drug in pregnant women may be acceptable despite its potential risks.
- X: Studies in animals or humans have demonstrated fetal abnormalities, and there is positive evidence of fetal risk based on adverse reaction reports from investigational or marketing experience, or both, and the risk of the use of the drug in a pregnant woman clearly outweighs any possible benefit.

Q: Describe the American Society of Anesthesiologists (ASA) classification.

The ASA physical status classification system is used by clinicians to assess the fitness of patients before surgery. The categories are:

- 1: Normal, healthy patient
- 2: Patient with mild systemic disease
- 3: Patient with severe systemic disease
- 4: Patient with severe systemic disease that is a constant threat to life
- 5: Moribund patient who is not expected to survive without the surgery
- 6: Patient who has been declared brain-dead and whose organs are being removed for donation purposes

Systemic Antibiotics

Q: When should systemic antibiotics be prescribed in a dental practice?

- When there is an active infection (eg, acute periodontal abscess)
- As antibiotic prophylaxis
- When placing bone or a membrane in a surgical site[2]
- To treat aggressive periodontitis (*Aggregatibacter actinomycetemcomitans* bacteria invades the tissue and cannot be mechanically removed)
- In some cases when surgery is refused by the patient or is contraindicated
- In cases of recurrent or refractory periodontitis due to persistent subgingival pathogens and possibly weakened host resistance[3]

Q: How should a dentist choose the correct antibiotic to give a patient?

- Culture and sensitivity
- DNA probe

However, according to the 2003 periodontal workshop,[4] there is limited evidence to suggest that identification of bacteria and determination of susceptibility to antibiotics is helpful in the management of patients who do not respond to therapy.

Q: Describe the type and spectrum as well as the drug interactions, side effects, and contraindications of the most commonly prescribed antibiotics in dentistry.

Table 5-1 presents the antibiotics commonly prescribed in dentistry.

Table 5-1	Commonly prescribed antibiotics in dentistry		
Antibiotic	**Type**	**Spectrum**	**Drug interactions, side effects, and contraindications**
Tetracycline (minocycline and doxycycline)	Bacteriostatic	Broad: Many gram-positive and gram-negative bacteria, including anaerobes, rickettsiae, chlamydiae, mycoplasmas,[5] and some protozoa (amoebas)	- Should not be taken with warfarin. - Patients should not take antacids or consume dairy products. - Birth control pills may become less effective. - Patients with renal dysfunction should not take tetracycline.
Metronidazole	Bactericidal	Obligate anaerobes, *Porphyromonas gingivalis*, *Prevotella intermedia*; also treats acute necrotizing ulcerative gingivitis	- Patients should not consume alcohol. - May increase the effect of warfarin.
Amoxicillin	Bactericidal	Broad: Kills many gram-negative anaerobes and gram-positive bacteria	Can make birth control pills less effective.
Clindamycin	Bacteriostatic	Aerobic gram-negative and gram-positive cocci; anaerobic gram-negative rod-shaped bacteria, including some bacteroides, fusobacterium, and *Prevotella* species, although resistance is increasing in *Bacteroides fragilis*	- May cause pseudomembranous colitis. - Do not use in kidney transplant patients.
Amoxicillin and metronidazole	Bactericidal	Broad: Used for treating patients with localized aggressive periodontitis	- Patients should not consume alcohol. - May increase the effect of warfarin. - Can make birth control pills less effective.

Q: What is the dosage for each antibiotic?

- Metronidazole and amoxicillin: 250 to 500 mg three times a day for 8 days
- Amoxicillin: 250 to 500 mg three times a day for 7 days
- Clindamycin: 300 mg three times a day for 8 days for advanced periodontitis
- Metronidazole: 500 mg three times a day for 8 days for advanced periodontitis
- Augmentin: 500 mg three times a day for 7 days

Q: What are common drug interactions with antibiotics?

See Table 5-2 below.

Table 5-2	Common drug interactions with antibiotics
Antibiotic	**Interacting drug**
Antibiotics in general	Oral contraceptives
β-lactams (penicillins and cephalosporins)	Allopurinol Beta blockers Bacteriostatic antibiotics and tetracyclines
Metronidazole	Ethanol Lithium
Tetracyclines	Antacids Insulin
Macrolides	Benzodiazepines Carbamazepines Cyclosporine H1 histamine blockers Statins Prednisone, methylprednisolone Theophylline
Cephalosporins, erythromycin, clarithromycin, metronidazole	Warfarin
Erythromycin and tetracyclines	Digoxin

Data from Blicher et al.[6]

Q: **What is the effect of systemically administered antibiotics on clinical measures of attachment level in patients with periodontitis as compared with controls?**

According to a systematic review by Haffajee et al,[7] one can expect about a 0.5-mm improvement in attachment level with scaling and root planing (SRP). They reported greater improvement in clinical attachment levels when systemically administered adjunctive antibiotics were used with and without SRP and/or surgery compared with treatment that did not include their use.

Sgolastra et al[8] demonstrated that full-mouth SRP in addition to systemic use of amoxicillin and metronidazole treatment was effective therapy in patients with generalized aggressive periodontitis.

López et al[9] studied the effect of metronidazole plus amoxicillin as the sole therapy for chronic periodontitis. Twenty-two patients with untreated chronic periodontitis were randomly assigned to a group that received systemically administered 250 mg metronidazole plus 500 mg amoxicillin three times a day for 7 days or to a group receiving SRP and two placebos. The study found similar changes in clinical and microbiologic parameters in both groups. However, there is still insufficient evidence supporting the use of systemic antibiotics as a monotherapy and regarding optimal dosage and duration of systemic antibiotics.

Casarin et al[10] also did a study on metronidazole and amoxicillin and found that the regimen decreased pocket depth and the amount of *A acti-nomycetemcomitans* when performing full-mouth ultrasonic debridement in generalized aggressive periodontitis patients.

Q: **Which patients need antibiotic prophylaxis?**

Antibiotic prophylaxis is required for:

1. Patients with heart conditions

The American Heart Association[11] recommends the use of preventive antibiotics before certain dental procedures for people with:

- A prosthetic heart valve or who have had a heart valve repaired with prosthetic material
- A history of endocarditis
- A heart transplant with abnormal heart valve function
- Certain congenital heart defects including:
  - Cyanotic congenital heart disease (birth defects with oxygen levels lower than normal) that has not been fully repaired, including children who have had surgical shunts and conduits. →

- A congenital heart defect that has been completely repaired with prosthetic material or a device for the first 6 months after the repair procedure.
- Repaired congenital heart disease with residual defects, such as persisting leaks or abnormal flow at or adjacent to a prosthetic patch or prosthetic device.

Prophylactic antibiotics were formerly but are no longer recommended for certain patients, including those with mitral valve prolapse, rheumatic heart disease, bicuspid valve disease, calcified aortic stenosis, and congenital (ie, present from birth) heart conditions such as ventricular septal defect, atrial septal defect, and hypertrophic cardiomyopathy.

2. Patients with joint replacement

According to the American Dental Association Council on Scientific Affairs:

> In general, for patients with prosthetic joint implants, prophylactic antibiotics are not recommended prior to dental procedures to prevent prosthetic joint infection. The practitioner and patient should consider possible clinical circumstances that may suggest the presence of a significant medical risk in providing dental care without antibiotic prophylaxis, as well as the known risks of frequent or widespread antibiotic use. As part of the evidence-based approach to care, this clinical recommendation should be integrated with the practitioner's professional judgment and the patient's needs and preference.[12]

Q: What is the regimen for antibiotic prophylaxis?

According to the American Dental Association (ADA),[13] the suggested antibiotic regimen is as follows:

- Patients not allergic to penicillin: Cephalexin, cephradine, or amoxicillin 2 g orally 1 hour prior to the dental procedure
- Patients not allergic to penicillin, cefazolin, or ampicillin and unable to take oral medications: Cefazolin 1 g or ampicillin 2 g intramuscularly or intravenously (IV) 1 hour prior to the dental procedure
- Patients allergic to penicillin: Clindamycin 600 mg orally 1 hour prior to the dental procedure
- Patients allergic to penicillin and unable to take oral medications: Clindamycin 600 mg IV 1 hour prior to the dental procedure

Locally Delivered Antibiotics

Q: What are locally delivered antibiotics?

Locally delivered antibiotics are those placed in a periodontal pocket with a delivery system and released in a controlled manner, allowing minimum inhibitory concentration for 7 days.

Q: What are the indications for the use of locally delivered antibiotic therapy?

The indication for the use of locally delivered antibiotic therapy is when local sites with inflammation have not responded to periodontal or maintenance therapy.

Q: List the common locally delivered antibiotics and their properties.

Figure 5-1 presents the properties of the common locally delivered antibiotics.

Actisite (Procter & Gamble/Alza)	Atridox (Atrix)	PerioChip (PerioChip)	Arestin (OraPharma)
• Tetracycline fiber. • Jeffcoat et al[14] found that the adjunctive use of the chlorhexidine chip results in a significant reduction of probing depth when compared with both SRP alone and the adjunctive use of a placebo chip. The chlorhexidine chip is a safe and effective adjunctive chemotherapy for the treatment of adult periodontitis. • This product is no longer available.	• Doxycycline gel 10%. • Bioabsorbable mixture in a syringe. • Placed below the gingival margin, it flows to the bottom of the pocket and adapts to root morphology. • Controlled release over a period of 21 days. • The 2003 workshop on periodontics[15] found a statistically significant improvement in clinical attachment level (CAL) with adjunctive use of the chlorhexidine chip and the doxycycline gel combined with SRP.	• Chlorhexidine chip, 2.5 mg. • The 2003 workshop on periodontics[15] found a statistically significant improvement in CAL with adjunctive use of the chlorhexidine chip and the doxycycline gel combined with SRP.	• Minocycline microsphere (MM) 1 mg. • Bioabsorbable powder. • Grossi et al[16] found that, compared with SRP alone, MM combined with SRP significantly reduced red complex bacteria (RCB) in current smokers and caused a greater improvement in probing depth, bleeding on probing, and CAL regardless of smoking status.

Fig 5-1 Common locally delivered antibiotics and their properties.

Host Modulation

Q: What is host modulation?

Host modulation is adjusting the host response to a microbial challenge.

Q: List the host modulatory products used in periodontics and their properties and related research findings.

Table 5-3 presents the properties and research findings related to host modulatory products used in periodontics.

Table 5-3	Host modulatory products used in periodontics	
Product	**Properties**	**Studies**
Subantimicrobial dose doxycycline (SDD) (Periostat, CollaGenex)	• 20 mg doxycycline taken two times a day for 6 to 9 months • Adjunct to conventional treatment in management of chronic periodontitis • No antibacterial activity, but its low concentration blocks enzyme (matrix metalloproteinase) activity involved in tissue destruction	Preshaw et al[17] studied 266 patients over 9 months and found that patients who had SRP and SDD (40 mg) had significantly greater clinical benefits than those with SRP alone in the treatment of periodontitis. In deep sites at month 9, mean CAL gains from baseline were 19% greater with adjunctive once-daily 40-mg SDD than with placebo (2.62 mm versus 2.20 mm, respectively; $P < .01$).
Nonsteriodal anti-inflammatory drugs (NSAIDs)	Inhibit prostaglandins	Evidence shows promise that the use of NSAIDs can slow bone loss in chronic periodontitis. However, the safety profile does not support long-term ingestion due to potentially significant side effects.
Bisphosphonates	Inhibit osteoclasts and decrease bone turnover	Reddy et al[18] found that there is a potential role for these agents in periodontitis management.

Anti-Resorptive Medications

Q: What are some anti-resorptive medications?

See Table 5-4 below.

Table 5-4	Anti-resorptive medications
Drug (trade/generic); route of administration	**FDA-approved osteoporosis indications**
Bisphosphonates	
Alendronate sodium (Fosamax and Fosamax plus D [Merck], Binosto [Mission Pharmacal], generics); oral	• Prevention and treatment of postmenopausal osteoporosis • Increasing bone mass in men with osteoporosis • Treatment of osteoporosis in men and women taking glucocorticoids
Ibandronate sodium (Boniva [Hoffman La Roche], generics); oral, IV	Prevention and treatment of postmenopausal osteoporosis
Risedronate sodium (Actonel and Atelvia [Allergen], generics); oral	• Prevention and treatment of postmenopausal osteoporosis • Increasing bone mass in men with osteoporosis • Prevention and treatment of osteoporosis in men and women initiating or taking glucocorticoids
Zoledronic acid (Reclast [Novartis]); IV	• Prevention and treatment of postmenopausal osteoporosis • Increasing bone mass in men with osteoporosis • Prevention and treatment of osteoporosis in men and women expected to be on glucocorticoid therapy for at least 12 months • Prevention of new clinical fractures in both men and women who have recently had a low-trauma, osteoporosis-related hip fracture
RANK ligand inhibitor	
Denosumab (Prolia [Amgen]); subcutaneous	• Treatment of postmenopausal women with osteoporosis at high risk for fracture • Treatment to increase bone mass in men with osteoporosis at high risk for fracture • Treatment to increase bone mass in men at high risk for fracture receiving androgen deprivation therapy for nonmetastatic prostate cancer • Treatment to increase bone mass in women at high risk for fracture receiving adjuvant aromatase inhibitor therapy for breast cancer

Data from the American Dental Association.[19]

61

Q: What is currently known about the risk of periodontal surgery while patients are on bisphosphonate therapy?

Bisphosphonates are nonbiodegradable analogs of pyrophosphate with a high affinity for calcium, and they inhibit osteoclasts, thus decreasing bone turnover. Osteonecrosis can result from temporary or permanent loss of blood to the bone. Patients undergoing periodontal surgery who are taking bisphosphonates (especially IV bisphosphonates) have a higher risk of medication-related osteonecrosis of the jaw (MRONJ) following surgery. The incidence of MRONJ associated with parenteral administration has been reported between 1% and 10%.[20]

A systematic study found that osteoporosis is the most common reason for the prescription of bisphosphonates. Tooth extraction was the most frequent trigger for MRONJ. Of all patients studied after bisphosphonate treatment, only 24 out of 1442 (1.7%) developed bisphosponate-related ONJ (BRONJ).[21]

In a study of 30 patients with osteonecrosis, Marx et al[22] found alendronate (Fosamax) to be related to a higher incidence of the disease, which had a 94.7% predilection for the posterior mandible and a 50% (15 patients) spontaneous occurrence. The remaining 15 patients had osteonecrosis resulting from an oral surgical procedure, primarily extractions. There was a direct exponential relationship between the size of the exposed bone and the duration of oral bisphosphonate use. About 63% (19/30) of patients reported pain with the bone exposure. The incidence of IV bisphosphonate–induced osteonecrosis in women is 70%.

Q: What is the CTX test and is it reliable?

The morning fasting serum C-terminal telopeptide (CTX; the breakdown product of bone resorption) test correlates to the duration of oral bisphosphonate use and could indicate a recovery of bone remodeling with increased values if the oral bisphosphonate was discontinued. CTX values less than 100 pg/mL represent high risk, between 100 pg/mL and 150 pg/mL represent moderate risk, and above 150 pg/mL represent minimal risk. If CTX values are low, a drug holiday is recommended.

In 2008, the ADA released a statement that its expert panel could not recommend CTX testing and drug holidays for predicting and mitigating the risk of BRONJ until such measures had been supported by well-controlled, randomized clinical trials.[23] A systematic study discovered that CTX levels were not predictive of the development of MRONJ in patients taking bisphosphonates.[21]

Q: How should a dentist manage a patient on bisphosphonates?

- Oral bisphosphonates: According to the 2009 American Association of Oral and Maxillofacial Surgeons position paper,[24] although the risk of developing MRONJ with oral bisphosphonates is low, it appears to increase when therapy lasts more than 3 years or in a shorter period with certain comorbidities such as chronic use of corticosteroids. Therefore, they recommended that, systemic conditions permitting, the clinician consider discontinuing the use of oral bisphosphonates for a 3-month period before and after elective invasive dental surgery as a means of reducing the risk of MRONJ. The ADA recommends staging of non-critical dental treatment, allowing 2 months between sextants to assess for the development of MRONJ before the next one is treated.[25]
- IV bisphosphonates: If conditions permit, initiation of bisphosphonate therapy should be delayed until dental health has been optimized. This should be a collaborative decision by the treating physician, dentist, and other specialists involved in the care of the patient.

MRONJ development may be reduced by optimizing oral hygiene and postoperatively using topical and systemic antibiotics as appropriate.[26]

Q: What is the treatment if a patient develops MRONJ?

Table 5-5 presents treatment for patients with different stages of BRONJ.

Teriparatide may be helpful in healing BRONJ lesions and may be considered in osteoporosis patients at a high fracture risk when not contraindicated. Continuation of bisphosphonates following healing of BRONJ lesions is suggested, and there have not been accounts of subsequent local recurrence.[26]

Table 5-5	Treatment of patients with different stages of BRONJ	
Risk category	**Description**	**Treatment**
At risk	No apparent necrotic bone in patients who have been treated with either oral or IV bisphosphonates	• No treatment indicated • Patient education
Stage 0	No clinical evidence of necrotic bone, but nonspecific clinical findings and symptoms	Systemic management, including use of pain medication and antibiotics

⟶

Table 5-5 (cont)	Treatment of patients with different stages of BRONJ	
Risk category	**Description**	**Treatment**
Stage 1	Exposed and necrotic bone in asymptomatic patients without evidence of infection	• Antibacterial mouthrinse • Clinical follow-up on a quarterly basis • Patient education and review of indications for continued bisphosphonate use
Stage 2	Exposed and necrotic bone associated with infection as evidenced by pain and erythema in the region of exposed bone with or without purulent drainage	• Symptomatic treatment with oral antibiotics • Oral antibacterial mouthrinse • Pain control • Superficial debridement to relieve soft tissue irritation
Stage 3	Exposed and necrotic bone in patients with pain, infection, and one or more of the following: exposed and necrotic bone extending beyond the region of alveolar bone (ie, inferior border and ramus in the mandible; maxillary sinus and zygoma in the maxilla), resulting in pathologic fracture; extraoral fistula; oroantral/oronasal communication; or osteolysis extending to the inferior border of the mandible or the sinus floor	• Antibacterial mouthrinse • Antibiotic therapy and pain control • Surgical debridement/resection for longer-term palliation of infection and pain

Reprinted from Ruggiero et al[24] with permission.

Q: Describe receptor activator of nuclear factor kappa-B ligand (RANKL) inhibitors.

RANKL inhibitors are a new class of medications (eg, denosumab) with a shorter half-life. Studies suggests that the inhibition of RANKL could be a good therapeutic target to reduce the activity of osteoclasts, ultimately resulting in increased bone mineral density and preventing bone loss.[27] →

Denosumab has a more favorable adverse events profile than bisphospho-nates, with a lower likelihood of renal toxicity.[28] It was introduced with the hopes of avoiding MRONJ. However, some reports of osteonecrosis of the jaw after the use of RANKL inhibitors have been documented.[29]

Local Anesthetics

Q: Describe the local anesthetics used in dentistry.

Table 5-6 describes the different local anesthetics and their properties (see next page).[6]

- Procaine (esther; Novocaine, Hospira): Metabolized in the kidney and not the liver.
- Benzocaine (Orajel orabase, Church & Dwight): Topical anesthetic.

All local anesthetics are vasodilators. Epinephrine is added to the solution to slow diffusion from the sight of injection.

Q: In what conditions is epinephrine contraindicated?

- Pheochromocytoma
- Hyperthyroid crisis
- Supraventricular tachycardia
- Uncontrolled hyperthyroidism
- Recent myocardial infarction
- Unstable angina

Oral Sedation

Q: Describe the oral sedation medications (benzodiazepines) commonly used in dentistry.

Table 5-7 lists the medications commonly used in dentistry for oral sedation (see page 67).

Ehrich et al[30] found that 0.25 mg of triazolam was more effective than 5 mg of diazepam in relieving dental anxiety.

Table 5-6   Local anesthetics and their properties

Local anesthetic	Maximum dose (mg/kg)	Maximum dose for adults (mg)	Dose of local anesthetic per cartridge (mg)	Dose of vasoconstrictor per cartridge	Notes
0.5% bupivacaine 1:200,000 epinephrine	1.3	90	8.5	.0085	Amino acid; Marcaine, Hospira: Most cardiotoxic, highest lipid solubility and anesthetic potency, strongest vasodilator and longest lasting.
3% mepivacaine	6.6	400	51	Not applicable	Amide; Carbocaine, Hospira and Polocaine, Dentsply: Contains no epinephrine.
4% articaine 1:100,000 epinephrine	7.0	500	72	.017	Amide; Septocaine, Septodont: Some controversy regarding whether it can cause paresthesia when a block injection is given.
2% lidocaine 1:100,000 epinephrine	6.6	500	34	.017	Amino acid; Xylocaine, AstraZeneca: Anti-arrhythmic and local anesthetic.
4% prilocaine 1:200,000 epinephrine	6.0	400	72	.0085	Amide; Citanest, AstraZeneca: In some patients, a metabolite of prilocaine may cause the unusual side effect of methemoglobinemia.

Table 5-7	Oral sedation medications commonly used in dentistry		
Drug	**Dosage**	**Properties**	**Side effects**
Lorazepam (Ativan, Wyeth-Ayerst)	1 to 4 mg 1 hour prior to the procedure	• Does not convert to an active metabolite • Half-life is 12 hours • A sedative and anxiolytic • Has potent amnesic effect	• Adverse effects can include severe sedation and hypotension • Effects are increased in combination with other central nervous system depressant drugs
Diazepam (Valium, Roche)	2 to 10 mg 1 hour prior to the procedure	• Has an active metabolite • Half-life is greater than 20 hours • Used to treat anxiety and insomnia	Side effects include anterograde amnesia, confusion, and sedation
Alprazolam (Xanax, Pfizer)	0.25 to 0.5 mg 1 hour prior to the procedure	• Short-acting benzodiazepam • Used to treat anxiety and panic disorders • Half-life is 11 hours	Adverse effects include change in libido, ataxia, and slurred speech
Triazolam (Halcion, Pfizer)	0.0125 to 0.25 mg 1 hour prior to the procedure	• Half-life is 1.5 to 5 hours • Possesses hypoxic, amnesic, anxiolytic, sedative, anti-convulsant, and muscle relaxant properties	Side effects include somnolence, dizziness, feeling of lightness, and altered coordination

Nitrous Oxide

Q: Describe the properties and advantages of nitrous oxide.

Properties:

- An inorganic gas
- Very low solubility
- An analgesic and a sedative at the concentrations used in dentistry
- Safe, effective, and reliable

Advantages[31]:

- Quick onset of action.
- Ability to be titrated for a rapid recovery.
- No risk of motor or sensory impairment following administration.
- Low cardiovascular and respiratory depression.
- Stanley et al found that administration of 30% to 50% nitrous oxide resulted in a statistically significant increase in the success of the inferior alveolar nerve block compared with room air/oxygen.[32]

IV Sedation

Q: What are the important instructions to communicate to patients about IV sedation?

- Do not eat or drink 6 to 8 hours prior to IV sedation.
- You must have a ride home; you cannot drive after IV sedation.

Q: Describe the IV conscious sedation medications commonly used for periodontal procedures.

Below are the conscious sedation IV medications commonly used for periodontal procedures. It is important to give a test dose (one drop) of any of these medications before administering the recommended dosage to ensure that the patient has no adverse reactions.

Midazolam (Versed, Roche)
- Benzodiazepine
- Metabolized in the liver and water soluble →

- Available in 10-mL vials and given 1 mg/mL
- Lacks active metabolites
- Greater amnesia than diazepam but less duration of clinical effects
- Three times as potent as diazepam
- Half-life is 1.8 to 6 hours

Diazepam (Valium)

- Benzodiazepine
- Ceiling dose is 20 mg
- Most patients need 0.6 to 1 mg
- Not water soluble; IV should be run for a period of time before administering
- Needle should not be inserted on the dorsum of the hand because of the risk of venous irritation
- Half-life is 20 to 100 hours

Fentanyl

- Narcotic analgesic
- 100 times more potent than morphine
- 25 to 50 mg
- Half-life is 2.5 minutes

Meperidine (Demerol, Hospira)

- Opioid analgesic
- Ceiling dose is 50 to 100 mg
- Harder to titrate; better for longer procedures
- Must dilute because of strong histamine reaction
- Half-life is 3 to 5 hours

Q: What are the contraindications for benzodiazepines?

- Use of monoamine oxidase (MAO) inhibitors
- Use of Prozac (Eli Lily)
- Narrow angle glaucoma
- Myasthenia gravis
- Bronchospasm

Q: What medication is given for a benzodiazepine overdose? Opioid overdose?

- Benzodiazepine overdose: Flumazenil is given 0.2 mg/mL; most patients need 0.6 to 1 mg. Its half-life is 20 to 80 minutes. It is important to note →

that the half-life of flumazenil is shorter than the half-life of midazolam. The patient's vitals must be continually monitored.

▪ Opioid overdose: Naloxone should be diluted to 1 mg/mL and given 0.1 to 0.2 mg IV every 2 to 3 minutes. Maximum dose is 10 mg. Half-life is 1 to 1.5 hours.

Q: What should be in the IV bag?

Dextrose should be used because distilled water could fractionize. Every 15 drops emitted is approximately 1 mL.

Q: What are some complications that can result from IV sedation?

Figure 5-2 presents the possible complications associated with IV sedation.
    For management of complications from IV sedation, please see Becker and Haas.[33]

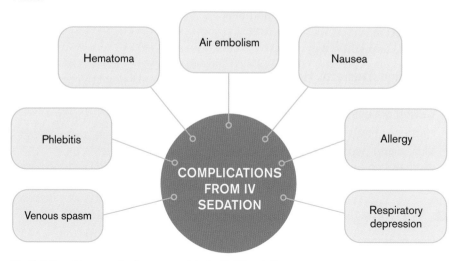

Fig 5-2 Possible complications associated with IV sedation.

Pain Relievers

Q: What medications are given for pain?

Analgesic drugs exert their effects by different mechanisms. Ibuprofen, an NSAID, blocks the cyclooxygenase 1 and 2 enzymes, thus preventing the production of prostaglandins. Acetaminophen has antipyretic and analgesic →

effects comparable to aspirin. Its mechanism of action is inhibition of pros-taglandin synthesis as well as interactions with both the cannabinoid and serotonergic systems. Narcotics, which should only be used to treat severe pain, assert their effects on central μ and κ opioid receptors.[6] Table 5-8 lists pain medications and prescriptions.

Table 5-8	Pain medications
Medication	**Prescription**
Ibuprofen	200–800 mg: 1 tablet every 4–6 hours
Tylenol with Codeine No. 3 (McNeil)	Acetaminophen 300 mg, codeine 30 mg: 1 tablet every 8 hours
Vicodin (AbbVie)	Hydrocodone 5 mg, acetaminophen 325 mg: 1–2 tablets every 4–6 hours
Percocet (Endo)	Oxycodone 5 mg, acetaminophen 325 mg: 1–2 tablets every 4–6 hours
Percodan (Endo)	Oxycodone 4.88 mg, aspirin 325 mg: 1 tablet every 6 hours

Q: What are common drug-drug interactions with analgesics?[6]

See Table 5-9 below.

Table 5-9	Drug interactions with analgesics
Analgesic	**Interacting drug**
Acetaminophen	Alcohol
Aspirin	Oral hypoglycemic agents (sulfonylureas, glyburide, chlorpropamide)
Aspirin and NSAIDs	Alcohol and anticoagulants
NSAIDs	β-blockers, ACE inhibitors, lithium, methotrexate

Q: Is there an association between low-dose aspirin and periodontal disease?

Results from the continuous National Health and Nutrition Examination Survey (NHANES) 2011–2012 concluded that low-dose aspirin is not associated with prevalent periodontal status.[34]

Q: What are the recent recommendations by the US Centers for Disease Control and Prevention (CDC)[35] for opioid use?

1. Non-opioid therapy is preferred for chronic pain outside of active cancer, palliative, and end-of-life care. Opioids should only be used when their benefits are expected to outweigh their substantial risks.
2. When opioids are used, the lowest possible effective dosage should be prescribed to reduce risks of opioid use disorder and overdose. Clinicians should start low and go slow.
3. Providers should always exercise caution when prescribing opioids and monitor all patients closely. Clinicians should minimize risk to patients by utilizing their state prescription drug monitoring program, or having an "off-ramp" plan to taper.

Anticoagulation and Antiplatelet Medications

Q: What is anticoagulation therapy?

Anticoagulation therapy is used to prevent heart attack, stroke, and other embolic complications in patients with pulmonary embolism, deep vein thrombosis, history of stroke, atrial fibrillation, and mechanical heart valves.

Q: What medications are anticoagulant? Antiplatelet? Direct-acting oral anticoagulants?

See Table 5-10 on next page.

Table 5-10	Drug classes and names
Drug class	**Drug names**
Anticoagulant	Warfarin (Coumadin, Bristol-Myers Squibb)
Antiplatelet agents	• Clopidogrel (Plavix, Bristol-Myers Squibb) • Ticlopidine (Ticlid, Apotex) • Prasugrel (Effient, Eli Lilly) • Ticagrelor (Brilinta, AstraZeneca) • Aspirin
Direct-acting oral anticoagulants	• Dabigatran (Pradaxa, Boehringer Ingleheim)—Direct thrombin inhibitor • Rivaroxaban (Xarelto, Janssen)—Direct factor Xa inhibitor • Apixaban (Eliquis, Bristol-Myers Squibb)—Direct factor Xa inhibitor • Edoxaban (Savaysa, Daiichi Sankyo)—Reduced production of vitamin K–dependent factors

From the American Dental Association.[36]

Q: How does direct anticoagulation therapy differ from traditional oral anticoagulant therapy (ie, warfarin)?

Many patients have been treated exclusively with dicumarinic anticoagulant agents (warfarin and acenocoumarol), but the dose for these medications must be adjusted specifically for each patient. They interact with many other drugs and with certain foods, and their use necessitates periodic monitoring using the International normalized ratio (INR).[37]

Direct-acting oral anticoagulants contrast from traditional oral anticoagulant therapy in that they are targeted in action; are given as fixed doses; have more predictable pharmacokinetics and shorter half-lives; necessitate little to no routine monitoring; and have fewer drug or food interactions.[36]

Q: Is there a consensus on how to manage patients on anticoagulation therapy?

When patients receiving anticoagulation therapy undergo dental surgery (eg, extractions, implants, osseous surgery), the dentist must decide to continue anticoagulation therapy and risk bleeding complications or suspend anticoagulation therapy and risk embolic complications. There is now near consensus that anticoagulation therapy including either warfarin (Coumadin)

$\rightarrow$

73

or direct oral anticoagulation therapy with dabigatran (Pradaxa), apixaban (Eliquis), rivaroxaban (Xarelto), or edoxaban (Savaysa) should not be suspended for most dental surgical patients because the increased danger of developing bleeding complications (which are typically easy to treat and have not been shown to be terminal) with continuation is overshadowed by the increased risk of developing embolic complications (which often are debilitating and sometimes deadly) with interruption.[38]

Another review found that in addition to local measures to control bleeding, low-risk procedures such as scaling and/or root planing, restorative or endodontic treatment, simple extractions, or surgery lasting less than 45 minutes do not seem to necessitate interruption of therapy with the new anticoagulants. For procedures linked with increased risk of bleeding, such as surgical extractions, multiple extractions, or more complex oral surgery, the authors recommend a multidisciplinary preoperative approach that includes consultation with the patient's physician regarding potentially stopping anticoagulant medications 2 to 5 days before surgery.[39]

Side Effects of Medications

Q: What medications can cause gingival enlargement?

Gingival enlargement is associated with the medications listed in Fig 5-3.[40]

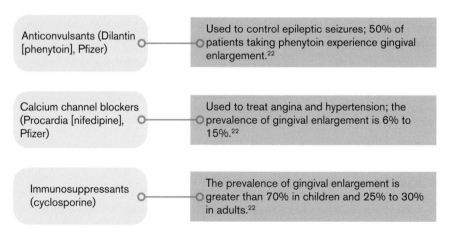

Anticonvulsants (Dilantin [phenytoin], Pfizer)	Used to control epileptic seizures; 50% of patients taking phenytoin experience gingival enlargement.[22]
Calcium channel blockers (Procardia [nifedipine], Pfizer)	Used to treat angina and hypertension; the prevalence of gingival enlargement is 6% to 15%.[22]
Immunosuppressants (cyclosporine)	The prevalence of gingival enlargement is greater than 70% in children and 25% to 30% in adults.[22]

Fig 5-3 Medications associated with gingival enlargement, with prevalence according to position papers by the American Academy of Periodontology.[40]

Q: What are some commonly prescribed medications that can cause dry mouth (xerostomia)? What medications can be dispensed to manage dry mouth?

Xanax, Prozac, Lasix (Sanofi Aventis), and antihistamines can cause dry mouth. Radiation and chemotherapy can also contribute to xerostomia.

Biotene gel (GlaxoSmithKline) can be applied to the tongue to relieve dry mouth for up to 8 hours. Another option is Moi-Stir moistening solution (Kingswood Laboratories), which is sprayed directly in the mouth.[41]

Q: What dental conditions are associated with inhalation steroids?

Gingivitis, dental caries, and oral candidiasis are associated with the use of inhalation steroids.

Q: In what situations is it recommended to increase the dosage of a steroid?

Patients with adrenal insufficiency following the use of exogenous gluco-corticosteroid hormones are less able to acclimatize to stressful situations. Typically, a two- to fourfold increase in glucocorticosteroid dosage on the day of dental treatment will allow the patient to cope with a dental visit. To determine if a patient has adrenal insufficiency, follow the rule of twos[42]:

- A dose of 20 mg or more of cortisone
- For a continuous period of 2 weeks or longer
- In a 2-year time frame

Toothpastes and Mouthrinses

Q: What is triclosan and its mechanism of action?

Triclosan is a phenol nonionic antimicrobial and antifungal agent. Triclosan has the ability to inhibit both the cyclooxygenase and lipoxygenase pathways of arachidonic acid metabolism. As a result, triclosan can inhibit formation of several important mediators of gingival inflammation.

Zambon et al[43] found an association between triclosan and beneficial changes to the bacterial composition of supragingival dental plaque. Colgate Total toothpaste (Colgate-Palmolive) contains triclosan. →

Pera et al[44] demonstrated in a double-masked randomized clinical trial that triclosan/copolymer dentifrices allow greater clinical benefits (improved clinical attachment level) following full-mouth debridement in the treatment of generalized severe chronic periodontitis.

Q: What is the spectrum of chlorhexidine (0.12% chlorhexidine gluconate)?

Chlorhexidine is antibacterial (effective on gram-positive and gram-negative bacteria), antifungal, and antiviral. It causes membrane disruption and is found in mouthrinses. It exhibits substantivity, which is the ability to adhere to soft and hard tissues and then be released over time. With continued use, it can cause staining of the teeth, altered taste sensation, and increased supragingival calculus formation.

In a meta-analysis, Gunsolley[45] found seven studies reporting that mouthrinses with 0.12% chlorhexidine had a strong antiplaque, antigingivitis effect.

Q: What are the active ingredients in Listerine antiseptic rinse and Crest Pro-Health rinse?

- Listerine (McNeil): Methyl salicylate (0.060%) and essential oils (phenolytic compounds, thymol) (0.064%), menthol (0.042%), and eucalyptol (0.092%). The antiplaque efficacy of mouthrinses with essential oils was corroborated by the largest number of studies (21) in the meta-analysis by Gunsolley.[45]
- Crest Pro-Health (Procter & Gamble): Cetylpyridinium chloride (0.07%) (no alcohol).

Q: What are the three major components in toothpaste?

1. Abrasives: Hydrated silica, calcium carbonate, and alumina
2. Therapeutic: Potassium nitrate and sodium fluoride
3. Foaming agents: Sodium lauryl sulfate and hydrogen peroxide

Q: What is the active ingredient in Prevident? Sensodyne?

- PreviDent (Colgate-Palmolive): Sodium fluoride 1.1%
- Sensodyne (GlaxoSmithKline): Potassium nitrate 5% and sodium fluoride 0.15%

Q: What is stannous fluoride?

- Stannous fluoride is a chemical compound with the formula SnF_2. It is a colorless solid used as an ingredient in toothpastes as an alternative to sodium fluoride.
- It is an antibacterial agent that can protect against gingivitis, plaque and tooth sensitivity.[46,47]

Miscellaneous

Q: What prescription would a dentist write for a patient with oral candidiasis?

The patient should take 1 teaspoon nystatin 300 mL and rinse for 2 minutes four times a day. Another option is Mycelex troches (Bayer), 10 mg given four times per day for 10 days (dissolves in 30 minutes). It should be noted that Mycelex troches contain sucrose and therefore are associated with a risk of caries.

Q: What medication is prescribed for a patient with an oral viral infection?

The following medications are prescribed for patients with oral viral infections[41]:

- Topical: Acyclovir ointment 5%, 15 g. Patient should be instructed to apply a thin layer to the lesion six times a day for 7 days.
- Systemic: Acyclovir 200 mg, 70 tablets. Patient should be instructed to take one capsule every 4 hours for 2 weeks (maximum of five tablets a day).

References

1. Food and Drug Administration, Department of Health and Human Services. Content and Format for Labeling Human Prescription Drug and Biological Products; Requirements for Pregnancy and Lactation Labeling. http://edocket.access.gpo.gov/2008/pdf/E8-11806.pdf. Accessed 18 September 2012.
2. Sanders JJ, Sepe WW, Bowers GM, et al. Clinical evaluation of freeze-dried bone allografts in periodontal osseous defects. Part III. Composite freeze-dried bone allografts with and without autogenous bone grafts. J Periodontol 1983;54:1–8.

3. Slots J; Research, Science and Therapy Committee. Systemic antibiotics in periodontics. J Periodontol 2004;75:1553–1565.

4. Listgarten MA, Loomer PM. Microbial identification in the management of periodontal diseases. A systematic review. Ann Peridontol 2003;8:182–192.

5. Eliopoulos GM, Roberts MC. Tetracycline therapy: Update. Clin Infect Dis 2003;36:462–467.

6. Blicher B, Pryles RL, Lin J. Endodontics Review: A Study Guide. Chicago: Quintessence, 2016.

7. Haffajee AD, Socransky SS, Gunsolley JC. Systemic anti-infective periodontal therapy. A systematic review. Ann Periodontol 2003;8:115–181.

8. Sgolastra F, Petrucci A, Gatto R, Monaco A. Effectiveness of systemic amoxicillin/metronidazole as an adjunctive therapy to full-mouth scaling and root planing in the treatment of chronic periodontitis: A systematic review and meta-analysis. J Periodontol 2012;83:731–743.

9. López NJ, Socransky SS, Da Silva I, Japlit MR, Haffajee AD. Effects of metronidazole plus amoxicillin as the only therapy on the microbiological and clinical parameters of untreated chronic periodontitis. J Clin Periodontol 2006;33:648–660.

10. Casarin RC, Peloso Ribeiro ED, Sallum EA, Nociti FH Jr, Gonçalves RB, Casati MZ. The combination of amoxicillin and metronidazole improves clinical and microbiologic results of one-stage, full-mouth, ultrasonic debridement in aggressive periodontitis treatment. J Periodontol 2012;83:988–998.

11. American Heart Association. Infective Endocarditis. https://www.heart.org/en/health-topics/infective-endocarditis. Accessed 16 August 2018.

12. Sollecito TP, Abt E, Lockhart PB, et al. The use of prophylactic antibiotics prior to dental procedures in patients with prosthetic joints: Evidence-based clinical practice guideline for dental practitioners—A report of the American Dental Association Council on Scientific Affairs. J Am Dent Assoc 2015;146:11–16.e8.

13. American Dental Association. Antibiotic Prophylaxis for Dental Patients with Total Joint Replacements. aae.org/specialty/wp-content/uploads/sites/2/2017/07/antibioticprophylaxisfordentalpatientswithtotaljointreplacements.pdf. Accessed 12 December 2019.

14. Jeffcoat MK, Bray KS, Ciancio SG, et al. Adjunctive use of a subgingival controlled-release chlorhexidine chip reduces probing depth and improves attachment level compared with scaling and root planing alone. J Periodontol 1998;69:989–997.

15. Hanes PJ, Purvis JP. Local anti-infective therapy: Pharmacological agents. A systematic review. Ann Periodontol 2003;8:79–98.

16. Grossi SG, Goodson JM, Gunsolley JC, et al. Mechanical therapy with adjunctive minocycline microspheres reduces red-complex bacteria in smokers. J Periodontol 2007;78:1741–1750.

17. Preshaw PM, Novak MJ, Mellonig J, et al. Modified-release subantimicrobial dose doxycycline enhances scaling and root planing in subjects with periodontal disease. J Periodontol 2008;79:440–452.

18. Reddy MS, Geurs NC, Gunsolley JC. Periodontal host modulation with antiproteinase, anti-inflammatory, and bone-sparing agents. A systematic review. Ann Periodontol 2003;8:12–37.

19. American Dental Association. Osteoporosis Medications and Medication-Related Osteonecrosis of the Jaw. https://www.ada.org/en/member-center/oral-health-topics/osteoporosis-medications. Accessed 1 October 2019.

20. McLeod NM, Brennan PA, Ruggiero SL. Bisphosphonate osteonecrosis of the jaw: A historical and contemporary review. Surgeon 2012;10:36–42.

21. Dal Prá KJ, Lemos CA, Okamoto R, Soubhia AM, Pellizzer EP. Efficacy of the C-terminal telopeptide test in predicting the development of bisphosphonate-related osteonecrosis of the jaw: A systematic review. Int J Oral Maxillofac Surg 2017;46:151–156.

22. Marx RE, Cillo JE Jr, Ulloa JJ. Oral bisphosphonate-induced osteonecrosis: Risk factors, prediction of risk using serum CTX testing, prevention, and treatment. J Oral Maxillofac Surg 2007;65:2397–2410.

23. Edwards BJ, Hellstein JW, Jacobsen PL, et al. Updated recommendations for managing the care of patients receiving oral bisphosphonate therapy: An advisory statement from the American Dental Association Council on Scientific Affairs. J Am Dent Assoc 2008;139:1674–1677.

24. Ruggiero SL, Dodson TB, Assael LA, et al. American Association of Oral and Maxillofacial Surgeons position paper on bisphosphonate-related osteonecrosis of the jaw—2009 update. Aust Endod J 2009;35:119–130.

25. Patel V, McLeod NM, Rogers SN, Brennan PA. Bisphosphonate osteonecrosis of the jaw—A literature review of UK policies versus international policies on bisphosphonates, risk factors and prevention. Br J Oral Maxillofac Surg 2011;49:251–257.

26. Khan AA, Morrison A, Kendler DL, et al. Case-based review of osteonecrosis of the jaw (ONJ) and application of the international recommendations for management from the international task force on ONJ. J Clin Densitom 2017;20:8–24.

27. George S, Brenner A, Sarantopoulos J, Bukowski RM. RANK ligand: Effects of inhibition. Curr Oncol Rep 2010;12:80–86.

28. Epstein MS, Ephros HD, Epstein JB. Review of current literature and implications of RANKL inhibitors for oral health care providers. Oral Surg Oral Med Oral Pathol Oral Radiol 2013;116:e437–e442.

29. Qaisi M, Hargett J, Loeb M, Brown J, Caloss R. Denosumab related osteonecrosis of the jaw with spontaneous necrosis of the soft palate: Report of a life threatening case. Case Rep Dent 2016;2016:5070187.

30. Ehrich DG, Lundgren JP, Dionne RA, Nicoll BK, Hutter JW. Comparison of triazolam, diazepam, and placebo as outpatient oral premedication for endodontic patients. J Endod 1997;23:181–184.

31. Newman MG, Takei H, Klokkevold PR, Carranza FA. Carranza's Clinical Periodontology, ed 11. St Louis: Elsevier Saunders, 2012:543.

32. Stanley W, Drum M, Nusstein J, Reader A, Beck M. Effect of nitrous oxide on the efficacy of the inferior alveolar nerve block in patients with symptomatic irreversible pulpitis. J Endod 2012;38:565–569.

33. Becker DE, Haas DA. Management of complications during moderate and deep sedation: Respiratory and cardiovascular considerations. Anesth Prog 2007;54:59–68.

34. Kotsakis GA, Thai A, Ioannou AL, Demmer RT, Michalowicz BS. Association between low-dose aspirin and periodontal disease: Results from the continuous National Health and Nutrition Examination Survey (NHANES) 2011–2012. J Clin Periodontol 2015;42:333–341.

35. Dowell D, Haegerich TM, Chou R. CDC Guideline for Prescribing Opioids for Chronic Pain—United States, 2016. MMWR Recomm Rep 2016;65;1–49 [erratum 2016;65:295].

36. American Dental Association. Anticoagulant and Antiplatelet Medications and Dental Procedures. https://www.ada.org/en/member-center/oral-health-topics/anticoagulant-antiplatelet-medications-and-dental-. Accessed 1 October 2019.

37. Curto A, Albaladejo A. Implications of apixaban for dental treatments. J Clin Exp Dent 2016;8:e611–e614.

38. Wahl MJ. The mythology of anticoagulation therapy interruption for dental surgery. J Am Dent Assoc 2018;149:e1–e10.

39. Thean D, Alberghini M. Anticoagulant therapy and its impact on dental patients: A review. Aust Dent J 2016;61:149–156.

40. Dongari-Bagtzoglu A; Research, Science and Therapy Committee of the American Academy of Periodontology. Drug-assisted gingival enlargement. J Periodontol 2004;75:1424–1431.

41. Newland JR, Meiller TF, Wynn RL, Crossley HL. Oral Soft Tissue Diseases: A Reference Manual for Diagnosis and Management, ed 2. Hudson, Ohio: Lexi-Comp, 2002.

42. Malamed S. Medical Emergencies in the Dental Office, ed 5. St Louis: Mosby, 2000:149.

43. Zambon JJ, Reynolds HS, Dunford RG, et al. Microbial alterations in supragingival dental plaque in response to a triclosan-containing dentifrice. Oral Microbiol Immunol 1995;10:247–255.

44. Pera C, Ueda P, Casarin RC, et al. Double-masked randomized clinical trial evaluating the effect of a triclosan/copolymer dentifrice on periodontal healing after one-stage full-mouth debridement. J Periodontol 2012;83:909–916.

45. Gunsolley JC. A meta-analysis of six-month studies of antiplaque and antigingivitis agents. J Am Dent Assoc 2006;137:1649–1657.

46. Cannon M, Khambe D, Klukowska M, et al. Clinical effects of stabilized stannous fluoride dentifrice in reducing plaque microbial virulence II: Metabonomic changes. J Clin Dent 2018;29:1–12.
47. Xie S, Haught JC, Tansky CS, et al. Clinical effects of stannous fluoride dentifrice in reducing plaque microbial virulence III: Lipopolysaccharide and TLR2 reporter cell gene activation. Am J Dent 2018;31:215–224.

Diagnosis

6

Background

Q: What is the definition of gingivitis?

Gingivitis is a nonspecific gingival inflammation resulting from interactions between dental plaque and the host's immune response without loss of periodontal attachment (cementum, periodontal ligament [PDL], alveolar bone).

Plaque-induced gingivitis can be reversed once the dental biofilm is removed. Gingivitis is a major risk factor, and a necessary prerequisite, for periodontitis.[1]

Q: Describe the clinical and biologic signs of gingivitis.[1]

- Swelling
- Erythema
- Edema
- Bleeding and discomfort on gentle probing
- Redness and/or bleeding gingiva (metallic/altered taste)
- Halitosis
- Pain or soreness

Q: What are the histopathologic changes of gingivitis? Clinical signs?

Histopathologic changes[2]:

- Elongation of rete ridges into the gingival connective tissue
- Vasculitis of blood vessels adjacent to the junctional epithelium
- Progressive destruction of the collagen fiber network (alterations in fibroblasts and collagen types)
- Progressive inflammatory and immune cellular infiltrate

Clinical signs:

- Erythema, bleeding, tenderness, edema, and enlargement

Q: What is periodontitis?

Periodontitis is gingival inflammation at sites where there has been loss of collagen fibers from cementum and the junctional epithelium has migrated apically. Periodontitis results from the advancement of gingivitis.[3]
   Periodontal disease is not just a simple bacterial infection. It is a complex disease involving interactions between subgingival bacteria, inflammatory responses, the host immune system, and the environmental modifying factors.[4]
   Primary features:

1. Loss of periodontal tissue support
2. Radiographically assessed alveolar bone loss
3. Periodontal pocketing and gingival bleeding

Q: How do you diagnose a patient as having periodontitis?

A patient is diagnosed with periodontitis if:

1. Interdental clinical attachment loss (CAL) is detectable at ≥ 2 nonadjacent teeth or
2. Buccal or lingual/palatal CAL ≥ 3 mm with pocketing ≥ 3 mm is detectable at ≥ 2 teeth
3. The observed CAL cannot be ascribed to non-periodontal causes (eg, fracture, caries).[5]

Q: What is clinical attachment level?

Clinical attachment level is the distance from the cementoenamel junction (CEJ) to the tip of the periodontal probe during normal probing.

Q: What is probing depth?

Probing depth is the distance from the soft tissue margin to the tip of the periodontal probe.

Q: What can affect probing depth?

The following factors may influence probing depth:

- Insertion force
- Size of the probe tip
- Inflammatory status of the tissues

In health, the probe should stop within the junctional epithelium. In patients with periodontitis, it may stop in connective tissue or bone.

Classification of Periodontal and Peri-implant Diseases and Conditions

An overview of the classification is presented in the appendix. This section will go into further detail.

Please note the new vocabulary in the new classification:

> Periodontal biotype $\longrightarrow$ Periodontal phenotype
> Excessive occlusal force $\longrightarrow$ Traumatic occlusal force
> Biologic width $\longrightarrow$ Supracrestal tissue attachment
> Chronic periodontitis, aggressive periodontitis $\longrightarrow$ Periodontitis

The classification presented in the following answers is taken directly from the 2017 World Workshop Classification of Periodontal and Peri-implant Diseases and Conditions.[6] See the appendix for the full classification.

Q: On a site level, how is clinical gingival health classified?

I. Periodontal health, gingival diseases/conditions
  A. Periodontal health and gingival health
    1. Clinical gingival health on an intact periodontium (bleeding on probing [BOP] < 10% without attachment loss, erythema, edema, and radiographic bone loss, no probing depths of 4 mm or greater with BOP)
    2. Clinical gingival health on a reduced periodontium $\rightarrow$

    a. Stable periodontitis patient (no BOP, erythema, and edema in the presence of reduced bone and clinical attachment levels, no probing depths of 4 mm or greater with BOP)

    b. Non-periodontitis patient

Clinical gingival health is associated with a host response and an inflammatory infiltrate consistent with homeostasis.[1]

Q: What are the gingival diseases/conditions?

B. Gingivitis, dental biofilm-induced
1. Associated with dental biofilm alone
    a. Plaque-induced gingivitis on an intact periodontium
      1) Localized: BOP ≥ 10% and ≤ 30% without attachment loss and radiograghic bone loss
      2) Generalized: BOP score > 30% without attachment loss and radiographic bone loss
    b. Plaque-induced gingivitis on a reduced periodontium (criteria: without a history of periodontitis, possible radiographic bone loss, all probing depths ≤ 3 mm)[7]
      1) Non-periodontitis patient (eg, recession, crown lengthening)
        a) Localized: BOP ≥ 10% and ≤ 30%
        b) Generalized: BOP > 30%
      2) Successfully treated periodontitis patient
        a) Localized: BOP ≥ 10% and ≤ 30%
        b) Generalized: BOP > 30%
2. Mediated by systemic or local risk factors
    a. Systemic risk factors (modifying factors)
      1) Smoking
      2) Hyperglycemia
      3) Nutritional factors
      4) Pharmacologic agents
      5) Sex steroid hormones
        a) Puberty (inflammation in presence of small amounts of plaque during adolescence)
        b) Menstrual cycle
        c) Pregnancy (inflammation in presence of small amounts of plaque during pregnancy)
        d) Oral contraceptives
      6) Hematologic conditions
    b. Oral factors enhancing plaque accumulation
      1) Prominent subgingival restoration margins
      2) Hyposalivation
3. Drug-influenced gingival enlargement (Fig 6-1) →

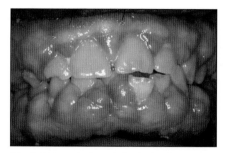

Fig 6-1 Drug-induced gingival enlargement.

C. Gingival diseases, non–dental biofilm–induced[8] (not caused by plaque and do not resolve following plaque removal)
   1. Genetic/developmental disorders
      a. Hereditary gingival fibromatosis
   2. Specific infections
      a. Bacterial origin
         1) Necrotizing periodontal disease (*Treponema* spp, *Selenomonas* spp, *Fusobacterium* spp, *Prevotella intermedia*, and others)
         2) *Neisseria gonorrhoeae* (gonorrhea)
         3) *Treponema pallidum* (syphilis)
         4) *Myobacterium tuberculosis* (tuberculosis)
         5) *Streptococcal gingivitis* (strains of streptococcus)
      b. Viral origin
         1) Coxsackie virus (hand-foot-and-mouth disease)
         2) Herpes simplex 1/2 (primary or recurrent)
         3) Varicella-zoster virus (chicken pox or shingles affecting V nerve)
         4) Molluscum contagiosum virus
         5) Human papilloma virus (squamous cell papilloma, condyloma acuminatum, verrucca vulgaris, and focal epithelial hyperplasia)
      c. Fungal
         1) Candidosis
         2) Other mycoses (eg, histoplasmosis, aspergillosis)
   3. Inflammatory and immune conditions
      a. Hypersensitivity reactions
         1) Contact allergy
         2) Plasma cell gingivitis
         3) Erythema multiforme
      b. Autoimmune diseases of skin and mucous membranes (See chapter 16 for more detail)
         1) Pemphigus vulgaris
         2) Pemphigoid
         3) Lichen planus →

       4) Lupus erythematosus
         a) Systemic lupus erythematosus
         b) Discoid lupus erythematosus
     c. Granulomatous inflammatory condition (orofacial granulomatosis)
       1) Crohn disease
       2) Sarcoidosis
  4. Reactive processes
    a. Epulides
       1) Fibrous epulis
       2) Calcifying fibroblastic granuloma
       3) Pyogenic granuloma (vascular epulis)
       4) Peripheral giant cell granuloma (or central)
  5. Neoplasms
    a. Premalignant
       1) Leukoplakia
       2) Erythroplakia
    b. Malignant
       1) Squamous cell carcinoma
       2) Leukemia
       3) Lymphoma
         a) Hodgkin
         b) Non-Hodgkin
  6. Endocrine, nutritional, and metabolic diseases
    a. Vitamin deficiencies
       1) Vitamin C deficiency (scurvy)
  7. Traumatic lesions
    a. Physical/mechanical insults
       1) Frictional keratosis
       2) Mechanically (toothbrushing) induced gingival ulceration
       3) Factitious injury (self-harm)
    b. Chemical (toxic) insults
       1) Etching
       2) Chlorhexidine
       3) Acetylsalicyclic acid
       4) Cocaine
       5) Hydrogen peroxide
       6) Dentifrice detergents
       7) Paraformaldehyde or calcium hydroxide
    c. Thermal insults
       1) Burns of mucosa →

8. Gingival pigmentation
   a. Gingival pigmentation/melanoplakia
   b. Smoker's melanosis
   c. Drug-induced pigmentation (antimalarials; minocycline)
   d. Amalgam tattoo

BOP is the primary parameter to set thresholds for gingivitis. The authors decided that a patient with gingivitis can revert to health, but a patient with periodontitis has the condition for life.[6]

Q: What determines clinical periodontal health?

Determinants of periodontal health fall into three categories (Fig 6-2):

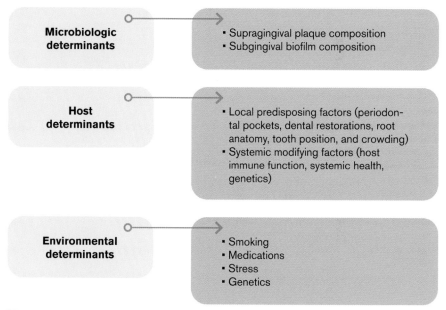

Fig 6-2 Determinants of periodontal health. From Lang and Bartold.[9]

Please note: A controlled patient with periodontitis remains at higher risk for recurrent disease compared to a patient with gingivitis or a healthy patient.[1]

Q: Is there BOP in periodontal health? Gingivitis? Periodontitis (reduced periodontium)?

See Table 6-1 on next page. →

| Table 6-1 | BOP in periodontal health, gingivitis, and periodontitis |

Health status	BOP	Normal gingival sulcus depth	Normal base heights	Modifying factors (cigarette smoking, hyperglycemia)	Predisposing factors
Pristine periodontal health (not likely observed clinically)	No	Yes	Yes	Controlled	Controlled
Clinical periodontal health (intact periodontium)	No/minimal	Yes	Yes	Controlled	Controlled
Gingivitis	Yes	Yes	Yes	May be present	May be present
Periodontitis (reduced periodontium and stable)	No/minimal	No	No	Controlled	Controlled
Periodontitis (reduced periodontium and remission/ control)	Significantly reduced	No	No	Not fully controlled	Not fully controlled

From Lang and Bartold.[9]

Q: Describe the difference between health and gingivitis in an intact periodontium and reduced periodontium (non-periodontitis and successfully treated stable periodontitis patient).[1]

See Table 6-2 on next page. →

Table 6-2	Health and gingivitis in intact periodontium and reduced periodontium	
	Health	**Gingivitis**
Intact periodontium		
Probing attachment loss	No	No
Probing pocket depths	≤ 3 mm	≤ 3 mm
BOP	< 10%	≥ 10%
Radiographic bone loss	No	No
Reduced periodontium in a non-periodontitis patient		
Probing attachment loss	Yes	Yes
Probing pocket depths	≤ 3 mm	≤ 3 mm
BOP	< 10%	≥ 10%
Radiographic bone loss	Possible	Possible
Successfully treated stable periodontitis patient		
Probing attachment loss	Yes	Yes
Probing pocket depths	≤ 4 mm (no site ≥ 4 mm with BOP)	≤ 3 mm
BOP	< 10%	≥ 10%
Radiographic bone loss	Yes	Yes

Q: Describe the characteristics of drug-induced gingival enlargement, a dental biofilm–induced gingivitis.[2]

1. Occurs mostly in the anterior gingiva
2. Higher prevalence in the younger age groups
3. Symptoms within 3 months of use
4. No tooth mortality or tooth loss
5. First observed at the papilla

It is characterized by non-reversible tissue destruction resulting in progressive attachment loss, eventually leading to tooth loss.[10]

Q: Which different forms of periodontitis are recognized in the revised classification?[11]

1. Necrotizing periodontitis
2. Periodontitis as a direct manifestation of systemic diseases
3. Periodontitis

Q: What is the classification of periodontitis?[6]

II. Periodontitis
  A. Staging based on severity, complexity, extent, and distribution
    1. Stage 1: Slight (Fig 6-3)
      ▪ Interdental CAL 1 to 2 mm at site of greatest loss
      ▪ Radiographic bone loss < 15% in coronal third of the root, mostly horizontal
      ▪ Probing depths 3 to 4 mm
    2. Stage 2: Moderate (Fig 6-4)
      ▪ Interdental CAL 3 to 4 mm at site of greatest loss
      ▪ Radiographic bone loss 15% to 33% in coronal third of root, mostly horizontal
      ▪ Probing depths 4 to 5 mm

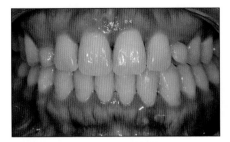

Fig 6-3 Stage 1 periodontitis.[11]

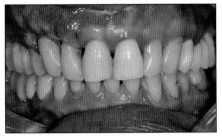

Fig 6-4 Stage 2 periodontitis.[11]

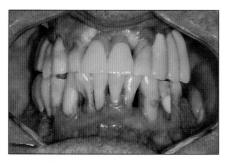

Fig 6-5 Stage 3 periodontitis.[14]

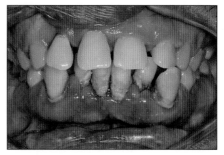

Fig 6-6 Stage 4 periodontitis.[14]

3. Stage 3: Severe (Fig 6-5)
   - Interdental CAL ≥ 5 mm
   - Radiographic bone loss, extending to middle third of root
   - Vertical defects ≥ 3 mm
   - Probing depths ≥ 6 mm
   - Furcation involvement grade II and III
   - Masticatory function is preserved
   - Moderate ridge defect
   - Periodontal tooth loss ≤ 4 teeth
4. Stage 4: Very severe (Fig 6-6)
   - Interdental CAL ≥ 5 mm
   - Radiographic bone loss extending to middle third of root and beyond
   - Vertical defects ≥ 3 mm
   - Probing depths ≥ 6 mm
   - Furcation involvement grade II and III
   - Masticatory dysfunction—need for complex rehabilitation
   - Secondary occlusal trauma, mobility ≥ 2
   - Bite collapse
   - Less than 20 remaining teeth
   - Severe ridge defect
   - Periodontal tooth loss ≥ 5 teeth

B. Grading based on past progression, risk of future progression, anticipated treatment outcome, and general health status
   1. Grade A: Slow rate of progression
   2. Grade B: Moderate rate of progression
   3. Grade C: Rapid rate of progression

Q: Explain staging of periodontitis.

There is only one stage per patient, and it is keyed to the worst tooth (eg, interdental CAL at site of greatest loss). See Table 6-3 below. →

Table 6-3 Staging of periodontitis

	Stage 1	Stage 2	Stage 3	Stage 4
Severity				
▪ CAL interproximal (gold standard for diagnosis)	1–2 mm	3–4 mm	≥ 5 mm	≥ 5 mm
▪ Radiographic bone loss	Coronal 1/3 < 15%	Coronal 1/3 15%–33%	Middle 1/3 +	Middle 1/3 +
▪ Periodontal tooth loss (TL) (only if cause of tooth loss is known)	No perio TL	No perio TL	Perio TL ≤ 4	Perio TL ≥ 5
Complexity	Horizontal bone loss (BL) Probing depth (PD) ≤ 4 mm	Horizontal BL PD ≤ 5 mm	Vertical BL ≥ 3 mm, furcation grade II or III, PD ≥ 6 mm, moderate ridge defects	In addition to stage 3 complexity; need for complex rehabilitation due to: ▪ Bite collapse, drifting, flaring ▪ Less than 20 teeth ▪ Secondary occlusal trauma (tooth mobility ≥ 2) ▪ Severe ridge defects ▪ Masticatory dysfunction
Extent	Local: < 30% teeth; general: ≥ 30% teeth; molar/incisor pattern			

From Caton and Greenwell.[12]

Severity based on:

1. CAL at site with greatest loss
2. Radiographic bone loss
3. Tooth loss

Complexity of management based on: ridge defects, probing depths, furcation lesions, pattern of bone loss, number of remaining teeth, masticatory dysfunction, and tooth mobility

Extent: Localized means < 30% of teeth are involved, and generalized means ≥ 30% of teeth are involved.

Please note the following:

- Vertical bone loss ≥ 3 mm: automatic stage 3 or 4.
- Furcation involvement grade II or III: automatic stage 3 or 4.
- < 20 teeth remaining: automatic stage 4.
- Removing teeth for periodontal reasons and leaving only relatively healthy teeth should not move the diagnosis to an earlier stage (for example, if six periodontally compromised teeth are removed, leaving only healthy teeth, then the diagnosis is still stage 4).

Figure 6-7 shows examples of different stages.

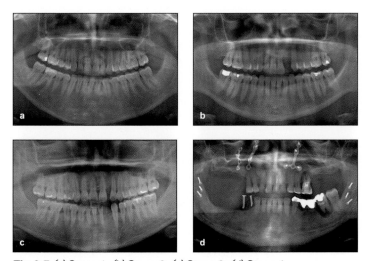

Fig 6-7 *(a)* Stage 1. *(b)* Stage 2. *(c)* Stage 3. *(d)* Stage 4.

Q: Explain grading of periodontitis.

Only one grade is used per patient, and it is keyed to the worst grade assignment. The idea is to predict progression based on past progression or the presence of risk factors. See Table 6-4 on the next page. →

Table 6-4	Grading of periodontitis		
Parameter	Grade A: Slow	Grade B: Moderate	Grade C: Rapid
Progression			
Radiographic BL or CAL over 5 years*	None	< 2 mm	≥ 2 mm
%BL/age† (see Table 6-5)	< 0.25/year	0.25–1.0/year	> 1.0/year
Plaque/BL†	Heavy biofilm with low levels of destruction	Destruction commensurate with biofilm deposits	Destruction exceeds expectations given biofilm deposit
Risk factors			
Smoking (cigarettes/day)	Nonsmoker	< 10	≥ 10
Diabetes	No diabetes diagnosis, normoglycemic	Diabetes diagnosis, HbA1c < 7%	Diabetes diagnosis, HbA1c ≥ 7%
Systemic impact (inflammation)			
hsCRP (mg/L)	< 1	1–3	> 3
BOP (%)	0–25	26–75	> 75

BL, bone loss; hsCRP, high-sensitivity C-reactive protein.
*Direct evidence of progression (preferred).
†Indirect evidence of progression (use only if direct evidence not available).

Clinicians should initially assume grade B disease and seek specific evidence to shift to grade A or C. Whenever available, direct evidence should be used.

Grading adds dimensions beyond periodontitis as an isolated oral disease:

- Progression rate (multiple influences)
- Influence of risk factors on periodontitis progression
- Systemic impact of periodontitis on other body systems

Table 6-5 shows the percent bone loss by age for each grade.

Table 6-5	Percent bone loss divided by age		
Age (years)	Grade A: Slow (< 0.25/year)	Grade B: Moderate (0.25–1.0/year)	Grade C: Rapid (> 1.0/year)
30	< 7.5%	7.5%–30%	> 30%
40	< 10%	10%–40%	> 40%
50	< 12.5%	12.5%–50%	> 50%
60	< 15%	15%–60%	> 60%

Given a grade C diagnosis for parameters 1–4 presented in Table 6-4, the following recommendation can be made:

- Grade 1C: Radiographic bone loss or CAL shows rapid progression; focus on periodontal treatment/maintenance to slow progression.
- Grade 2C: Smoking favors rapid progression; focus on smoking cessation, utilize co-therapist if needed.
- Grade 3C: Diabetes favors rapid progression; focus on utilizing a co-therapist to improve diabetes control.
- Grade 4C: Systemic impact favors rapid progression; focus on decreasing inflammatory burden.

Q: What is the classification of systemic diseases associated with loss of periodontal supporting tissues?

III. Systemic diseases associated with loss of periodontal supporting tissues
    A. Systemic disorders that have a major impact on the loss of periodontal supporting tissues by influencing periodontal inflammation
        1. Genetic disorders
            a. Diseases associated with Immunologic disorders
                1) Down syndrome
                2) Leukocyte adhesion deficiency syndromes
                3) Papillon-Lefèvre syndrome
                4) Haim-Munk syndrome
                5) Chediak-Higashi syndrome
                6) Congenital neutropenia (Kostmann syndrome)
                7) Primary immunodeficiency diseases
                    a) Chronic granulomatous disease
                    b) Hyperimmunoglobulin E syndromes
                8) Cohen syndrome
            b. Diseases affecting the oral mucosa and gingival tissue
                1) Epidermolysis bullosa
                    a) Dystrophic epidermolysis bullosa
                    b) Kindler syndrome
                2) Plasminogen deficiency
            c. Diseases affecting the connective tissues
                1) Ehlers-Danlos syndromes (types IV, VIII)
                2) Angioedema (C1-inhibitor deficiency)
                3) Systemic lupus erythematosus
            d. Metabolic and endocrine disorders
                1) Glycogen storage disease
                2) Gaucher disease
                3) Hypophosphatasia
                4) Hypophosphatemic rickets
                5) Hajdu-Cheney syndrome
         2. Acquired immunodeficiency diseases
            a. Acquired neutropenia
            b. Human immunodeficiency virus infection
         3. Inflammatory immune diseases
            a. Epidermolysis bullosa acquisita
            b. Inflammatory bowel disease
    B. Other systemic disorders that influence the pathogenesis of periodontal diseases
        1. Diabetes mellitus →

  2. Obesity
  3. Osteoporosis
  4. Arthritis
     a. Rheumatoid arthritis
     b. Osteoarthritis
  5. Emotional stress and depression
  6. Smoking (nicotine dependence)
  7. Medications
C. Systemic disorders that can result in loss of periodontal tissues independent of periodontitis
  1. Neoplasms
     a. Primary neoplastic diseases of the periodontal tissues
        1) Squamous cell carcinoma
        2) Odontogenic tumors
        3) Other primary neoplasms
     b. Secondary metastatic neoplasms of the periodontal tissues
  2. Other disorders that may affect the periodontium
     a. Granulomatosis with polyangiitis
     b. Langerhans cell histiocytosis
     c. Giant cell granulomas
     d. Hyperparathyroidism
     e. Systemic sclerosis (scleroderma)
     f. Gorham-Stout disease (vanishing bone disease)

It is recommended to follow the classification of the primary disease according to the International Statistical Classification of Diseases and Related Health Problems (ICD) codes.[5]

Q: Describe Papillon-Lefèvre syndrome.

Papillon-Lefèvre syndrome is an autosomal recessive syndrome characterized by hyperkeratosis of the soles of the feet, palms, knees, and elbows. Most patients also have severe periodontitis that leads to early loss of primary and permanent teeth. Neutrophil dysfunction is believed to be the cause of the disease.[13]

Q: What is the classification of necrotizing periodontal diseases?

IV. Necrotizing periodontal diseases
  A. In severely compromised patients (eg, HIV+/AIDS, with CD4 counts < 200 and detectable viral load in adults, malnutrition and viral infections in kids) →

1. Necrotizing gingivitis (presence of necrosis/ulcer of the interdental papillae, gingival bleeding, and pain)
2. Necrotizing periodontitis (presence of necrosis/ulcer of the interdental papillae, gingival bleeding, halitosis, pain, and rapid bone loss)
3. Necrotizing stomatitis (severe inflammatory condition with soft tissue necrosis extending beyond the gingiva and bone denudation with formation of bone sequestrum)
4. Noma (cancrum oris)

B. In moderately/temporarily compromised patients (eg, uncontrolled factors, stress, nutrition, smoking)
1. Necrotizing gingivitis
2. Necrotizing periodontitis

Q: Describe the clinical symptoms of necrotizing periodontitis.

It is characterized by[5]:

1. History of pain
2. Presence of ulceration and bleeding of the gingival margin/fibrin deposits
3. Papilla necrosis
4. In some cases, exposure of the marginal alveolar bone

Q: Describe the classification for periodontal abscesses.[14]

A. In periodontitis patients (in a preexisting periodontal pocket)
1. Acute exacerbation
    a. Untreated periodontitis
    b. Non-responsive to therapy
    c. Supportive periodontal therapy
2. After treatment
    a. Post-scaling
    b. Postsurgery (eg, foreign body sutures or membranes)
    c. Post-medication (eg, systemic antimicrobials)

B. In non-periodontitis patients (not mandatory to have a preexisting pocket)
1. Impaction (eg, dental floss, rubber dam)
2. Harmful habits (eg, nail biting)
3. Orthodontic factors (eg, crossbite)
4. Gingival overgrowth
5. Alteration of the root surface
    a. Severe anatomical alterations (eg, invaginated tooth)
    b. Minor anatomical alterations (eg, cemental tears, enamel pearls)
    c. Iatrogenic conditions (eg, perforations)
    d. Severe root damage (eg, fissure or fracture)
    e. External root resorption →

Periodontal abscesses are characterized by localized accumulation of pus within the gingival wall of the periodontal pocket/sulcus, resulting in a significant tissue breakdown.[14] It can cause tissue destruction, which may compromise the prognosis of the tooth.

Q: What is the differential diagnosis for a periodontal abscess?[1]

1. Tumor lesions (eg, non-Hodgkin lymphoma, myxoma, squamous cell carcinoma)
2. Sickle cell anemia
3. Surgical procedures causing abscesses
4. Other oral lesions (eg, osteomyelitis, pyogenic granuloma, eosinophilic granuloma)
5. Odontogenic abscesses (dentoalveolar abscesses, pericoronitis, lateral periapical cyst, endoperiodontal abscess)

Q: How is a periodontal abscess distinguishable from a pulpal abscess?

Differences between a periodontal and pulpal abscess are shown in Fig 6-8.

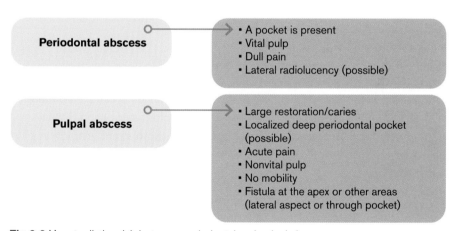

Fig 6-8 How to distinguish between periodontal and pulpal abscesses.

Q: How can a gingival abscess be distinguished from a periodontal abscess?

A gingival abscess is more superficial than a periodontal abscess. It is painful and expands rapidly.

Q: What causes a periodontal abscess and how is it treated?

The causes and treatment for periodontal abscesses are presented in Fig 6-9.

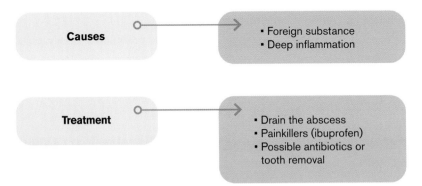

Causes	→	• Foreign substance • Deep inflammation

Treatment	→	• Drain the abscess • Painkillers (ibuprofen) • Possible antibiotics or tooth removal

Fig 6-9 Causes and treatment for periodontal abscesses.

Q: What is a pericoronal abscess?

A pericoronal abscess occurs when the gingiva associated with erupting third molars becomes inflamed. It may occur because of foreign substance entrapment under the gingiva. The pain may spread to the ear or throat and may worsen into Ludwig angina. The treatment includes irrigating the site under anesthesia, antibiotics if there are systemic factors, and extraction if indicated.[15]

Q: What is an endo-periodontal lesion (EPL)?

It is a pathologic communication between the pulpal and periodontal tissues at a given tooth that may occur in an acute or chronic form.

Q: Describe the classification of periodontitis associated with endodontic lesions.

    A. Endodontic-periodontal lesion (pathologic communication between the pulpal and periodontal tissues at a given tooth) →

1. With root damage (pain)
   a. Root fracture/cracking
   b. Root canal or pulp chamber perforation
   c. External root resorption
2. Without root damage
   a. In periodontitis site (slow and chronic without evident symptoms)
      1) Grade 1: Narrow deep periodontal pocket in one tooth surface
      2) Grade 2: Wide deep periodontal pocket in one tooth surface
      3) Grade 3: Deep periodontal pockets in more than one tooth surface
   b. In non-periodontitis site
      1) Grade 1: Narrow deep periodontal pocket in one tooth surface
      2) Grade 2: Wide deep periodontal pocket in one tooth surface
      3) Grade 3: Deep periodontal pockets in more than one tooth surface

Q: What are signs and symptoms of a tooth affected by an EPL?

An EPL may be acute or chronic, and it can involve both the pulp and the periodontal tissues.[1]

1. Abscess accompanied by pain
2. Deep periodontal pockets close or reaching the apex
3. Altered or negative pulp response
4. Bone resorption in the furcation area
5. Spontaneous pain or pain on palpation and percussion
6. Purulent exudate
7. Tooth mobility
8. Sinus tract
9. Crown and gingival color changes

Q: What is the etiology associated with EPLs?

EPLs are always linked to microbial contamination. This may be associated with[1]:

1. Periodontal/endodontic infections

▪ A caries lesion that affects the pulp
▪ Periodontal destruction that affects the root canal
▪ Both of the above events occurring at the same time (combined lesion) →

2. Iatrogenic/trauma factors[1]

- Furcation perforation
- Root fracture or cracking
- Pulp necrosis
- External root resorption

Q: Describe the prognosis of a tooth with an EPL.

An EPL caused by trauma or iatrogenic factors is usually hopeless. The prognosis of a tooth with a periodontal and endodontic lesion ranges depending on the severity of periodontal destruction.

Q: Describe the classification of developmental or acquired deformities and conditions.

A. Prostheses and tooth-related factors that modify or predispose to plaque-induced gingival diseases/periodontitis[16]
   1. Localized tooth-related factors
      a. Tooth anatomical factors
      b. Root fractures
      c. Cervical root resorption, cemental tears
      d. Root proximity
      e. Altered passive eruption
   2. Localized dental prostheses–related factors
      a. Restoration margins placed within the supracrestal attached tissues
      b. Loss of periodontal supporting tissues caused by fabrication of indirect restoration
      c. Hypersensitivity/toxicity reactions to dental materials
B. Mucogingival deformities and conditions around teeth
   1. Gingival phenotype
      a. Thin scalloped (Fig 6-10)
      b. Thick scalloped (Fig 6-11)
      c. Thick flat
   2. Gingival/soft tissue recession
      a. Facial or lingual surfaces
      b. Interproximal (papillary)
      c. Severity of recession[17] (Fig 6-12)

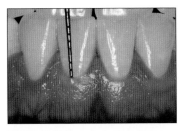

Fig 6-10 Thin periodontal phenotype.

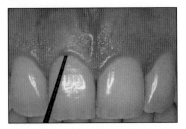

Fig 6-11 Thick periodontal phenotype.

$\rightarrow$

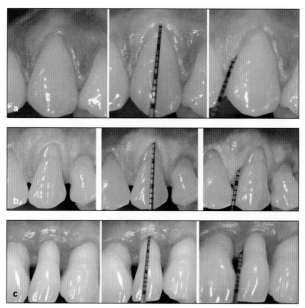

Fig 6-12 *(a)* RT1. *(b)* RT2. *(c)* RT3.[12]

    1) Recession type 1: Gingival recession with no loss of interproximal attachment. Interproximal CEJ is clinically not detectable at both mesial and distal aspects of the tooth.
    2) Recession type 2: Gingival recession associated with loss of interproximal attachment. The amount of interproximal attachment loss (measured from the interproximal CEJ to the depth of the interproximal sulcus/pocket) is less than or equal to the buccal attachment loss (measured from the buccal CEJ to the apical end of the buccal sulcus/pocket).
    3) Recession type 3: Gingival recession associated with loss of interproximal attachment. The amount of interproximal attachment loss (measured from the interproximal CEJ to the apical end of the sulcus/pocket) is greater than the buccal attachment loss (measured from the buccal CEJ to the apical end of the buccal sulcus/pocket).
  d. Gingival thickness
  e. Gingival width
  f. Presence of noncarious cervical lesions (NCCLs)/cervical caries
  g. Patient esthetic concern (smile esthetic index)
  h. Presence of hypersensitivity
3. Lack of keratinized gingiva →

4. Decreased vestibular depth
5. Aberrant frenum/muscle position
6. Gingival excess
   a. Pseudopocket
   b. Inconsistent gingival margin
   c. Excessive gingival display
   d. Gingival enlargement
7. Abnormal color
8. Surface condition
C. Traumatic occlusal forces
   1. Primary occlusal trauma
   2. Secondary occlusal trauma
   3. Orthodontic forces

A diagnostic approach to classifying gingival phenotype[16] is based on the CEJ (A: detectable; B: undetectable) and a cervical step (+: presence of a cervical step > 0.5 mm; −: absence of a cervical step > 0.5 mm). For example, class A+ would indicate a detectable CEJ and a cervical step > 0.5 mm.

Q: Describe cemental tears.

A cemental tear is a unique type of surface fracture that may cause periodontal and periapical tissue destruction. Cemental tears are noted in males (77.5%), older than 60 (73.2%), maxillary and mandibular incisors (76.1%), and vital teeth (65.3%). Treatment options include nonsurgical scaling and root planing, surgical debridement with guided tissue regeneration or combined with a bone graft, and extraction. The authors found that surgical technique was more effective than nonsurgical technique. Most teeth can be retained to function by nonsurgical and surgical periodontal and endodontic treatment.[18]

Q: What are peri-implant diseases and conditions?

A. Peri-implant health (no erythema, no BOP, no inflammation, the probing depth is less than 5 mm, changes ≥ 2 mm during or after the first year should be considered pathologic, and the mucosa forms a tight seal around the implant)[15]
   1. Normal bone height
   2. Reduced bone height
B. Peri-implant mucositis (disease that includes inflammation of the soft tissues surrounding a dental implant without additional bone loss after

→

the initial bone remodeling that may occur during healing following
implant placement)[15]

C. Peri-implantitis (an inflammatory process affecting the tissue around
an implant in function that has resulted in loss of supporting bone)

D. Peri-implant soft and hard tissue deficiencies

1. Soft tissue deficiencies
   a. Thin peri-implant mucosa
   b. Lack of keratinized peri-implant mucosa
   c. Reduced papilla height
   d. Peri-implant frenum attachments
2. Hard tissue deficiencies
   a. Horizontal ridge deficiency
   b. Vertical ridge deficiency
   c. Pneumatization of maxillary sinus
   d. Thin/absent buccal and lingual bone plates

**Q: What is the classification system that the American
Academy of Periodontology (AAP) has developed for
periodontal diseases (mostly for insurance purposes)?**

- Case Type I: Gingivitis
- Case Type II: Early periodontitis–mild bone loss with no furcation invasion
- Case Type III: Moderate periodontitis–moderate bone loss with early furcation invasion
- Case Type IV: Advanced periodontitis–severe bone loss with far-reaching furcation invasion

Predictors of Diagnosis

**Q: Is BOP a reliable predictor of periodontal disease
progression?**

The following studies investigated the reliability of BOP as a predictor of
periodontal disease progression:

- Lang et al[19] evaluated 41 patients using BOP at each maintenance visit
  and found a 6% positive predictive value and a 98% negative predictive
  value for disease progression. They concluded that BOP is a reliable
  predictor of periodontal health maintenance. →

- Lang et al[20] conducted a retrospective study to evaluate the prognostic value of BOP in identifying sites at risk for periodontal breakdown during the maintenance phase of periodontal therapy. Pockets with an incidence of BOP of 4/4 had a 30% chance of losing attachment. As BOP decreased, the chance of attachment loss also decreased: BOP of 3/4—14%, 2/4—6%, 1/4—3%, and 0/4—1.5%.
- The absence of BOP at 0.25 N is a reliable parameter to indicate periodontal stability with a negative predictive value of 98% to 99%.[21]
- A study by Greenstein et al[22] found that while both inflammation and BOP could be used to identify gingival inflammatory lesions, in areas where observation of inflammatory signs was not possible, BOP using controlled pressure on insertion served as an objective method of diagnosis of inflammatory lesions.
- Haffajee et al[23] evaluated the sensitivity of clinical measurements of gingival redness, plaque, suppuration, and BOP. Because no clinical parameter demonstrated high sensitivity and high specificity values, none of the clinical parameters used individually or in combination were found useful in predicting disease activity at individual sites.
- A retrospective study found that the mean percentage of BOP in patients enrolled in supportive periodontal therapy was statistically significantly increased with initial disease severity and periodontal instability irrespective of the smoking status. Over an average period of 11.9 years, periodontally unstable patients demonstrated a mean BOP > 20%, while periodontally stable patients presented with a mean BOP < 20%, reaching statistical significance.[24]

Q: How much pressure should be applied to a probe when measuring BOP?

According to Gerber et al,[25] false-positive BOP results around teeth could be minimized by using a probing pressure of 0.25 N, and around implants a threshold pressure of 0.15 N could reduce false positives.

Q: Is suppuration a predictor of periodontal disease?

Suppuration is found in 3% to 5% of sites with periodontal disease.

Q: **Are CAL measurements, ie, the distance from the CEJ to the base of the probable crevice, a good predictor of periodontal disease?**

Clinical attachment loss is difficult to accurately measure, but it gives a better overall estimate of the amount of damage to the periodontium compared with probing depth measurements. In prospective studies, CAL measurements are the most valid method of assessing treatment outcomes.[1]

Q: **Is probing depth a good predictor of periodontal disease?**

In terms of disease progression, Isidor et al[26] found a low positive predictive value for deep probing depth but a very high negative predictive value for absence of probing depth.

Armitage et al[27] concluded the following from studies in beagle dogs:

- Periodontal probes do not precisely measure connective tissue attachment levels.
- Inflammation has a significant influence on the degree of probe penetration.
- Histologic and clinical sulcus depths differ significantly.

Q: **Are there any host-based tests for susceptibility to periodontitis?**

There is a test for the interleukin 1 gene cluster available to practitioners. According to the position paper by the AAP,[3] individuals with this composite genotype may have an increased risk of BOP, severe chronic periodontitis, tooth loss, and diminished stability of clinical attachment gain following guided tissue regeneration.

Q: **Is increased tooth mobility a sign of disease?**

Increased tooth mobility in conjunction with a widening of the PDL is most likely a sign of occlusal trauma. Furthermore, an increase in tooth mobility is not a sign of disease for a tooth with a reduced but healthy periodontium. Due to reduced periodontal support, the tooth has increased mobility. Consequently, tooth mobility should not be used as a sign of disease or health status.[9]

Diagnostic Process

Q: What are some important factors when determining a diagnosis?

The medical history questionnaire and examination are vital and should include the factors[28] listed in Fig 6-13.

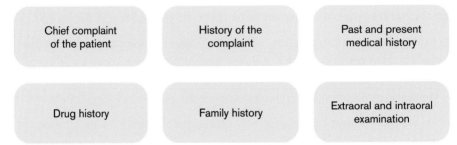

| Chief complaint of the patient | History of the complaint | Past and present medical history |
| Drug history | Family history | Extraoral and intraoral examination |

Fig 6-13 Factors to be included in a medical health questionnaire. The medical doctor may need to be contacted to determine if there is a possible dental contraindication.

Q: In which situations are biopsies required?

- A cancerous lesion is suspected
- A positive histologic diagnosis has implications for other body systems
- The lesion being diagnosed has variable clinical histologic features.

  If in doubt, the dentist should always refer.

Radiographs

Q: What may be some important signs seen in radiographs that suggest periodontal disease?

Radiographic signs of periodontal disease may include:

- Break/fuzziness in the crestal lamina dura
- Wedge-shaped radiolucency
- Crestal fuzziness may be an early sign of angular bone loss
- Bone loss in furcation areas

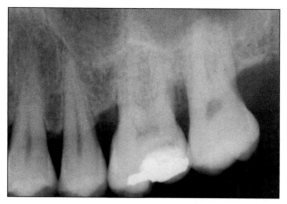

Fig 6-14 Radiograph of a patient with bone loss.

Q: Are radiographs an accurate method of diagnosing periodontal disease?

Ortman et al[29] found that the unaided eye is able to detect radiographic changes when approximately 50% of the bone has been lost (Fig 6-14).

Deas et al[30] found that the furcation arrow is an accurate predictor of furcation invasion 70% of the time. However, when furcation invasions are known to be present, the furcation arrow is seen in less than 40% of sites.

Q: What alveolar crest level represents bone loss on a bitewing radiograph?

Hausmann et al[31] suggested that the radiographic threshold for crestal bone loss is greater than 2 mm from the CEJ to the alveolar crest on bitewing radiographs.

Q: Are digital radiographs equivalent to conventional radiographs in revealing bone loss?

Digital radiographs have dose advantages and are able to enhance images. Khocht et al[32] noted that digital radiographs showed a higher number of sites with bone loss than did conventional radiographs. Bruder et al[33] found that digital radiographs saved time, exposed the patient to less radiation (50% to 60%), allowed versatility in viewing the image, and produced no chemical waste.

Q: When should CBCT be used?

The AAP found limited evidence supporting the utilization of CBCT for diagnosis of intrabony and furcation defects. There are still no current evidence-based guidelines on its need and use for periodontal treatment planning. In selective cases, however, limited field of view CBCT may be beneficial for periodontal disease diagnoses due to decreased radiation dosage to the patient, higher spatial resolution, and shorter volumes to be interpreted.[34]

According to the American Dental Association,[35] "clinicians should perform radiographic imaging, including CBCT, only after professional justification that the potential clinical benefits will outweigh the risks associated with exposure to ionizing radiation. All radiographic examinations should be indicated clinically and justified appropriately."

Miscellaneous

Q: Is rheumatoid arthritis (RA) a predictor of periodontal disease?

Pischon et al[36] found that study participants with RA had significantly increased periodontal attachment loss and a significant 8.05-fold increased odds of periodontitis compared with control participants. They stated that this association may be only partially accounted for by oral hygiene.

Gleissner et al[37] suggested that patients with long-term active RA present a substantially higher degree of periodontal disease, including loss of teeth, compared with controls.

See chapter 14 for more on RA.

References

1. Chapple ILC, Mealey BL, Van Dyke TE, et al. Periodontal health and gingival diseases and conditions on an intact and a reduced periodontium: Consensus report of workgroup 1 of the 2017 World Workshop on the Classification of Periodontal and Peri-Implant Diseases and Conditions. J Periodontol 2018;89(suppl 1):S74–S84.
2. Murakami S, Mealey BL, Mariotti A, Chapple ILC. Dental plaque-induced gingival conditions. J Periodontol 2018;89(suppl 1):S17–S27.
3. Armitage GC; Research, Science and Therapy Committee of the American Academy of Periodontology. Diagnosis of periodontal diseases. J Periodontol 2003;74:1237–1247 [erratum 2004;75:779].

4. Bartold PM, Van Dyke TE. Periodontitis: A host-mediated disruption of microbial homeostasis. Unlearning learned concepts. Periodontol 2000 2013;62:203–217.

5. Tonetti MS, Greenwell H, Kornman KS. Staging and grading of periodontitis: Framework and proposal of a new classification and case definition. J Periodontol 2018;89(suppl 1):S159–S172.

6. Caton JG, Armitage G, Berglundh T, et al. A new classification scheme for periodontal and peri-implant diseases and conditions—Introduction and key changes from the 1999 classification. J Periodontol 2018;89(suppl 1):S1–S8.

7. Trombelli L, Farina R, Silva CO, Tatakis DN. Plaque-induced gingivitis: Case definition and diagnostic considerations. J Periodontol 2018;89(suppl 1):S46–S73.

8. Holmstrup P, Plemons J, Meyle J. Non-plaque-induced gingival diseases. J Periodontol 2018;89(suppl 1):S28–S45.

9. Lang NP, Bartold PM. Periodontal health. J Periodontol 2018;89(suppl 1):S9–S16.

10. Tonetti MS, Eickholz P, Loos BG, et al. Principles in prevention of periodontal diseases: Consensus report of group 1 of the 11th European Workshop on Periodontology on effective prevention of periodontal and peri-implant diseases. J Clin Periodontol 2015;42(suppl 16):S5–S11.

11. Froum S. The new classification of periodontal disease that you, your patient, and your insurance company can understand. Perio-Implant Advisory website. https://www.perioimplantadvisory.com/clinical-tips/article/16412257/the-new-classification-of-periodontal-disease-that-you-your-patient-and-your-insurance-company-can-understand. Accessed 18 Oct 2019.

12. Caton J, Greenwell H. Joint pre- and postdoctoral educators workshop: Findings from the World Workshop: A Perspective for educators. Presented at the 10th Annual Meeting of the American Academy of Periodontology, Vancouver, 29 Oct 2018.

13. Van Dyke TE, Taubman MA, Ebersole JL, et al. The Papillon-Lefèvre syndrome: Neutrophil dysfunction with severe periodontal disease. Clin Immunol Immunopathol 1984;31:419–429.

14. Papapanou PN, Sanz M, Buduneli N, et al. Periodontitis: Consensus report of workgroup 2 of the 2017 World Workshop on the Classification of Periodontal and Peri-Implant Diseases and Conditions. J Periodontol 2018;89(suppl 1):S173–S182.

15. Renvert S, Persson GR, Pirih FQ, Camargo PM. Peri-implant health, peri-implant mucositis, and peri-implantitis: Case definitions and diagnostic considerations. J Periodontol 2018;89(suppl 1):S304–S312.

16. Jepsen S, Caton JG, Albandar JM, et al. Periodontal manifestations of systemic diseases and developmental and acquired conditions: Consensus report of workgroup 3 of the 2017 World Workshop on the Classification of Periodontal and Peri-Implant Diseases and Conditions. J Periodontol 2018;89(suppl 1):S237–S248.

17. Cairo F, Nieri M, Cincinelli S, Mervelt J, Pagliaro U. The interproximal clinical attachment level to classify gingival recessions and predict root coverage outcomes: An explorative and reliability study. J Clin Periodontol 2011;38:661–666.

18. Lin HJ, Chang MC, Chang SH, et al. Treatment outcome of the teeth with cemental tears. J Endod 2014;40:1315–1320.

19. Lang NP, Adler R, Joss A, Nyman S. Absence of bleeding on probing. An indicator of periodontal stability. J Clin Periodontol 1990;17:714–721.

20. Lang NP, Joss A, Orsanic T, Gusberti FA, Siegrist BE. Bleeding on probing. A predictor for the progression of periodontal disease? J Clin Periodontol 1986;13:590–596.

21. Lang NP, Joss A, Tonetti MS. Monitoring disease during supportive periodontal treatment by bleeding on probing. Periodontol 2000 1996;12:44–48.

22. Greenstein G, Caton J, Polson AM. Histologic characteristics associated with bleeding after probing and visual signs of inflammation. J Periodontol 1981;52:420–425.

23. Haffajee AD, Socransky SS, Goodson JM. Clinical parameters as predictors of destructive periodontal disease activity. J Clin Periodontol 1983;10:257–265.

24. Ramseier CA, Mirra D, Schütz C, et al. Bleeding on probing as it relates to smoking status in patients enrolled in supportive periodontal therapy for at least 5 years. J Clin Periodontol 2015;42:150–159.

25. Gerber JA, Tan WC, Balmer TE, Salvi GE, Lang NP. Bleeding on probing and pocket probing depth in relation to probing pressure and mucosal health around oral implants. Clin Oral Implants Res 2009;20:75–78.

26. Isidor F, Karring T, Attström R. Reproducibility of pocket depth and attachment level measurements when using a flexible splint. J Clin Periodontol 1984;11:662–668.

27. Armitage GC, Svanberg GK, Löe H. Microscopic evaluation of clinical measurements of connective tissue attachment levels. J Clin Periodontol 1977;4:173–190.

28. Clerehugh V, Tugnait A, Genco RJ. Periodontology at a Glance. West Sussex, UK: Wiley-Blackwell, 2009:32.

29. Ortman LF, McHenry K, Hausmann E. Relationship between alveolar bone measured by 125I absorptiometry with analysis of standardized radiographs: 2. Bjorn technique. J Periodontol 1982;53:311–314.

30. Deas DE, Moritz AJ, Mealey BL, McDonnell HT, Powell CA. Clinical reliability of the "furcation arrow" as a diagnostic marker. J Periodontol 2006;77:1436–1441.

31. Hausmann E, Allen K, Clerehugh V. What alveolar crest level on a bite-wing radiograph represents bone loss? J Periodontol 1991;62:570–572.

32. Khocht A, Janal M, Harasty L, Chang KM. Comparison of direct digital and conventional intraoral radiographs in detecting alveolar bone loss. J Am Dent Assoc 2003;134:1468–1475.

33. Bruder GA, Casale J, Goren A, Friedman S. Alteration of computer dental radiography images. J Endod 1999;25:275–276.

34. Kim DM, Bassir SH. When is cone-beam computed tomography imaging appropriate for diagnostic inquiry in the management of inflammatory periodontitis? An American Academy of Periodontology best evidence review. J Periodontol 2017;88:978–998.

35. The American Dental Association Council on Scientific Affairs. The use of cone-beam computed tomography in dentistry: An advisory statement from the American Dental Association Council on Scientific Affairs. J Am Dent Assoc 2012;143:899–902.

36. Pischon N, Pischon T, Kröger J, et al. Association among rheumatoid arthritis, oral hygiene, and periodontitis. J Periodontol 2008;79:979–986.

37. Gleissner C, Willershausen B, Kaesser U, Bolten WW. The role of risk factors for periodontal disease in patients with rheumatoid arthritis. Eur J Med Res 1998;3:387–392.

Prognosis

Background

Q: What is prognosis?

Prognosis is a forecast of probable outcome of disease based on the experience of a large number of other patients with similar disease progression.

Q: Describe what Hirschfeld and Wasserman[1] and McFall[2] found in their studies on tooth loss over time?

Hirschfeld and Wasserman[1] used three categories to classify the amount of tooth loss that could be expected. They studied 600 patients over 22 years in which 39% received surgical care. They found a rate of 7.1% overall tooth loss (0.08 teeth per patient per year), and 31% of the teeth that were lost had furcations. Table 7-1 presents a summary of their findings.

Table 7-1	Hirschfeld and Wasserman[1] findings on tooth loss over time		
Maintenance	**Teeth lost (no.)**	**Population (%)**	**Teeth lost (%)**
Well-maintained	0–3	83.6%	2.6%
Downhill	4–9	12.6%	22.7%
Extreme downhill	10–23	4.2%	55.4%

$\rightarrow$

McFall[2] studied 100 patients over 19 years in which 63% received surgical care. He found that 9.8% of all surgically treated teeth were lost, and 7.1% of nonsurgically treated teeth were lost. He also found that 56.9% of teeth with furcations were lost. His findings are presented in Table 7-2.

Table 7-2	McFall[2] findings on tooth loss over time	
Maintenance	Teeth lost (no.)	Population (%)
Well-maintained	0–3	77%
Downhill	4–9	15%
Extreme downhill	10–23	3%

Based on the above studies, the following conclusions can be made:

- Furcation-involved teeth are lost three to five times as often as other teeth.
- Maxillary molars are most often lost, and mandibular canines are more frequently retained.
- Periodontal disease is bilateral and symmetric.
- Periodontal therapy has 87% to 92% tooth retention.

Q: What are the most relevant tooth-related factors for loss of molars?

A recent study found grade III furcation involvement is the most relevant tooth-related factor for loss of molars during supportive periodontal therapy. In addition to furcation involvement, advanced bone loss (> 60%) at the onset of periodontal therapy and endodontic treatment are significant tooth-related aspects with a negative impact on survival of molars. Interestingly, about 63% of molars with grade III furcation involvement were still present after 10 years with a mean survival time of 11.8 years. The study also found that increased age, females, patients with diabetes, and smokers lost more molars.[3]

Miller et al[4] reported that of all the prognostic factors evaluated for the periodontal prognosis of molars, smoking had the most negative impact, far exceeding the impact of probing depth, mobility, or furcation involvement. Molar type had a lesser impact, while age had the least impact. Finally, treating moderate to severe periodontal disease can result in an excellent long-term prognosis regardless of the patient's age.

Q: What amount of tooth loss is expected if patients do not comply with a recommended compliance schedule?

Becker et al[5] found the following amount of tooth loss over 5 years. Treated groups received pocket reduction and scaling and root planing in two quadrants.

- 0.36 teeth lost per year for patients who were not treated
- 0.22 teeth lost per year for patients who were treated but not maintained
- 0.11 teeth lost per year for patients who were treated and maintained

Classification

Q: Describe the McGuire[6] classification of prognosis. What categories were considered?

The McGuire[6] classification, based on tooth loss, is presented in Fig 7-1 (see next page).

   A study by McGuire and Nunn[7] showed a 5- to 8-year prediction accuracy of the above classification of 80%. That decreased to 50% or less when the good prognosis category was removed. As a result, assigning prognoses is ineffective for teeth with an initial prognosis of less than good. Although this system was based on tooth loss, critics believed that the status of the remaining teeth is variable and should be based on periodontal stability (clinical attachment level and radiographic bone measurements). Furthermore, tooth extraction is usually performed by the dentist rather than the patient and may be done for other non-periodontal reasons. $\rightarrow$

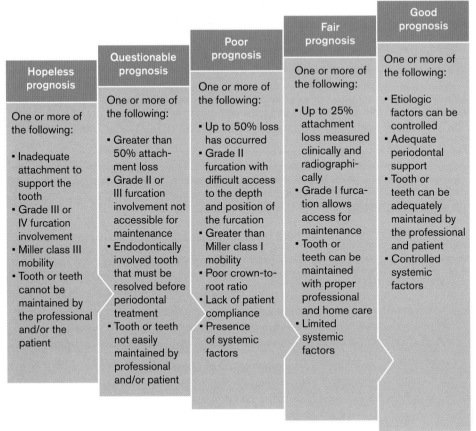

Fig 7-1 McGuire[4] classification.

Q: What amount of time is indicated by short- and long-term prognosis?

Short-term prognosis is fewer than 5 years, and *long-term prognosis* is considered greater than 5 years. However, Kwok and Caton[8] believed "periodontal prognostication" to be dynamic, suggesting that it should be reevaluated throughout treatment and maintenance.

Q: Describe the prognostic classification by Kwok and Caton.[8]

The Kwok and Caton[8] classification system is based on the probability of disease progression. The four proposed classifications are shown in Fig 7-2.

→

Hopeless
The tooth must
be extracted.

Unfavorable
The periodontal status
of the tooth is
influenced by local
and/or systemic
factors that cannot be
controlled.

Questionable
The periodontal status
of the tooth is
influenced by local
and/or systemic
factors that may or
may not be controlled.

Favorable
The periodontal
status of the tooth
can be stabilized
with comprehensive
periodontal treat-
ment and periodontal
maintenance.

Fig 7-2 Kwok and Caton[8] classification.

They identified the following general factors:

- Amount of patient compliance.
- Cigarette smoking: Smokers have a greater prevalence of periodontal disease and bone loss.
- Diabetes mellitus: Patients with diabetes have a greater prevalence of peri-odontal disease and attachment loss.
- Other systemic conditions (neutrophil dysfunction, Papillon-Lefèvre syndrome, Down syndrome, and immunologic dysfunctions).

They further identified the following local factors:

- Deep probing depths and attachment loss
- Anatomical plaque-related factors (furcation involvement, enamel pearls, cervical enamel projections, open contacts, crowding, root proximity, and overhanging restorations)
- Trauma from occlusion and parafunctional habits
- Root fractures (Fig 7-3)
- Mobility

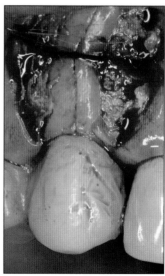

Fig 7-3 Hopeless tooth with a vertical root fracture.

117

Periodontitis and Its Effect on Prognosis

Q: Describe the prognosis of stage 1, 2, 3, and 4 of periodontitis.

See Table 7-3 below.

Table 7-3	Stages of periodontitis
Stage	**Prognosis**
I	Early diagnosis can allow for early intervention and can be cost-effective.
II	Standard treatment principles and regular professional maintenance is expected to arrest disease progression.
III	Management is complicated, and tooth loss may occur.
IV	Considerable damage and significant tooth loss, which means loss of masticatory function.

Data from Tonetti et al.[9]

Past Periodontitis and Its Effect on Prognosis

Q: Is there any harm in not extracting hopeless teeth when treating a periodontitis patient?

DeVore et al[10] studied 17 patients who received open flap debridement with frequent maintenance on retained hopeless teeth. The study found that retained hopeless and periodontally compromised teeth have no effect on the proximal periodontium of adjacent teeth prior to and following periodontal therapy.

Machtei et al[11] studied 145 teeth and concluded that retained hopeless teeth (with severe periodontal breakdown) without periodontal treatment had a negative effect on the adjacent teeth. They found that it was 10 times more likely for the adjacent teeth to have bone loss.

Q: Does a history of periodontal disease predispose to future disease?

McGuire and Nunn[12] found a strong association between prognosis and initial probing depth, furcation involvement, and mobility.

Prognosis of Different Diseases and Therapies

Q: What is the prognosis of a patient with necrotizing gingivitis? Necrotizing periodontitis?

- Necrotizing gingivitis: Good prognosis with the control of plaque and secondary factors.
- Necrotizing periodontitis: Many are immunocompromised; prognosis depends on systemic factors.

Q: What is the prognosis of a tooth that has been diagnosed with a furcation lesion?

Cobb[13] reported that over a 15-year period, 19% to 57% of teeth with furcation lesions and only 5% to 10% of teeth without furcation lesions were lost.

Ramfjord et al[14] discovered that 16 of 17 teeth extracted in 5 years during maintenance and following active treatment initially presented with furcation involvement.

Q: Describe the prognosis of a tooth with a tooth fracture and/or root fracture.

The 2017 World Workshop[15] found that if a tooth fracture occurred coronal to the gingival margin and does not extend to parts of the tooth surrounded by periodontal tissues, it does not initiate gingivitis or periodontitis.

The location of the root fracture had a strongly significant effect on tooth survival. The 10-year tooth survival of apical root fractures was 89%, of mid-root fractures 78%, of cervical mid-root fractures 67%, and of cervical fractures 33%.[16] Cervical fractures are more likely to be colonized by subgingival plaque and can cause gingivitis and periodontitis.

Q: **Compare the prognosis of implant therapy and endodontic therapy.**

It is important to note that there are many variables to consider when reviewing these articles. For example, some of the articles may be comparing surface characteristics of implants that are no longer used.

According to Christensen,[17] there are many factors to consider when comparing the prognosis of implant and endodontic therapy, most of which are listed below:

- Cost: The implant-supported alternative can be twice as expensive as the endodontic alternative, which may influence a patient's decision.
- Coronal breakdown of the tooth: If endodontic therapy is questionable, extraction of the tooth may be a better alternative.
- Type of supporting bone around the tooth: The quality of the bone in the anterior maxilla and mandible is better for implant placement than that in the posterior maxilla.
- The tooth's ability to support a single crown or fixed prosthesis: Questionable nonvital teeth planned for a fixed prosthesis should be replaced with implants.
- Occlusion: Because of increased chewing forces, endodontic and restorative treatment has a questionable prognosis in bruxers and clenchers. Patients who are bruxers and receive implants require a splint and occlusal equilibration.
- Periodontal condition: The periodontal condition of the teeth needs to be addressed before any decision can be made about treatment.
- Patient's perception of treatment: Each treatment should be thoroughly discussed with patients, because how they perceive the psychologic and physiologic trauma associated with different treatment options may greatly influence their decision.
- Overall health: Considerations include smoking and systemic conditions.
- Time needed for treatment: Implant therapy may take longer because of the time needed for implants to osseointegrate.
- Potential esthetic result: If esthetics would be compromised with an implant, retention of the tooth may be a better option.

Iqbal and Kim[18] did a systematic review and found no differences in survival when comparing teeth with treated root canals and single-tooth implants.

Table 7-4 describes the success rate of different endodontic treatment modalities. →

Table 7-4	Prognostic values for endodontic treatment modalities
Treatment	**Successful outcome**
Nonsurgical root canal therapy	97% (Salehrabi and Rotstein) 88% (de Chevigny et al)
Nonsurgical retreatment	89% (Salehrabi and Rotstein) 86% (Fristad et al) 83% (de Chevigny et al)
Surgical root canal therapy	89% (Tsesis et al) 96% (Rubinstein and Kim)
MTA pulp capping	37% (Barthel et al) 80% (Mente et al)

MTA, mineral trioxide aggregate.
Data from Blicher et al.[19]

Q: Does tooth/root position affect the prognosis of the patient?

Misalignment/rotation of a tooth, crossbite, and crowding of the mandibular and maxillary anterior teeth have been associated with gingivitis, attachment loss, increased plaque retention, and greater pocket depth.[15]

An interradicular distance of < 0.8 mm is a significant local risk factor for alveolar bone loss in mandibular anterior teeth.[20]

Q: What are some considerations to recognize when deciding to save or extract a tooth?

According to Tarnow,[21] the dentist should consider the following:

- Restorative needs of the patient
- Size of the defect
- Endodontic status of the tooth or teeth
- History of periodontal disease
- Decay rate (may be related to the drugs the patient is taking)
- Esthetics in the area
- Anatomical considerations
- Status of the adjacent teeth
- Economic situation of the patient
- Patient's emotions

Figure 7-4 presents factors to consider when deciding whether to extract or save a tooth.[14] →

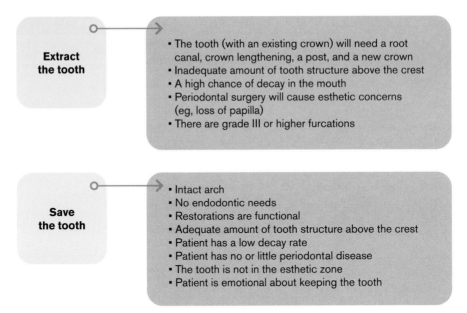

Extract the tooth
- The tooth (with an existing crown) will need a root canal, crown lengthening, a post, and a new crown
- Inadequate amount of tooth structure above the crest
- A high chance of decay in the mouth
- Periodontal surgery will cause esthetic concerns (eg, loss of papilla)
- There are grade III or higher furcations

Save the tooth
- Intact arch
- No endodontic needs
- Restorations are functional
- Adequate amount of tooth structure above the crest
- Patient has a low decay rate
- Patient has no or little periodontal disease
- The tooth is not in the esthetic zone
- Patient is emotional about keeping the tooth

Fig 7-4 Considerations when deciding to extract or save a tooth.

Q: Is there a correlation between periodontitis and pulpal changes?

Bender and Seltzer[22] found that teeth with restorations or caries and periodontal disease had a higher likelihood of atrophic pulps than teeth with restorations or caries that did not have periodontal disease.

Giovanella et al[23] found oxygen saturation was lower in the pulp of permanent teeth with periodontal attachment loss, periodontal pockets, and gingival recession, indicating that periodontal disease correlates with the level of oxygen saturation in the pulp.

Mazur and Massler[24] studied 106 periodontally involved teeth from patients aged 19 to 70 years. The study failed to confirm a correlation between periodontal disease and pulp tissue changes.

Q: Describe the prognosis of implant therapy versus root resection in molars.

Fugazzotto[25] found the lowest success rate (85%) among single implants in second molar positions, while all other implant treatment in molar sites had a success rate of 97.0% to 98.6%. Molars with root resection and molar implants had the highest failure rate when they were single terminal abutments.

Q: **Does a fixed partial denture or single implant have a better prognosis?**

According to Lindh et al,[26] in the short term (after 1 year), the success rate is 85.7% for fixed partial dentures and 97.2% for implants with single crowns. After 6 to 7 years, the success rate is 93.6% for fixed partial dentures and 97.5% for implants with single crowns.

Q: **Can removable partial dentures (RPDs) affect the periodontal status of the patient?**

Zlatarić et al[27] found that RPDs do affect the health of the periodontium. There were significant differences in plaque and gingival indices as well as probing depth, mobility, and gingival recession between abutment and nonabutment teeth. It is important for the RPD to be located as far as possible from the gingival margin because its coverage had a negative effect on gingival health.

According to a literature review by Petridis and Hempton,[28] if good periodontal health is established and maintained through oral hygiene measures prior to prosthetic treatment, RPDs do not cause any harm to the periodontium.

A recent study found abutment teeth presented higher values of gingival recession when compared with nonabutment or antagonist teeth. No significant differences were found between teeth that supported RPDs and teeth that did not regarding bleeding on probing or probing depth over time.[29]

References

1. Hirschfeld L, Wasserman B. A long-term survey of tooth loss in 600 treated periodontal patients. J Periodontol 1978;49:225–237.
2. McFall WT Jr. Tooth loss in 100 treated patients with periodontal disease. A long-term study. J Periodontol 1982;53:539–549.
3. Dannewitz B, Zeidler A, Hüsing J, et al. Loss of molars in periodontally treated patients: Results 10 years and more after active periodontal therapy. J Clin Periodontol 2016;43:53–62.
4. Miller PD Jr, McEntire ML, Marlow NM, Gellin RG. An evidenced-based scoring index to determine the periodontal prognosis on molars. J Periodontol 2014;85:214–225.
5. Becker W, Becker BE, Berg LE. Periodontal treatment without maintenance. A retrospective study in 44 patients. J Periodontol 1984;55:505–509.
6. McGuire MK. Prognosis versus actual outcome: A long-term survey of 100 treated periodontal patients under maintenance care. J Periodontol 1991;62:51–58.
7. McGuire MK, Nunn ME. Prognosis versus actual outcome. II. The effectiveness of clinical parameters in developing an accurate prognosis. J Periodontol 1996;67:658–665.

8. Kwok V, Caton JG. Commentary: Prognosis revisited: A system for assigning periodontal prognosis. J Periodontol 2007;78:2063–2071.
9. Tonetti MS, Greenwell H, Kornman KS. Staging and grading of periodontitis: Framework and proposal of a new classification and case definition. J Periodontol 2018;89(suppl 1):S159–S172.
10. DeVore CH, Beck FM, Horton JE. Retained "hopeless" teeth. Effects on the proximal periodontium of adjacent teeth. J Periodontol 1988;59:647–651.
11. Machtei EE, Zubrey Y, Ben Yehuda A, Soskolne WA. Proximal bone loss adjacent to periodontally "hopeless" teeth with and without extraction. J Periodontol 1989;60:512–515.
12. McGuire MK, Nunn ME. Prognosis versus actual outcome. III. The effectiveness of clinical parameters in accurately predicting tooth survival. J Periodontol 1996;67:666–674.
13. Cobb CM. Non-surgical pocket therapy: Mechanical. Ann Periodontol 1996;1:443–490.
14. Ramfjord SP, Caffesse RG, Morrison EC, et al. Four modalities of periodontal treatment compared over 5 years. J Clin Periodontol 1987;14:445–452.
15. Ercoli C, Caton JG. Dental prostheses and tooth-related factors. J Periodontol 2018;89(suppl 1):S223–S236.
16. Andreasen JO, Ahrensburg SS, Tsilingaridis G. Root fractures: The influence of type of healing and location of fracture on tooth survival rates—An analysis of 492 cases. Dent Traumatol 2012;28:404–409.
17. Christensen GJ. Implant therapy versus endodontic therapy. J Am Dent Assoc 2006;137:1440–1443.
18. Iqbal MK, Kim S. For teeth requiring endodontic treatment, what are the differences in outcomes of restored endodontically treated teeth compared to implant-supported restorations? Int J Oral Maxillofac Implants 2007;22(suppl):96–116.
19. Blicher B, Pryles RL, Lin J. Endodontics Review: A Study Guide. Chicago: Quintessence, 2016:256.
20. Kim T, Miyamoto T, Nunn ME, Garcia RI, Dietrich T. Root proximity as a risk factor for progression of alveolar bone loss: The Veterans Affairs Dental Longitudinal Study. J Periodontol 2008;79:654–659.
21. Tarnow DP. When to retain the compromised tooth: Point-counterpoint. Presented at the 98th Annual Meeting of the American Academy of Periodontology, Los Angeles, California, 1 Oct 2012.
22. Bender IB, Seltzer S. The effect of periodontal disease on the pulp. Oral Surg Oral Med Oral Pathol 1972;33:458–474.
23. Giovanella LB, Barletta FB, Felippe WT, Bruno KF, de Alencar AH, Estrela C. Assessment of oxygen saturation in dental pulp of permanent teeth with periodontal disease. J Endod 2014;40:1927–1931.
24. Mazur B, Massler M. Influence of periodontal disease on the dental pulp. Oral Surg Oral Med Oral Pathol 1964;17:592–603.
25. Fugazzotto PA. A comparison of the success of root resected molars and molar position implants in function in a private practice: Results of up to 15-plus years. J Periodontol 2001;72:1113–1123.
26. Lindh T, Gunne J, Tillberg A, Molin M. A meta-analysis of implants in partial edentulism. Clin Oral Implants Res 1998;9:80–90.
27. Zlatarić DK, Celebić A, Valentić-Peruzović M. The effect of removable partial dentures on periodontal health of abutment and non-abutment teeth. J Periodontol 2002;73:137–144.
28. Petridis H, Hempton TJ. Periodontal considerations in removable partial denture treatment: A review of the literature. Int J Prosthodont 2001;14:164–172.
29. Costa L, do Nascimento C, de Souza VO, Pedrazzi V. Microbiological and clinical assessment of the abutment and non-abutment teeth of partial removable denture wearers. Arch Oral Biol 2017;75:74–80.

Occlusion

8

Background

Q: What is excessive occlusal force? Occlusal trauma?

Excessive occlusal force is defined as occlusal force that exceeds the reparative capacity of the periodontal attachment apparatus, which results in occlusal trauma and/or causes excessive tooth wear.[1]

Occlusal trauma is injury resulting in tissue changes within the attachment apparatus (including periodontal ligament [PDL], supporting alveolar bone, and cementum) because of occlusal forces. It can occur in an intact periodontium or in a reduced periodontium caused by periodontal disease.

Primary occlusal trauma is injury resulting in tissue changes from excessive occlusal forces applied to a tooth with normal support.

Secondary occlusal trauma is injury resulting in tissue changes from normal to excessive occlusal forces applied to a tooth or teeth with reduced support.

Reinhardt et al[2] found in a bench study using finite element analysis that a "reduction of alveolar bone height had little effect on the degree of periodontal ligament stress until 60% of bone support had been lost."

Q: What are the definitions of *abrasion*, *attrition*, and *abfraction*?

The definitions of *abrasion*, *attrition*, and *abfraction* are provided in Fig 8-1 (see next page).

Abfraction is one of the proposed etiologies for noncarious cervical lesions (NCCLs). NCCLs may also result from abrasion, erosion, or corrosion.

Although some studies have suggested an association between the progression of NCCLs and excessive occlusal forces, a causal relationship is uncertain.[1]

> **Abrasion:** Loss of tooth substance by mechanical wear other than mastication

> **Attrition:** Occlusal wear from functional contacts with opposing teeth

> **Abfraction:** Occlusal loading on surfaces causing tooth flexure (in the cervical area)

Fig 8-1 Definitions of *abrasion*, *attrition*, and *abfraction*.

Q: What are some clinical signs of trauma to the periodontium?

- Tooth fracture
- Increased tooth mobility
- Increased PDL space (radiographically)
- Tooth migration
- Pain on chewing
- Occlusal prematurities
- Fremitus
- Hypertrophy of muscles of mastication
- Temporomandibular joint dysfunction
- Wear facets
- Thermal sensitivity
- Root resorption
- Cemental tear

Mobility

Q: Describe the Miller classification[3] of mobility.

The Miller classification[3] of mobility:

- Class I: First sign of movement greater than normal.
- Class II: The tooth can be moved up to 1 mm in a buccolingual or mesiodistal direction but does not exhibit abnormal mobility in an occlusoapical direction. →

- Class III: The tooth can be moved 1 mm or more in either buccolingual or mesiodistal and occlusoapical directions.

Q: What are the causes of increased mobility of the teeth?

- Any functional or parafunctional force that cannot be dissipated by the PDL and nearby bone and that causes adaptive changes to nearby bone (that result in increased mobility)
- Loss of osseous support
- Trauma from occlusion
- Parafunctional habits
- Short root
- Orthodontic movement
- Periodontal procedures, including closed procedures that disrupt gingival fibers and nearby bone, but more often flap surgery (usually temporary)
- Hormonal changes (eg, pregnancy or portions of the menstrual cycle) may cause small transient increases in mobility
- Other pathologic processes in underlying bone
- PDL atrophy

Q: Is there a relationship between mobile teeth and success of periodontal treatment?

Fleszar et al[4] studied 82 patients for 8 years and found that pockets of clinically mobile teeth do not respond as well to periodontal treatment as do those of immobile teeth exhibiting the same initial disease severity.

Grant et al[5] found significantly higher proportions of *Campylobacter rectus* and *Peptostreptococcus micros* in pockets around mobile teeth compared with those adjacent to nonmobile teeth. Elevated levels of *Porphyromonas gingivalis* were also found around mobile teeth, but the difference was not statistically significant. The authors concluded that tooth mobility and its associated increase in subgingival levels of periodontopathogens may present a periodontal risk.

McGuire and Nunn[6] reported increased probing depth, initial furcation involvement, initial mobility, initial percent bone loss, parafunctional habit with no bite guard, and smoking were all related to the risk of tooth loss.

Fan and Caton[1] found that reduction of tooth mobility may enhance the effect of periodontal therapy.

Q: Is there an association between tooth mobility and gingival recession?

There is no significant correlation between gingival recession and tooth mobility.[7]

Q: What is fremitus?

Fremitus is a palpable or visible movement of a tooth when it is subjected to occlusal forces.

Types of Occlusion

Q: What is group function? Canine-guided occlusion?

During lateral movement, if there is simultaneous contact of the posterior teeth of the working side, it is called *group function*. In the same situation, if the canine alone contacts, then it is called *canine-guided occlusion* or *canine protection*.

Q: What percentage of the population has canine protection? Group function?

Goldstein[8] found that 14% of study participants exhibited canine protection, 46% had group function, and 24% demonstrated a different disocclusion pattern on each side.

Implants

Q: What type of occlusion is ideal for patients with implants?

Sheridan et al[9] found that:

> …occlusal schemes for single implants or fixed partial denture supported by implants include a mutually protected occlusion with anterior guidance and evenly distributed contacts with wide freedom in centric relation. Suggestions to reduce occlusal overload include reducing cantilevers, increasing the number of implants, increasing contact points, monitoring

→

for parafunctional habits, narrowing the occlusal table, decreasing cuspal inclines, and using progressive loading in patients with poor bone quality.

Q: What can cause occlusal overload? What is the effect of occlusal overload for implants?

Causes of occlusal overload:

- Large cantilevers
- Parafunctional habits/bruxism
- Steep cusp inclines
- Poor distribution of forces (limited contacts)
- Interferences
- Poor quality bone

Occlusal overload effects:
- Screw loosening
- Prosthesis failure
- Screw fracture
- Implant fixture fracture
- Implant failure

Sheridan et al[9] found that:

Occlusal overload has been regarded as a major cause of biomechanical complications, including screw loosening, prosthesis failure, and the fracture of screws, veneering material, or the implant. This is significant because these complications can be costly, time consuming, and some complications, such as implant fixture fracture, can lead to implant failure.

Kozlovsky et al[10] reported that overloading the implant aggravated the plaque-induced bone resorption when peri-implant inflammation was present.

Fu et al[11] found occlusal overloading to be positively associated with peri-implant marginal bone loss.

Theories of Occlusion

Q: Describe the classic animal studies in the United States and Sweden.

- In a cadaver study, Glickman[12] defined the term *co-destruction,* naming two regions in the periodontium: a zone of irritation (marginal and interdental gingiva and gingival and transseptal fibers) and the zone of co-destruction (PDL, alveolar bone, cementum, and transseptal and alveolar crest fibers). He speculated that inflammation in the presence of occlusal trauma alters the alignment of the transseptal fibers, thus allowing inflammation to spread to the PDL space with resultant intrabony pocket formation.
- Based on a cadaver study, Waerhaug[13] believed bacterial plaque in conjunction with local anatomy was the primary cause of intrabony defect formation, not occlusal trauma.
- In Sweden, a series of studies by Lindhe and Svanberg and others[14,15] used a jiggling force produced via a permanently affixed cap-splint apparatus in dogs. The studies' key findings were that trauma from occlusion alone did not appear to cause loss of connective tissue attachment and that trauma combined with induced periodontitis caused ample attachment and bone loss.
- At Rochester, Kennedy and Polson[16] used nonjiggling forces on wooden wedges in squirrel monkeys. They found that trauma alone caused loss of bone height that was largely reversible when trauma was removed, and a reduction of coronal bone but no loss of attachment.

The Americans' and Swedes' results were similar in the following ways[1]:

1. In animals without periodontitis, occlusal trauma resulted in increased mobility and loss of bone density without apparent loss of connective tissue attachment.
2. If trauma was removed from animals without periodontitis, the loss of bone density was largely reversible.
3. In the presence of periodontitis and occlusal trauma, there was greater loss of bone volume and increased mobility.
4. The studies found that without plaque-induced inflammation, occlusal trauma does not cause irreversible bone loss of connective tissue attachment. Occlusal trauma alone did not appear to cause periodontitis, but it may be a cofactor that can accelerate periodontal breakdown in the presence of periodontitis. →

Ramfjord and Ash[17] found that traumatic occlusion does not initiate or aggravate gingivitis or initiate pockets, but it can increase mobility and may accelerate bone loss and pocket formation, depending on the presence of inflammation. Bruxism can perpetuate trauma. Splinting is not indicated in self-limiting trauma from occlusion but is indicated in conjunction with occlusal adjustment when trauma from occlusion is progressive.

Q: Does traumatic occlusal force or occlusal trauma cause periodontal attachment loss in humans? Inflammation? NCCLs?

There is no clear evidence that traumatic occlusal forces alone cause periodontal attachment loss in humans or cause NCCLs. Occlusal trauma does not appear to initiate periodontitis, and there is weak evidence that it alters the progression of the disease. There is no clear evidence to support the etiologies of abfractive lesions or that implicate abfraction as a cause of gingival recession. There are limited data that traumatic occlusal forces can cause inflammation in the periodontal ligament.[1,18]

Occlusal Discrepancies

Q: Do uneven marginal ridges increase attachment loss?

Blieden[19] found that poor restorative contouring and/or interdental marginal discrepancies can increase the risk for periodontal infections.

Kepic and O'Leary[20] did not report increased attachment loss with uneven marginal ridges.

Q: Do teeth with occlusal contacts in excursive positions exhibit any greater severity of periodontitis?

Yuodelis and Mann[21] found that 53% of nonworking contacts had greater pocket depth and greater mobility. However, this study had no controls. Nunn and Harrel[22] found teeth with initial occlusal discrepancies to have significantly deeper initial probing depths, significantly worse prognoses, and significantly worse mobility than teeth without initial occlusal discrepancies.

Pihlstrom et al[23] found that teeth with occlusal contacts in centric relation and working, nonworking, or protrusive positions did not exhibit any greater severity of periodontitis than teeth without these contacts. Shefter and $\rightarrow$

McFall[24] found that nonfunctional contacts are common and that occlusal disharmonies do not have a significant harmful impact on periodontal health.

Q: Do occlusal discrepancies affect gingival recession?

According to Harrel and Nunn,[25] there is no statistically significant relationship between the presence of occlusal discrepancies and initial width of the gingival tissue or between occlusal treatment and changes in the width of the gingiva.

Bruxism

Q: What is bruxism or tooth grinding?

It is a habit of grinding, clenching, or clamping the teeth. The habit damages the teeth and attachment apparatus.[1]

Q: What are symptoms of bruxism?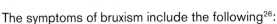

The symptoms of bruxism include the following[26]:

- Increased mobility
- Pulpal sensitivity
- Bite tenderness
- Excessive occlusal wear
- Muscle tenderness
- Temporomandibular joint pain
- Audible sounds

Q: Can periodontal disease be affected by bruxism?

Hanamura et al[27] found significantly greater alveolar bone loss, attachment loss, and tooth mobility in patients with moderate to severe periodontitis than in patients with bruxism, while more tooth attrition was found in the bruxism patients. In most cases, periodontal disease and bruxism did not coexist in the same individual, and the authors concluded that in general there was no close association between the two conditions.

Occlusal Adjustment

Q: What is occlusal adjustment?

Occlusal adjustment is the intentional, professional alteration to occlusal surfaces of teeth to create a balanced relationship between the maxillary and mandibular teeth. It is important to remove centric prematurities, preserve the supporting cusps, and remove lateral contacts.

Q: What are the indications and contraindications for occlusal adjustment?

Figure 8-2 presents the indications and contraindications for occlusal adjustment. Note that according to Lindhe et al,[28] occlusal adjustment is effective against tooth mobility when mobility is caused by a loss of bony support often detected as what appears to be an increased width of the PDL.

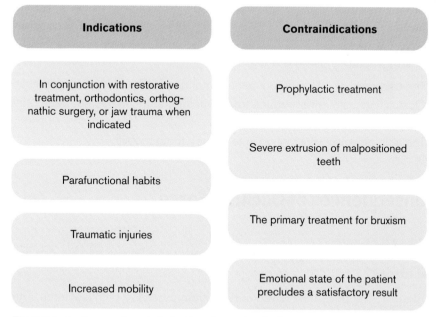

Fig 8-2 Indications and contraindications for occlusal adjustment.

Q: Is there greater gain of clinical periodontal attachment in patients who received occlusal adjustment compared with those who did not?

According to Burgett et al,[29] there was a significant gain in attachment of 0.4 mm in patients who received occlusal adjustment. Pocket depth was not affected by occlusal adjustment, and the response to occlusal adjustment was not impacted by initial tooth mobility or periodontal disease severity.

Splinting

Q: When should splinting be done?

Splinting should be done[30]:

- Following trauma
- For comfort
- To prevent drifting of the teeth
- To prevent or limit tooth mobility

Q: What are contraindications to splinting?

Splinting is contraindicated when[31]:

- The treatment of inflammatory periodontal disease has not been addressed
- Occlusal adjustment to reduce trauma or interferences has not been previously considered
- The sole objective of splinting is to reduce tooth mobility

Consequences of Occlusal Force

Q: What are the stages of tissue response to excessive occlusal forces?

- Stage 1: The body tries to repair injury from excessive occlusal force. The area most susceptible to injury is the furcation.
- Stage 2: Repair is constantly occurring in the normal periodontium. Trauma from occlusion stimulates increased reparative activity. The damaged →

tissues are removed, and new connective tissue cell fibers, bone, and cementum may be formed.

- Stage 3: Adaptive remodeling occurs. If a tooth remains in traumatic occlusion, the PDL becomes wider, and vascularization is temporarily increased. If a tooth moves out of traumatic occlusion (eg, orthodontic movement), normal anatomy results following healing.

Orthodontics

Q: How does orthodontics help a periodontal patient?

- Aligns the teeth and helps the patient with oral hygiene
- Can improve osseous defects (decrease need for resective surgery)
- Can force eruption to align the gingiva
- Can force eruption of a cracked tooth (at least 1:1 crown-to-root ratio)
- Closes open embrasures
- Improves adjacent tooth position before implant placement

Q: What are the risks of orthodontic treatment?

- Recession
- Cemental resorption
- Root resorption (shortened root length)
- Loss of attachment
- Loss of tooth vitality
- Tooth relapse
- Caries

A systematic review[32] found weak evidence from one randomized study and 11 nonrandomized studies suggesting that orthodontic therapy was associated with averages of 0.03 mm of gingival recession, 0.13 mm of alveolar bone loss, and 0.23 mm of increased pocket depth when compared with no treatment. The existing evidence suggests that orthodontic therapy results in small disadvantageous effects to the periodontium.

Q: Under what circumstances should extrusion be done?

- Increasing bone height prior to extraction of a hopeless tooth and subsequent implant placement. Amato et al[33] found that forced eruption was able to regenerate 70% of bone and augment the gingiva by 60%.
- Crown lengthening (may still need surgery because the bone moves with the tooth).
- Filling intraosseous defects.
- Leveling and aligning the gingival margin for esthetic harmony.

Q: Can tooth movement into adjacent defects be accomplished successfully?

In a study with a monkey model, Polson et al[34] established that orthodontic tooth movement into intrabony periodontal defects with a reduced but healthy periodontium was not damaging to the connective tissue attachment.

Q: Should orthodontics be used to upright a molar?

A study by Lang[35] demonstrated a 0.6-mm decrease in pocket depth and a 0.4-mm gain in attachment level following uprighting of mandibular tipped molars in advance of prosthetic treatment. He concluded that this technique was a simple and predictable method that would improve the prognosis of the treated teeth.

Kessler[36] pointed out the risks of uprighting mesially tipped second molars. Bone loss and furcation involvement may be caused by the uprighting as a periodontal osseous lesion is widened when the tooth is uprighted. A study by Lundgren et al[37] concluded that a mesially tipped molar does not increase the risk for periodontal disease compared with an upright molar and therefore did not support the use of orthodontic uprighting to prevent the initiation or advancement of periodontal disease.

Q: Can orthodontics worsen the prognosis of a patient with periodontitis?

The lack of periodontal support may reduce resistance to unwanted tooth movement (anchorage problems) and can increase the risk of root resorption due to reduced available root surface area and decreased vascularity.[38]

A study of periodontal health during orthodontic treatment by Boyd et al[39] included 20 adults (10 of whom received treatment for generalized →

periodontitis prior to orthodontic treatment) and 20 adolescents. The study found that during fixed orthodontic treatment:

- No significant increase in loss of attachment occurs in patients with a reduced but healthy periodontium.
- Tooth loss may occur in adults with advanced periodontal disease, including pocket depths > 6 mm or advanced furcation involvements.
- Significantly more plaque accumulation and gingival inflammation can be expected in adolescents than in adults.

References

1. Fan J, Caton JG. Occlusal trauma and excessive occlusal forces: Narrative review, case definitions, and diagnostic considerations. J Periodontol 2018;89(suppl 1):S214–S222.
2. Reinhardt RA, Pao YC, Krejci RF. Periodontal ligament stresses in the initiation of occlusal traumatism. J Periodontal Res 1984;19:238–246.
3. Miller SC. Textbook of Periodontia. Philadelphia: Blakiston, 1938.
4. Fleszar TJ, Knowles JW, Morrison EC, Burgett FG, Nissle RR, Ramfjord SP. Tooth mobility and periodontal therapy. J Clin Periodontol 1980;7:495–505.
5. Grant DA, Grant DA, Flynn MJ, Slots J. Periodontal microbiota of mobile and non-mobile teeth. J Periodontol 1995;66:386–390.
6. McGuire MK, Nunn ME. Prognosis versus actual outcome. III. The effectiveness of clinical parameters in accurately predicting tooth survival. J Periodontol 1996;67:666–674.
7. Bernimoulin J, Curilovié Z. Gingival recession and tooth mobility. J Clin Periodontol 1977;4:107–114.
8. Goldstein GR. The relationship of canine-protected occlusion to a periodontal index. J Prosthet Dent 1979;41:277–283.
9. Sheridan RA, Decker AM, Plonka AB, Wang HL. The role of occlusion in implant therapy: A comprehensive updated review. Implant Dent 2016;25:829–838.
10. Kozlovsky A, Tal H, Laufer BZ, et al. Impact of implant overloading on the peri-implant bone in inflamed and non-inflamed peri-implant mucosa. Clin Oral Implants Res 2007;18:601–610.
11. Fu JH, Hsu YT, Wang HL. Identifying occlusal overload and how to deal with it to avoid marginal bone loss around implants. Eur J Oral Implantol 2012;5(suppl):S91–S103.
12. Glickman I. Inflammation and trauma from occlusion. Co-destructive factors in chronic periodontal disease. J Periodontol 1963;34:5–10.
13. Waerhaug J. The infrabony pocket and its relationship to trauma from occlusion and subgingival plaque. J Periodontol 1979;50:355–365.
14. Lindhe J, Svanberg G. Influence of trauma from occlusion on progression of experimental periodontitis in the beagle dog. J Clin Periodontol 1974;1:3–14.
15. Ericsson I, Lindhe J. Effect of longstanding jiggling on experimental marginal periodontitis in the beagle dog. J Clin Periodontol 1982;9:497–503.
16. Kennedy JE, Polson AM. Experimental marginal periodontitis in squirrel monkeys. J Periodontol 1973;44:140–144.
17. Ramfjord SP, Ash MM Jr. Significance of occlusion in the etiology and treatment of early, moderate, and advanced periodontitis. J Periodontol 1981;52:511–517.
18. Jepsen S, Caton JG, Albandar JM, et al. Periodontal manifestations of systemic diseases and developmental and acquired conditions: Consensus report of workgroup 3 of the 2017 World Workshop on the Classification of Periodontal and Peri-Implant Diseases and Conditions. J Periodontol 2018;89(suppl 1):S237–S248.

19. Blieden TM. Tooth-related issues. Ann Periodontol 1999;4:91–97.
20. Kepic TJ, O'Leary TJ. Role of marginal ridge relationships as an etiologic factor in periodontal disease. J Periodontol 1978;49:570–575.
21. Yuodelis RA, Mann WV Jr. The prevalence and possible role of nonworking contacts in periodontal disease. Periodontics 1965;3:219–223.
22. Nunn ME, Harrel SK. The effect of occlusal discrepancies on periodontitis. I. Relationship of initial occlusal discrepancies to initial clinical parameters. J Periodontol 2001;72:485–494.
23. Pihlstrom BL, Anderson KA, Aeppli D, Schaffer EM. Association between signs of trauma from occlusion and periodontitis. J Periodontol 1986;57:1–6.
24. Shefter GJ, McFall WT Jr. Occlusal relations and periodontal status in human adults. J Periodontol 1984;55:368–374.
25. Harrel SK, Nunn ME. The effect of occlusal discrepancies on gingival width. J Periodontol 2004;75:98–105.
26. Raigrodski AJ. Cosmetic dentistry: The full mouth fixed rehabilitation of the bruxing patient—Achieving function and esthetics. https://www.oralhealthgroup.com/features/cosmetic-dentistry-the-full-mouth-fixed-rehabilitation-of-the-bruxing-patient-achieving-function-an/. Accessed 25 November 2019.
27. Hanamura H, Houston F, Rylander H, Carlsson GE, Haraldson T, Nyman S. Periodontal status and bruxism. A comparative study of patients with periodontal disease and occlusal parafunctions. J Periodontol 1987;58:173–176.
28. Lindhe J, Nyman S, Ericsson I. Trauma from occlusion: Periodontal tissues. In: Lindhe J, Lang NP, Karring T (eds). Clinical Periodontology and Implant Dentistry, ed 5. Oxford, UK: Blackwell Munksgaard, 2008:359.
29. Burgett FG, Ramfjord SP, Nissle RR, Morrison EC, Charbeneau TD, Caffesse RG. A randomized trial of occlusal adjustment in the treatment of periodontitis patients. J Clin Periodontol 1992;19:381–387.
30. Lemmerman K. Rationale for stabilization. J Periodontol 1976;47:405–411.
31. Rupprecht R. Trauma from occlusion: A review. Navy Med 2004;26:25–27.
32. Bollen AM, Cunha-Cruz J, Bakko DW, Huang GJ, Hujoel PP. The effects of orthodontic therapy on periodontal health: A systematic review of controlled evidence. J Am Dent Assoc 2008;139:413–422.
33. Amato F, Mirabella AD, Macca U, Tarnow DP. Implant site development by orthodontic forced extraction: A preliminary study. Int J Oral Maxillofac Implants 2012;27:411–420.
34. Polson A, Caton J, Polson AP, Nyman S, Novak J, Reed B. Periodontal response after tooth movement into intrabony defects. J Periodontol 1984;55:197–202.
35. Lang NP. Preprosthetic straightening of tilted lower molars with reference to the condition of the periodontium [in German]. SSO Schweiz Monatsschr Zahnheilkd 1977;87:560–569.
36. Kessler M. Interrelationships between orthodontics and periodontics. Am J Orthod 1976;70:154–172.
37. Lundgren D, Kurol J, Thorstensson B, Hugoson A. Periodontal conditions around tipped and upright molars in adults. An intra-individual retrospective study. Eur J Orthod 1992;14:449–455.
38. Clerehugh V, Tugnait A, Genco R.J. Periodontology at a Glance. West Sussex, UK: Wiley-Blackwell, 2009:58.
39. Boyd RL, Leggott PJ, Quinn RS, Eakle WS, Chambers D. Periodontal implications of orthodontic treatment in adults with reduced or normal periodontal tissues versus those of adolescents. Am J Orthod Dentofacial Orthop 1989;96:191–198.

Nonsurgical Therapy

9

Background

Q: What treatment does nonsurgical therapy include?

- Plaque control
- Supra- and subgingival scaling and root planing (SRP)
- Use of chemical agents
- Local delivery of antimicrobials
- Oral hygiene instruction
- Recontouring/replacing defective restorations
- Occlusal therapy

Q: What is scaling?

Scaling is instrumentation of the crown and root surfaces of the teeth to remove plaque, calculus, and staining from the teeth.

Q: What is root planing?

Root planing is instrumentation to remove cementum or surface dentin that is rough, impregnated with calculus, or contaminated with toxins or microorganisms.

Q: What are the endpoints to successful nonsurgical therapy?

- Oral hygiene/plaque control compatible with health $\rightarrow$

- Pink and firm gingival tissue
- Pocket depth reduction (pocket depth < 5 mm)
- No bleeding on probing (BOP)
- No calculus detected
- Decreased mobility of the teeth
- Clinical attachment gain

Effectiveness of Scaling and Root Planing

Q: What studies show the effectiveness of SRP?

- A literature review by Cobb[1] found pocket depth reduction of 1.29 mm and attachment gain of 0.55 mm in 4- to 6-mm pockets and pocket depth reduction of 2.16 mm and attachment gain of 1.79 mm in pockets greater than 7 mm. Stambaugh et al[2] found curette efficacy of 3.73 mm (plaque- and calculus-free surface) when SRP was performed by hygienists with the patient under local anesthesia. The effective instrumentation limit was 6.21 mm. The average time working on each tooth was 35 minutes.
- Buchanan and Robertson[3] noted that premolars and molars are more difficult to clean without a flap. They found that more than 60% of molar sites had residual calculus.
- Waerhaug[4] found that after SRP was performed, more than 90% of cases had deposits of plaque and calculus remaining in sites with pocket depths greater than 5 mm.

Q: What are some factors that can limit the effectiveness of root planing?

Many anatomical factors can limit the effectiveness of root instrumentation[5]:

- Deep probing depths
- Root concavities and grooves
- Furcations
- Root proximity

Host response may also limit the effectiveness of wound healing after root instrumentation:

- Diabetes
- Pregnancy →

140

- Stress
- AIDS
- Immunodeficiencies
- Blood dyscrasias
- Tobacco use

Q: Is root debridement equally effective in molars and nonmolars?

Loos et al[6] found that, following full-mouth root debridement, more molar furcation sites (25%) lost probing attachment compared with nonmolar sites (7%) and molar flat-surface sites (10%).

Q: Are more experienced practitioners more effective at SRP?

Brayer et al[7] showed no difference in the effectiveness of SRP in shallow (1- to 3-mm) pockets based on the experience level of the practitioner or type of procedure. However, in moderate (4- to 6-mm) and deep (> 6-mm) periodontal pockets, a significantly higher number of calculus-free root surfaces were produced by practitioners with greater experience, and SRP was more effective when combined with an open flap procedure.

Q: Is open flap or closed flap SRP more effective?

Caffesse et al[8] found that residual calculus was greatest following scaling with no flap (Table 9-1; see next page) and at the cementoenamel junction or in association with grooves, fossae, or furcations. No differences were noted between anterior and posterior teeth or between different tooth surfaces.

Lindhe et al[9] monitored patients for 5 years following nonsurgical or surgical therapy. A high frequency of plaque-free tooth surfaces was associated with a lack of evidence of recurrent periodontal disease, whereas patients with a high frequency of surfaces with plaque had additional loss of attachment at a greater rate. Surgical and nonsurgical treatment were shown to be equally effective in sites with an initial pocket depth greater than 3 mm. The authors concluded that the quality of root surface debridement is a more important determinant in the success of periodontal therapy than the type of technique used (surgical versus nonsurgical). $\rightarrow$

Table 9-1	Percentage of calculus-free surface in different pocket depths following scaling with or without a flap		
Scaling	1- to 3-mm pockets	4- to 6-mm pockets	> 6-mm pockets
Without a flap	86%	43%	32%
With a flap	86%	76%	50%

Q: What are the consequences to patients with periodontitis who do not receive treatment?

Goodson et al[10] studied attachment level at two sites on each tooth in 22 untreated subjects with existing periodontal pockets for 1 year. They found no significant changes in 82.8% of the sites, significantly deeper pockets in 5.7% of the sites, and significantly shallower pockets in 11.5% of the sites. About half of the sites with increased pocket depth showed cycles of deepening pockets and spontaneous return to the original depth, suggesting that periodontal disease may be a dynamic condition characterized by periods of exacerbation, remission, and inactivity.

Löe et al[11] did a study on Sri Lankan laborers, who, in the absence of oral hygiene practices, presented with large amounts of plaque, calculus, and staining and widespread gingival inflammation. Using interproximal loss of attachment and rates of tooth loss, the authors identified three subpopulations:

- Individuals (approximately 8%) with rapid progression of periodontal disease
- Individuals with moderate progression of periodontal disease (approximately 81%)
- Individuals with no progression (approximately 11%) of periodontal disease beyond gingivitis

Q: What are the critical probing depths?

Using a split-mouth design, Lindhe et al[12] treated 15 patients with moderately advanced periodontal disease using SRP in combination with a modified Widman flap procedure on one side and SRP only on the contralateral side. The study found the following critical probing depths: →

- 2.9 mm: Attachment loss occurred in pockets < 2.9 mm when SRP was performed
- 4.2 mm: Attachment loss occurred in pockets < 4.2 mm if SRP and surgery were performed

Q: Is it more effective to do weekly SRP appointments or a single SRP appointment?

Quirynen et al[13] concluded that the use of antiseptics, as well as the completion of the SRP sessions within a short time frame, seems to have a beneficial effect in the treatment of moderate and severe periodontitis.

Greenstein[14] found that full-mouth therapy could reduce the number of patient visits and facilitate more efficient use of treatment time. In addition, he stated that there did not appear to be any major adverse reactions to full-mouth root planing whether or not it was paired with chemotherapy.

Q: Is full-mouth disinfection or SRP per quadrant more effective?

Patients treated by both SRP and full-mouth disinfection exhibited improvement in all periodontal clinical parameters (included probing depth, clinical attachment level, Plaque Index, and Gingival Index), with no significant differences between treatment groups.[15]

In moderate chronic periodontitis patients, SRP per quadrant and full-mouth disinfection provided periodontal clinical improvements and similar experiences of fear, anxiety, and pain.[16]

Q: Is removal of the cementum important?

Drisko and Killoy[17] suggested that while "thorough root debridement and planing are desirable treatment goals, not all would agree that complete cementum removal is either possible or desirable, or that the removal of calculus is more important than plaque or endotoxin removal in achieving clinical success."

In his literature review, Cobb[1] found that "given the fact that cementum is known to become contaminated when exposed in a periodontal pocket, the literature remains inconsistent concerning both the possibility or need to remove all cementum, and whether it is more important to remove plaque and calculus than 'diseased' cementum."

Q: How many strokes cause removal of the cementum?

Coldiron et al[18] reported that most teeth in groups treated with 20 to 70 strokes showed complete cementum removal, although fragments of cementum remained on the surface of the root in some sections of teeth from each of these treatment groups.

Ritz et al[19] investigated four methods of instrumentation: hand curette, ultrasonic scaler, air scaler, and fine-grit diamond bur. After 12 working strokes, the ultrasonic scaler removed only an 11.6-μm layer of root substance, while much larger amounts of 93.5 μm (air scaler), 108.9 μm (curette), and 118.7 μm (diamond bur) were removed by the other instruments.

Oral Hygiene

Q: How effective is brushing and flossing? What is the best sequence for brushing and flossing?

Graves et al[20] found that brushing decreases BOP by 35%, and additional flossing decreases BOP by 67%. Floss is the most widely used method of interdental cleaning, and the American Dental Association (ADA) reports that up to 80% of interdental plaque may be removed by this method, resulting in a significantly reduced incidence of caries and prevention of periodontal disease.[21]

Mazhari et al[22] found flossing followed by brushing is preferred to reduce interdental plaque and allow maximum fluoride concentration.

Q: How many adults report flossing daily?

About one-third of adults in the United States reported flossing daily.[23]

Q: What is the Bass technique?

In the *Bass technique*,[24] the bristles of a toothbrush are placed at 45 degrees to the tooth surface at the gingival margin. The bristles of the brush are moved in a back-and-forth motion.

Q: Is there a difference between the types of floss and their efficacy?

In a study that involved 24 dental hygiene students, Carr et al[25] tested four different floss types—waxed, unwaxed, woven, and shred-resistant—and reported minimal differences in the efficacy, comfort, and ease of use.

Q: Describe the effectiveness of interdental brushes.

In a single-blind, randomized controlled clinical trial, Jackson et al[26] reported that BOP and probing improved more in the interdental brush group than in the floss group at 6 weeks, and at 12 weeks, significantly greater changes in plaque, papillae level, and probing depths were found in the interdental brush group compared with the floss group.

Tu et al[27] used structural equation modeling to show a greater reduction in pocket depth and BOP with the use of interdental brushing compared with flossing. They attributed this difference primarily to plaque removal efficiency rather than interdental papillae compression.

Slot et al[28] did a systematic study and found interdental brushing (as an adjunct to brushing) removes more dental plaque than brushing alone. They found a positive significant difference using interdental brushes with respect to the plaque scores, bleeding scores, and probing pocket depth.

Q: If complete removal of plaque is not accomplished, how long does it take for gingivitis to develop?

Lang et al[29] found that intervals of 48 hours are compatible with gingival health; however, if intervals between complete removal of plaque exceed 48 hours, gingivitis develops. Plaque first appears on interproximal areas of premolars and last on the facial surfaces of molars and premolars.

Q: Is there a difference between an electric and manual brush?

Robinson et al[30] did a meta-analysis and found that powered toothbrushes with a rotation oscillation action reduce plaque and gingivitis more than manual toothbrushes.

Deery et al[31] did not find a statistically significant difference between the results of use of powered and manual brushes in general; however, they did report significant short- and long-term reduction of plaque and gingivitis with the use of rotation oscillation–powered brushes. →

Rapley and Killoy[32] compared a counter-rotational electric toothbrush and a manual toothbrush. The manual group had 30.57% plaque-free interproximal surfaces and the electric group had 53.23% plaque-free interproximal surfaces.

Q: How often should a toothbrush be replaced?

Glaze and Wade[33] found that after 10 weeks, significantly less plaque had formed in the participants who replaced their brushes every 2 weeks than in those who used the same toothbrush for the duration of the study. Deterioration of the brushes reduced their effectiveness, but differences in gingival health status were not detected.

Manual, Ultrasonic, and Sonic Instrumentation

Q: Are manual and ultrasonic/sonic instrumentation equally capable of improving clinical parameters?

- A study by Drisko[34] found that the unique ability of ultrasonic/sonic scalers to use water or other chemical irrigating solutions to flush pockets during subgingival instrumentation improves reduction of pocket depth and clinical attachment gain compared with hand scaling. In addition, they noted that power-driven scalers have better access to areas that are difficult to reach, such as deep narrow defects, root grooves, and furcations. They concluded that the improvements in clinical and microbial parameters achieved by ultrasonic or sonic scalers used for periodontal debridement should equal or surpass those achieved by hand scalers.
- Nishimine and O'Leary[35] found that endotoxin values were approximately eight times greater with ultrasonic scaling compared with hand scaling.
- Cobb[1] found that as probing depth increases, the power-driven instruments become less effective because of limitations of design. When comparing the manual curette and ultrasonic instruments, the curette appears slightly more efficient but requires more effort, time, and expertise. Newly designed ultrasonic inserts appear to overcome such inherent problems.
- Leon and Vogel[36] evaluated 33 furcated molars and found that, in terms of restoring healthy gingival fluid flow and bacterial composition, in grade I furcations hand scaling and ultrasonic debridement were equally effective,

$\rightarrow$

but in grade II and grade III furcations ultrasonic debridement was significantly more effective than hand scaling.

▪ Croft et al[37] found that patients have a strong preference for ultrasonic
instruments (74%).

▪ Dahiya et al[38] found that the greatest roughness was produced by the
Gracey curette, followed by the ultrasonic tip and rotary bur. However, it
took significantly longer to complete SRP procedures with the rotary bur
than with the Gracey curette and ultrasonic tip.

▪ Several studies have reported that the use of sonic or ultrasonic instruments can result in a 20% to 50% savings in time compared with manual
instrumentation when used for periodontal debridement procedures.[39]

▪ Kepic et al[40] did a study on teeth with "severe periodontal disease." Fourteen teeth (8 single-rooted, 6 multirooted) were treated by closed SRP
with an ultrasonic instrument, and 17 others (10 single-rooted, 7 multirooted) were treated with hand instruments. Twelve of the 14 teeth treated
by ultrasonics and 12 of the 17 treated by hand instruments retained
calculus. They concluded that complete removal of calculus from a periodontally diseased root surface is rare.

▪ Lastly, Bower[41] showed that the furcation entrance is 1 mm or less 81% of
the time and 0.7 mm or less 58% of the time. The ultrasonic (smaller) tip
would fit better in a grade II or grade III furcation than the tip of a Gracey
curette.

Q: What are the characteristics of ultrasonic and sonic scalers?

Figure 9-1 presents the characteristics of ultrasonic and sonic scalers.

Sonic	Ultrasonic	
	Magnetorestrictive	Piezoelectric
• 3,000 to 8,000 cycles/ second	• 1,800 to 4,500 cycles/ second	• 25,000 to 50,000 cycles/ second
• Tip moves in orbital direction	• Elliptical movement of tip	• Linear movement of tip
• Increased noise	• Faster than a sonic	• Faster than a sonic
	• Example: Cavitron	

Fig 9-1 Characteristics of ultrasonic and sonic scalers.

Q: Are sonic or ultrasonic instruments more efficient?

Cobb[1] found sonic instruments to be more efficient than ultrasonic instruments, while Drisko et al[42] found similar results with ultrasonic/sonic scalers and hand instruments for removal of plaque, calculus, and endotoxin. Less damage was found at the root surfaces with the use of ultrasonic scalers at medium power compared with hand or sonic scalers. The width of ultrasonic or sonic scalers may make them a better choice than manual scalers when accessing furcations. However, measures must be taken to ensure good infection control when using power-driven scalers, which produce contaminated aerosols. There may be some clinical benefit to adding certain antimicrobials to the lavage during ultrasonic instrumentation.

Q: Do ultrasonic devices interfere with pacemakers?

Miller et al[43] found inhibition of atrial and ventricular pacing with use of an electrosurgical unit up to a distance of 10 cm, ultrasonic bath cleaner up to 30 cm, and magnetostrictive ultrasonic scalers up to 37.5 cm. However, pacing rate and rhythm were unaffected by use of an amalgamator, electric pulp tester, composite curing light, dental handpieces, electric toothbrush, microwave oven, dental chair and light, radiography unit, and sonic scaler.

Roedig et al[44] noted interference of the ultrasonic scaler with the pacing activity of dual-chamber pacemakers (between 17 and 23 cm from the generator or leads), single-chamber pacemakers (15 cm from the generator or leads), and implantable cardioverter-defibrillators (ICDs) (7 cm from the leads). The ultrasonic cleaning system interfered with the activity of dual-chamber pacemakers (between 15 and 23 cm from the generator or leads) and single-chamber pacemakers (12 cm from the generator or leads). Pacing function was not altered by use of an electric toothbrush, electrosurgical unit, electric pulp tester, high- and low-speed handpieces, or amalgamator.

Q: Is there a difference between ultrasonic and sonic toothbrushes?

Costa et al[45] found that the use of both types of brushes resulted in significant decreases in plaque and gingival indices. However, the indices decreased more significantly in studies testing sonic brushes in orthodontic and dental implant patients. Gingival recession was not attributed to the use of the product.

Q: By how much is the blade of a Gracey curette offset?

A Gracey curette has a blade that is laterally offset by 70 degrees relative to the shank. The blade of the universal curette is situated perpendicular to the edge of the terminal shank.

Q: At what angle should the face of the curette be toward the root?

The face of the curette should be oriented at 60 degrees to the root surface.

Q: At what angle should the Gracey curette be held to the stone when sharpening the blade?

The curette should be held at an angle of 100 to 110 degrees to the stone.

Q: Is there any effect on the pulp from scaling?

Although Fischer et al[46] did not find any alteration to pulp sensitivity following scaling, dentin sensitivity to probe and/or air stimuli increased in a clinically significant manner in six patients, with five of them also experiencing sensitivity to daily stimuli. Desensitization seemed to occur naturally 2 weeks after subgingival debridement, indicating that supragingival and subgingival scaling might result in transient dentin hypersensitivity.

Reevaluation

Q: What is reevaluation and what is its purpose?

Reevaluation is defined as the evaluation or assessment of treatment. It is used to determine the effectiveness of SRP and to review the proficiency of home care/plaque control. Reevaluation "includes the following steps that are performed by the periodontist to determine the soft tissue results of scaling and root planing: bleeding on probing, probing depths, clinical attachment levels, pathologic tooth mobility, furcation involvement, assessment of local factors, Plaque Index, and review of oral hygiene. If needed, re-instrumentation is performed."[47]

Q: When is it an appropriate time to reevaluate a patient following SRP?

If a patient is reevaluated too soon, overtreatment may occur, but if a patient is reevaluated after too long a period, the disease might progress.

Proye et al[48] showed an initial improvement of clinical attachment at 3 weeks following SRP. No additional gain of clinical attachment occurred in the succeeding 3 months.[49] Similarly, Morrison et al[50] showed that the clinical severity of periodontitis is reduced 1 month following the "hygienic phase."

Lowenguth and Greenstein[51] concluded that prior to reevaluation following mechanical nonsurgical therapy, a minimum 3- to 4-week period should elapse, during which soft tissue healing and maturation can occur.

Longer than 2 months may be too long to wait for the reevaluation because pathogenic bacteria have already repopulated periodontal pockets.[47]

Q: When is it appropriate to reevaluate a patient following occlusal therapy for mobility?

The reevaluation of tooth mobility after occlusal therapy should occur after 6 to 12 months.[47]

Maintenance

Q: Does maintenance work?

Rosling et al[52] performed a study on 50 patients, distributed into five groups, with each group receiving one of the following treatments:

- Apically repositioned flap including elimination of bony defects
- Apically repositioned flap including curettage of the bony defects, without removal of bone
- Widman flap including elimination of bony defects through osseous surgery
- Widman flap including curettage of the bony defects, without removal of bone
- Gingivectomy including curettage of the bony defects, without removal of bone

Following treatment, oral hygiene instruction was provided, and professional dental cleanings were performed once every 2 weeks for 2 years. All surgical techniques for pocket elimination were effective in arresting →

periodontal disease and preventing further damage to the periodontal tissues.

Ramjford et al[53] reported that in patients who receive professional dental cleanings once every 3 months, posttreatment pocket depth and attachment levels could be maintained irrespective of personal oral hygiene (as expressed in plaque scores).

Q: **What are the endpoints to successful maintenance therapy?**

The endpoints to successful maintenance therapy are[54]:

- Prevent recurrence in patients who have been previously treated for gingivitis, periodontitis, and peri-implantitis
- Prevent the incidence of tooth or implant loss
- Increase the probability of diagnosis and treatment of other diseases/conditions

Q: **What is done during a maintenance visit?**

The steps taken during a maintenance visit[55] are shown in Fig 9-2.

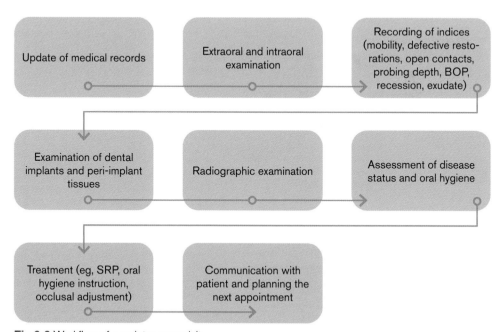

Fig 9-2 Workflow of a maintenance visit.

Q: What is the optimal frequency for maintenance visits?

Patients without additional attachment loss can have maintenance visits once every 6 months. However, most studies have reported that patients who have had a history of periodontal disease require maintenance visits at least four times per year.[55,56] Westfelt et al[57] found that the shorter the recall interval for maintenance visits following periodontal surgery, the better the surgical outcomes.

Q: What factors should be considered in developing an optimal maintenance schedule?

Figure 9-3 presents the factors that should be considered[58] when planning an optimal maintenance schedule.

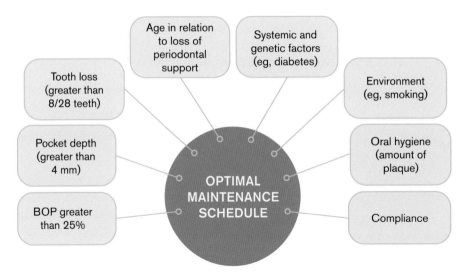

Fig 9-3 Factors to consider for an optimal maintenance schedule.

Q: What is the percentage of compliance by periodontal maintenance patients?

In a study of 961 patients, Wilson et al[59] found 16% full compliance, 49% erratic compliance, and 34% noncompliance with recommended maintenance schedules. The study found that the reasons for noncompliance included fear, lack of information, finances, and a lack of compassion from the practitioner.

In a subsequent study, Wilson et al[60] found that compliance increased from 16% in 1984 to 32% in 1991. The authors attributed this increase in patient compliance to factors such as efforts by office staff to educate patients, changes in dental hygiene practice laws, increased public awareness of the importance of dental care, and economic considerations. The authors concluded that compliance can be improved if patient awareness is increased and disease progression is recognized and addressed appropriately.

Q: What is the effect of compliance on BOP and Plaque Index?

Analysis by Miyamoto et al[61] of clinical parameters over a period of 15 years revealed that complete compliers to maintenance appointments tended to show reduction in BOP and Plaque Index compared with erratic compliers.

Q: What happens when there is a lack of supportive periodontal therapy?

In a study by Nyman et al,[62] all patients underwent presurgical treatment including case presentation and instruction in oral hygiene measures. Then patients were treated with one of the following surgical procedures:

- Apically repositioned flap including elimination of bony defects through osseous surgery
- Apically repositioned flap including curettage of bony defects, without removal of bone
- Widman flap including elimination of bony defects through osseous surgery
- Widman flap including curettage of bony defects, without removal of bone
- Gingivectomy including curettage of bony defects, without removal of bone

Patient assessment was performed 6, 12, and 24 months after treatment was complete. Renewed accumulation of plaque in the surgical areas resulted in recurrence of periodontal disease, including a significant further loss of attachment because the patients had poor oral hygiene and were not

$\rightarrow$

seen on a regular recall schedule (noncompliant). There was no difference in the results obtained with the various techniques; in the absence of periodontal maintenance, they were equally ineffective at preventing the recurrence of disease. Axelsson and Lindhe[63] conducted a study on 77 patients. One-third of the patients were sent to their general dentists (GP group), and two-thirds were in a well-organized maintenance program (recalled every 2 to 3 months). Patients in the GP group had increased plaque scores and 45% loss of attachment. Patients in the maintenance program had 99% improvement and no or less than 1% attachment loss.

Q: **What are some signs of disease recurrence?**

Signs of disease recurrence include[64]:

- Recurrence of BOP
- Increased probing depth
- Radiographic bone loss
- Progressive mobility

Surgical and Nonsurgical Therapy

Q: **What has been shown by studies comparing surgical and nonsurgical therapy?**

Table 9-2 presents the findings of studies comparing surgical and nonsurgical therapy. →

Table 9-2	Studies comparing surgical and nonsurgical therapy	
Study	**Design**	**Findings**
Kaldahl et al[65]	Split-mouth design involving 82 patients with periodontal disease; each quadrant received one of the following: coronal scaling, root planing, modified Widman surgery, or flap with osseous resection surgery	• All the therapies reduced the pocket depth. • Osseous resection was more effective at reducing pocket depth. • Osseous resection caused the most recession. • The deeper the initial probing depth, the greater was the mean reduction of probing depth. • Root planing and modified Widman surgery produced the greatest gain of mean probing attachment in the 5- to 6-mm probing depth category.
Brayer et al[7]	Random distribution of 114 periodontally involved, single-rooted teeth designated for extraction among four operators of various experience levels for either an open or closed session of SRP	In shallow pockets, no difference was found between the two procedures; in deeper pockets (4- to 6-mm and > 6 mm), open flap SRP was more effective than closed flap SRP.
Becker et al[66]	A longitudinal study comparing scaling, osseous surgery, and modified Widman procedures	• At 5 years, there were significant decreases in gingival and plaque scores. • For the three procedures, there were significant decreases in the depth of pockets with a baseline depth of 4 to 6 mm; however, there were no differences between the methods.
Serino et al[67]	Initial outcome and long-term effect of surgical and nonsurgical treatment of advanced periodontal disease	Surgical treatment provides better short- and long-term pocket depth reduction in patients with advanced periodontal disease and may result in a reduced need for additional adjunctive therapy.

Irrigation

Q: **What is the difference between supragingival and subgingival irrigation?**

Supragingival irrigation is used to remove bacteria coronal to the gingival margin and reduce the occurrence of gingivitis. *Subgingival irrigation* is used to reduce bacteria in the pocket and prevent the initiation of periodontal disease. Both techniques are aimed at reduction of the biofilm and bacterial load to a level compatible with health in the host.

Q: **Should supragingival irrigation be used as monotherapy?**

According to a position paper by the American Academy of Periodontology (AAP),[68] supragingival irrigation with water should not be used instead of toothbrushing.

Q: **Has supragingival irrigation been shown to be effective as an adjunct in oral hygiene?**

According to the AAP,[68] supragingival irrigation may not be required in patients with proficient toothbrushing skills and no gingivitis but can be of benefit in those with poor oral hygiene and/or gingivitis. Supragingival irrigation provides the greatest benefit to patients who do not perform adequate interproximal cleansing.

Greenstein[69] found that supragingival irrigation could enhance the oral hygiene efforts of patients not practicing optimal plaque control, but that generally no benefit beyond that provided by root planing alone could be achieved with subgingival irrigation.

Q: **Can supragingival irrigation with antimicrobial agents be useful?**

Newman et al[70] compared toothbrushing alone with adjunctive supragingival irrigation with 0.06% chlorhexidine gluconate and found the latter to significantly reduce gram-negative anaerobic rods and black-pigmented bacteroides. The effects of water irrigation on any of the assessed bacterial groups was limited. →

Aziz-Gandour and Newman[71] found that low concentrations of chlorhexidine (0.02%) and metronidazole (0.05%) as irrigants in patients with periodontitis did not induce clinically significant improvements.

Q: Can irrigation induce bacteremia?

According to a position paper by the AAP,[68] irrigation does not present any particular safety hazard to systemically healthy patients given that similar levels of bacteremia were detected following activities such as toothbrushing, flossing, periodontal dressing changes, scaling, root planing, and chewing. However, when providing instructions for home irrigation to individuals requiring premedication before periodontal treatment, clinicians should be cautious because there is no specific information available regarding risk associated with home irrigation for this population.

Q: What factors are important to consider when subgingival drug delivery and irrigation are used?

The position paper by the AAP[68] indicates that the following factors should be considered when providing subgingival drug delivery and irrigation:

- Circumferential application around the teeth.
- Teeth should be root planed because calculus can be an impediment and the diseased cementum harbors bacterial toxins.
- Either a side or end port cannula can be used.
- Low irrigation forces should be used (to minimize projection of bacteria to the tissues).

Q: Is subgingival irrigation effective?

The AAP position paper[68] states that although plaque indices were reduced by subgingival irrigation with medicaments, the technique did not completely eliminate inflammatory signs. When it was used alone, the number of sites with BOP was decreased. However, when it was used in conjunction with root planing, local effects were enhanced and bleeding points were fewer. Most studies demonstrated a reduction in mean probing depths of less than 1 mm with subgingival irrigation. On the other hand, if irrigation was preceded by root planing, probing depths decreased 2 to 3 mm, suggesting that root planing is indicated in the achievement of probing depth reduction, and subgingival irrigation may be of benefit as an adjunctive therapy, but not a stand-alone.

157

Q: How deep can supragingival and subgingival irrigation project?

The data indicate that supragingival irrigation does not routinely project solutions into deep pockets. However, subgingival irrigation via a cannula results in approximately 70% to 80% penetration of deep pockets.[68]

Pitcher et al[72] noted that solution did not routinely penetrate to the apical plaque border with mouthrinsing or direct irrigation. However, direct irrigation was partially effective, while no significant penetration of the pockets was achieved by mouthrinsing.

Q: Is there a difference between professional and personal subgingival irrigation?

There are no long-term studies comparing the benefit of personal versus professional administration of subgingival irrigation.

Root Conditioning

Q: Why is root surface modification done?

The demineralization agent removes the smear layer and facilitates new fibrous attachment and the exposure of collagen fibers to the dentin.

Q: Is root conditioning effective?

Chaves et al[73] used light microscopy to study the effects of SRP with and without citric acid application. They found that citric acid application did not alter the effects of SRP, and no effects to the diseased root surface were found with citric acid application as a monotherapy. Citric acid failed to penetrate the dentinal tubules and did not change the collagen content of the roots produced by SRP.

Gamal and Mailhot[74] noted that ethylenediaminetetraacetic acid (EDTA) gel conditioning for 4 minutes affords a root surface to which a maximum amount of periodontal ligament cells can adhere and propagate.

Nagata et al[75] reported root conditioning in monkeys with 10% tetracycline solution did not produce any additional new attachment in comparison to the controls.

Root Sensitivity

Q: **What part of the tooth experiences the most root sensitivity?**

The greatest amount of root sensitivity is experienced supragingival to the cementoenamel junction in the cervical region.

References

1. Cobb CM. Non-surgical pocket therapy: Mechanical. Ann Periodontol 1996;1:443–490.
2. Stambaugh RV, Dragoo M, Smith DM, Carasali L. The limits of subgingival scaling. Int J Periodontics Restorative Dent 1981;1:30–41.
3. Buchanan SA, Robertson PB. Calculus removal by scaling/root planing with and without surgical access. J Periodontol 1987;58:159–163.
4. Waerhaug J. Healing of the dento-epithelial junction following subgingival plaque control. II: As observed on extracted teeth. J Periodontol 1978;49:119–134.
5. Research, Science and Therapy Committee of the American Academy of Periodontology. Treatment of plaque-induced gingivitis, chronic periodontitis, and other clinical conditions. J Periodontol 2001;72:1790–1800 [erratum 2003;74:1568].
6. Loos B, Nylund K, Claffey N, Egelberg J. Clinical effects of root debridement in molar and non-molar teeth. A 2-year follow-up. J Clin Periodontol 1989;16:498–504.
7. Brayer WK, Mellonig JT, Dunlap RM, Marinak KW, Carson RE. Scaling and root planing effectiveness: The effect of root surface access and operator experience. J Periodontol 1989;60:67–72.
8. Caffesse RG, Sweeney PL, Smith BA. Scaling and root planing with and without periodontal flap surgery. J Clin Periodontol 1986;13:205–210.
9. Lindhe J, Westfelt E, Nyman S, Socransky SS, Haffajee AD. Long-term effect of surgical/non-surgical treatment of periodontal disease. J Clin Periodontol 1984;11:448–458.
10. Goodson JM, Tanner AC, Haffajee AD, Sornberger GC, Socransky SS. Patterns of progression and regression of advanced destructive periodontal disease. J Clin Periodontol 1982;9:472–481.
11. Löe H, Anerud A, Boysen H, Morrison E. Natural history of periodontal disease in man. Rapid, moderate and no loss of attachment in Sri Lankan laborers 14 to 46 years of age. J Clin Periodontol 1986;13:431–445.
12. Lindhe J, Socransky SS, Nyman S, Haffajee A, Westfelt E. "Critical probing depths" in periodontal therapy. J Clin Periodontol 1982;9:323–336.
13. Quirynen M, De Soete M, Boschmans G, et al. Benefit of "one-stage full-mouth disinfection" is explained by disinfection and root planing within 24 hours: A randomized controlled trial. J Clin Periodontol 2006;33:639–647.
14. Greenstein G. Full-mouth therapy versus individual quadrant root planing: A critical commentary. J Periodontol 2002;73:797–812.
15. Santuchi CC, Cortelli JR, Cortelli SC, et al. Scaling and root planing per quadrant versus one-stage full-mouth disinfection: Assessment of the impact of chronic periodontitis treatment on quality of life—A clinical randomized, controlled trial. J Periodontol 2016;87:114–123.
16. Santuchi CC, Cortelli SC, Cortelli JR, Cota LO, Alencar CO, Costa FO. Pre- and post-treatment experiences of fear, anxiety, and pain among chronic periodontitis patients treated by scaling and root planing per quadrant versus one-stage full-mouth disinfection: A 6-month randomized controlled clinical trial. J Clin Periodontol 2015;42:1024–1031.

17. Drisko CL, Killoy WJ. Scaling and root planing: Removal of calculus and subgingival organisms. Curr Opin Dent 1991;1:74–80.
18. Coldiron NB, Yukna RA, Weir J, Caudill RF. A quantitative study of cementum removal with hand curettes. J Periodontol 1990;61:293–299.
19. Ritz L, Hefti AF, Rateitschak KH. An in vitro investigation on the loss of root substance in scaling with various instruments. J Clin Periodontol 1991;18:643–647.
20. Graves RC, Disney JA, Stamm JW. Comparative effectiveness of flossing and brushing in reducing interproximal bleeding. J Periodontol 1989;60:243–247.
21. Warren PR, Chater BV. An overview of established interdental cleaning methods. J Clin Dent 1996;7(3 special issue):65–69.
22. Mazhari F, Boskabady M, Moeintaghavi A, Habibi A. The effect of toothbrushing and flossing sequence on interdental plaque reduction and fluoride retention: A randomized controlled clinical trial. J Periodontol 2018;89:824–832.
23. Fleming EB, Nguyen D, Afful J, Carroll MD, Woods PD. Prevalence of daily flossing among adults by selected risk factors for periodontal disease—United States, 2011–2014. J Periodontol 2018;89:933–939.
24. Bass CC. An effective method of personal oral hygiene. J LA State Med Soc 1954;106(2):57–73.
25. Carr MP, Rice GL, Horton JE. Evaluation of floss types for interproximal plaque removal. Am J Dent 2000;13:212–214.
26. Jackson MA, Kellett M, Worthington HV, Clerehugh V. Comparison of interdental cleaning methods: A randomized controlled trial. J Periodontol 2006;77:1421–1429.
27. Tu YK, Jackson M, Kellett M, Clerehugh V. Direct and indirect effects of interdental hygiene in a clinical trial. J Dent Res 2008;87:1037–1042.
28. Slot DE, Dörfer CE, Van der Weijden GA. The efficacy of interdental brushes on plaque and parameters of periodontal inflammation: A systematic review. Int J Dent Hyg 2008;6:253–264.
29. Lang NP, Cumming BR, Löe H. Toothbrushing frequency as it relates to plaque development and gingival health. J Periodontol 1973;44:396–405.
30. Robinson PG, Deacon SA, Deery C, et al. Manual versus powered toothbrushing for oral health. Cochrane Database Syst Rev 2005;(2):CD002281.
31. Deery C, Heanue M, Deacon S, et al. The effectiveness of manual versus powered toothbrushes for dental health: A systematic review. J Dent 2004;32:197–211.
32. Rapley JW, Killoy WJ. Subgingival and interproximal plaque removal using a counter-rotational electric toothbrush and a manual toothbrush. Quintessence Int 1994;25:39–42.
33. Glaze PM, Wade AB. Toothbrush age and wear as it relates to plaque control. J Clin Periodontol 1986;13:52–56.
34. Drisko CH. Root instrumentation. Power-driven versus manual scalers, which one? Dent Clin North Am 1998;42:229–244.
35. Nishimine D, O'Leary TJ. Hand instrumentation versus ultrasonics in the removal of endotoxins from root surfaces. J Periodontol 1979;50:345–349.
36. Leon LE, Vogel RI. A comparison of the effectiveness of hand scaling and ultrasonic debridement in furcations as evaluated by differential dark-field microscopy. J Periodontol 1987;58:86–94.
37. Croft LK, Nunn ME, Crawford LC, et al. Patient preference for ultrasonic or hand instruments in periodontal maintenance. Int J Periodontics Restorative Dent 2003;23:567–573.
38. Dahiya P, Kamal R, Gupta R, Pandit N. Comparative evaluation of hand and power-driven instruments on root surface characteristics: A scanning electron microscopy study. Contemp Clin Dent 2011;2:79–83.
39. Cobb CM. Clinical significance of non-surgical periodontal therapy: An evidence-based perspective of scaling and root planing. J Clin Periodontol 2002;29(suppl 2):6–16.
40. Kepic TJ, O'Leary TJ, Kafrawy AH. Total calculus removal: An attainable objective? J Periodontol 1990;61:16–20.
41. Bower RC. Furcation morphology relative to periodontal treatment. Furcation entrance architecture. J Periodontol 1979;50:23–27.

42. Drisko CL, Cochran DL, Blieden T, et al. Position paper: Sonic and ultrasonic scalers in periodontics. Research, Science and Therapy Committee of the American Academy of Periodontology. J Periodontol 2000;71:1792–1801.

43. Miller CS, Leonelli FM, Latham E. Selective interference with pacemaker activity by electrical dental devices. Oral Surg Oral Med Oral Pathol Oral Radiol Endod 1998;85:33–36.

44. Roedig JJ, Shah J, Elayi CS, Miller CS. Interference of cardiac pacemaker and implantable cardioverter-defibrillator activity during electronic dental device use. J Am Dent Assoc 2010;141:521–526.

45. Costa MR, Marcantonio RA, Cirelli JA. Comparison of manual versus sonic and ultrasonic toothbrushes: A review. Int J Dent Hyg 2007;5:75–81.

46. Fischer C, Wennberg A, Fischer RG, Attström R. Clinical evaluation of pulp and dentine sensitivity after supragingival and subgingival scaling. Endod Dent Traumatol 1991;7:259–265.

47. Segelnick SL, Weinberg MA. Reevaluation of initial therapy: When is the appropriate time? J Periodontol 2006;77:1598–1601.

48. Proye M, Caton J, Polson A. Initial healing of periodontal pockets after a single episode of root planing monitored by controlled probing forces. J Periodontol 1982;53:296–301.

49. Caton J, Proye M, Polson A. Maintenance of healed periodontal pockets after a single episode of root planing. J Periodontol 1982;53:420–424.

50. Morrison EC, Ramfjord SP, Hill RW. Short-term effects of initial, nonsurgical periodontal treatment (hygienic phase). J Clin Periodontol 1980;7:199–211.

51. Lowenguth RA, Greenstein G. Clinical and microbiological response to nonsurgical mechanical periodontal therapy. Periodontol 2000 1995;9:14–22.

52. Rosling B, Nyman S, Lindhe J, Jern B. The healing potential of the periodontal tissues following different techniques of periodontal surgery in plaque-free dentitions. A 2-year clinical study. J Clin Periodontol 1976;3:233–250.

53. Ramfjord SP, Morrison EC, Burgett FG, et al. Oral hygiene and maintenance of periodontal support. J Periodontol 1982;53:26–30.

54. Drisko CH. Nonsurgical periodontal therapy. Periodontol 2000 2001;25:77–88.

55. Cohen RE; Research, Science and Therapy Committee of the American Academy of Periodontology. Position paper: Periodontal maintenance. J Periodontol 2003;74:1395–1401.

56. Schallhorn RG, Snider LE. Periodontal maintenance therapy. J Am Dent Assoc 1981;103:227–231.

57. Westfelt E, Nyman S, Socransky S, Lindhe J. Significance of frequency of professional tooth cleaning for healing following periodontal surgery. J Clin Periodontol 1983;10:148–156.

58. Lang NP, Brägger U, Salvi GE, Tonetti MS. Supportive periodontal therapy (SPT). In: Lindhe J, Lang NP, Karring T (eds). Clinical Periodontology and Implant Dentistry, ed 5. Oxford, UK: Blackwell Munksgaard, 2008:1303.

59. Wilson TG Jr, Glover ME, Schoen J, Baus C, Jacobs T. Compliance with maintenance therapy in a private periodontal practice. J Periodontol 1984;55:468–473.

60. Wilson TG Jr, Hale S, Temple R. The results of efforts to improve compliance with supportive periodontal treatment in a private practice. J Periodontol 1993;64:311–314.

61. Miyamoto T, Kumagai T, Jones JA, Van Dyke TE, Nunn ME. Compliance as a prognostic indicator: Retrospective study of 505 patients treated and maintained for 15 years. J Periodontol 2006;77:223–232.

62. Nyman S, Lindhe J, Rosling B. Periodontal surgery in plaque-infected dentitions. J Clin Periodontol 1977;4:240–249.

63. Axelsson P, Lindhe J. The significance of maintenance care in the treatment of periodontal disease. J Clin Periodontol 1981;8:281–294.

64. Chace R. Retreatment in periodontal practice. J Periodontol 1977;48:410–412.

65. Kaldahl WB, Kalkwarf KL, Patil KD, Dyer JK, Bates RE Jr. Evaluation of four modalities of periodontal therapy. Mean probing depth, probing attachment level and recession changes. J Periodontol 1988;59:783–793.

66. Becker W, Becker BE, Caffesse R, et al. A longitudinal study comparing scaling, osseous surgery, and modified Widman procedures: Results after 5 years. J Periodontol 2001;72:1675–1684.

67. Serino G, Rosling B, Ramberg P, Socransky SS, Lindhe J. Initial outcome and long-term effect of surgical and non-surgical treatment of advanced periodontal disease. J Clin Periodontol 2001;28:910–916.

68. Greenstein G; Research, Science and Therapy Committee of the American Academy of Periodontology. Position paper: The role of supra- and subgingival irrigation in the treatment of periodontal diseases. J Periodontol 2005;76:2015–2027.

69. Greenstein G. Nonsurgical periodontal therapy in 2000: A literature review. J Am Dent Assoc 2000;131:1580–1592.

70. Newman MG, Flemmig TF, Nachnani S, et al. Irrigation with 0.06% chlorhexidine in naturally occurring gingivitis. II. 6 months microbiological observations. J Periodontol 1990;61:427–433.

71. Aziz-Gandour IA, Newman HN. The effects of a simplified oral hygiene regime plus supragingival irrigation with chlorhexidine or metronidazole on chronic inflammatory periodontal disease. J Clin Periodontol 1986;13:228–236.

72. Pitcher GR, Newman HN, Strahan JD. Access to subgingival plaque by disclosing agents using mouthrinsing and direct irrigation. J Clin Periodontol 1980;7:300–308.

73. Chaves E, Cox C, Morrison E, Caffesse R. The effect of citric acid application on periodontally involved root surfaces. 1. An in vitro light microscopic study. Int J Periodontics Restorative Dent 1992;12:219–229.

74. Gamal AY, Mailhot JM. The effects of EDTA gel conditioning exposure time on periodontitis-affected human root surfaces: Surface topography and PDL cell adhesion. J Int Acad Periodontol 2003;5:11–22.

75. Nagata MJ, Bosco AF, Leite CM, Melo LG, Sundefeld ML. Healing of dehiscence defects following root surface demineralization with tetracycline: A histologic study in monkeys. J Periodontol 2005;76:908–914.

Surgical Therapy

10

Gingivectomy

Q: **What are the indications for gingivectomy?**

Indications for gingivectomy include[1]:

- To treat horizontal bone loss with increased pocket depth
- To reduce gingival overgrowth from medications or genetics (Fig 10-1)
- To remove soft tissue craters resulting from surgical procedures
- To improve gingival esthetics in patients with delayed passive eruption
- For crown lengthening when ostectomy is not required (rare)

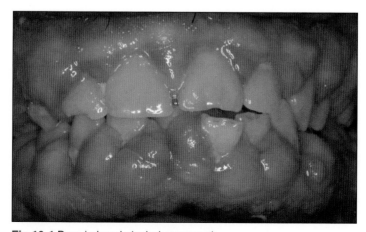

Fig 10-1 Drug-induced gingival overgrowth.

Q: What are the contraindications for a gingivectomy?

Contraindications for gingivectomy include[2]:

- Presence of osseous defects
- Inadequate keratinized gingiva
- Base of the pocket apical to the mucogingival junction
- Inadequate vestibular depth
- Inadequate oral hygiene

Q: Describe the gingivectomy procedure.

The goal of gingivectomy is to eliminate gingival pockets by the resection of gingival tissue. After probing the pocket to determine its base, a coronally directed external bevel incision is made using a suitable blade or knife at a 45-degree angle. The incision is made apical to the pocket but coronal to the mucogingival junction. Next, the interdental incisions are made with a sharp narrow knife. After these incisions, the excised tissue should be removed with a Prichard or periosteal elevator or surgical curettes.[1] Gingivoplasty may be performed with scissors, tissue nippers, or a rotary instrument under copious cooling. Scaling and root planing (SRP) should be performed, and hemostasis must be achieved.

Periodontal Flap and Osseous Surgery

Q: What are some general principles of periodontal surgery?

In 1977, Mörmann and Ciancio[3] outlined the following general principles of periodontal surgery:

- The flap should have a broad base to enable sufficient blood supply.
- The proportion of length to width should not exceed 2:1.
- The flap should be large enough to provide good access to the roots and bony defects.
- Partial-thickness flaps should not be too thin (to allow blood vessels to be part of the flap).
- The apical portion of periodontal flaps should be full thickness when possible. →

- Partial-thickness flaps should not be used in areas of thin connective tissue because necrosis of the soft tissue may occur. This can lead to bone exposure and bone necrosis.
- There should be minimal tension during suturing.

Q: What is the primary indication for periodontal flap surgery?

The primary indication for periodontal flap surgery is to gain access to the root surface and remove bacterial deposits and calculus that may have remained following nonsurgical therapy.

Q: Why is positive architecture important when performing osseous surgery?

Positive architecture (interproximal bone coronal to the facial or lingual bone) as opposed to negative architecture (interproximal bone apical to the facial or lingual bone) allows close adaptation of the gingival tissues to the bone, which results in minimum sulcus depth.

Q: What is osseous surgery? What are the indications for osseous surgery?

First outlined by Schluger in 1949,[4] *osseous surgery* was defined as the procedures to modify bone support altered by periodontal disease either by reshaping the alveolar process to achieve physiologic form without removal of supporting alveolar bone or by removing some supporting alveolar bone, thus changing the position of crestal bone relative to the tooth roots.
  Indications for osseous surgery, according to Schluger,[4] are:

- Presence of wide alveolar housing associated with increased pocket depth
- Existence of negative osseous architecture
- Failure of gingivectomy treatment
- Mesially tipped molars
- Deep isolated pockets
- Deep buccal and lingual pockets
- Saucer-shaped interproximal bone loss (craters)

Q: What is the rationale for osseous surgery?

- Establish access for root debridement
- Create physiologic osseous topology (positive bone architecture) →

- Decrease pocket depth
- Preserve the teeth
- Facilitate plaque control
- Improve prognosis
- Decrease bleeding on probing

Q: What are contraindications to osseous surgery?

- Proper follow-up and maintenance not possible
- Advanced bone loss (long-term prognosis and value of the tooth is questionable)
- Shallow pockets
- Three-wall defects (may be able to regenerate)
- Poor oral hygiene
- Medical contraindications
- Pockets in the esthetic zone
- Poor crown-to-root ratio

Q: What can lead to failure when performing osseous surgery?

- Poor operator technique
- Presence of calculus
- Reverse architecture
- Improper flap placement
- Failure to remove widow's peaks
- Inadequate maintenance

Q: What is osteoplasty? Ostectomy?

Both terms were first described by Friedman in 1955.[5] Friedman defined *osteoplasty* as a plastic procedure in which the periodontal pocket is eliminated and the bone reshaped to achieve physiologic contour of the bone and the gingiva overlying it. In this bone recontouring, the bone that is reshaped is not part of the attachment apparatus, thus no bony support of the tooth or teeth is lost. Friedman defined *ostectomy* as an operative procedure in which bone that is part of the attachment apparatus is removed to sustainably eliminate a periodontal pocket and establish gingival contours that will be maintained.

Q: What is the average amount of supporting bone loss following osseous surgery?

Selipsky[6] found that osseous surgery results in an average of 0.6 mm of supporting bone height loss. He also found that the maximum circumferential bone loss around a tooth is 1.5 mm.

Q: Where does the greatest amount of bone resection occur?

The greatest amount of bone resection occurs at the line angles and on the facial and lingual surfaces or both.[7]

Q: What determines the morphology of the defect?

- Radius of the inflammatory process
- Anatomy of the defect (thick/thin) periodontium
- Root anatomy (length and shape of the root)
- Root proximity

Q: Can angular defects worsen?

Papapanou and Wennström[8] found that angular defects do worsen and can be more challenging to treat if not detected early. An increased possibility of tooth loss was associated with teeth showing initial signs of angular defects.

Different Surgical Techniques

Q: What is the difference between a full-thickness and a partial-thickness flap?

The *full-thickness flap* includes the epithelium, connective tissue, and periosteum. In a *partial-thickness flap*, the mucosa is separated from the periosteum (which is attached to the alveolar bone). The periosteal blood supply is not disturbed.

Q: Describe the modified Widman flap.

The *modified Widman flap*, first described by Ramfjord and Nissle in 1974,[9] is a flap used to provide access for root planing. Following is the procedure:

$\rightarrow$

1. Initial inverse bevel incision parallel to the long axis of the teeth
2. Elevation of the mucoperiosteal flap only 2 to 3 mm from the alveolar crest
3. Crevicular incision around the neck of the teeth
4. Surgical excision of the collar of tissue around the teeth
5. Accentuated palatal scalloping for close interproximal flap adaptation
6. Osteoplasty for flap adaptation purposes

Q: Describe the apically repositioned flap.

First described by Nabers in 1954,[10] the *apically repositioned flap* is a full-thickness reverse-beveled scalloped incision with vertical releasing incisions to the mucogingival junction. The soft tissue is displaced in an apical direction. It allows preservation of the keratinized tissue while apically displacing the gingival margin following surgery.

Q: Describe the distal wedge excision.

With a *distal wedge excision*, excessive tissue distal to the last remaining tooth in the mouth can be excised to reduce the pocket. The flaps are raised, and a wedge of tissue is removed. Before suturing, the flaps are thinned, elevated, and approximated.

Q: What is an envelope flap?

In an *envelope flap*, the horizontal incision is made at the gingival margin away from the areas with pockets that are being treated and without any vertical incisions. The incision is used to create access.

Q: Describe the palatal approach to osseous surgery according to Ochsenbein and Bohannan.[11]

In 1963, Ochsenbein and Bohannan[11] described different types of defects (various interdental crater depths) and the approach that should be taken for each (Table 10-1; see next page). The majority of osteoplasty and ostectomy is done from the palatal aspect.

Ochsenbein and Bohannan[11] advocated the palatal approach for several reasons:

▪ Decreased ostectomy
▪ Increased embrasure space
▪ Less resorption—greater cancellous bone →

- Avoidance of exposure of the buccal furcation (maxilla root trunk is 3 mm)
- Apical slope of crest toward the palate
- Better esthetics

Table 10-1	Palatal approach to osseous surgery	
Class	Depth of the defect	Treatment
1	2 to 3 mm; thick facial and lingual tissue	10-degree palatal ramp
2 (most common)	4 to 5 mm	Facial and palatal ramp
3	6 to 7 mm	Facial and palatal ramp
4 (least common)	> 7 mm	Removal of facial and lingual tissue

Q: What were the advantages of the lingual approach to osseous surgery described by Tibbetts et al[12] in 1976?

- The external oblique ridge is avoided.
- The furcation on the lingual is in a more apical position.
- Craters are located more lingually.
- There is better access and wider embrasure.
- The defect is located more lingually because of the lingual incline of the molars.
- The root length on the facial aspect is shorter.
- The buccal furcation is avoided (mandible root trunk is about 4 mm).
- There is greater vestibular depth on the lingual aspect.

Q: What are options for pockets found in the anterior segment?

- Papilla preservation flap (see below), as described by Takei et al,[13] where a palatal incision is made to allow the papilla to move in a buccal direction. However, adequate width (> 2 mm) of the papilla is necessary as well as a sufficient embrasure space.
- Continuous SRP. →

- Perioscopy: Allows real-time indirect visualization of the root during SRP. According to Stambaugh,[14] it "can offer many patients an alternative to periodontal surgery in carefully selected sites."
- No treatment.

Q: Describe some minimally invasive surgical techniques

1. Minimally invasive surgery (MIS)[15] consists of an initial intrasulcular incision around the teeth neighboring the defect (Fig 10-2). The two initial incisions are connected on the surface (buccal or lingual) where the access flap will be elevated. This connecting incision is made apical to the col tissue. The col tissue and the papilla on the nonsurgical side remain intact and are not elevated. When the surgery is in an esthetic area, such as the maxillary anterior, this horizontal incision will usually be placed on the palatal aspect of the papilla. This will help to preserve the shape of the papilla as well as cover the grafted site with soft tissue. In a nonesthetic area, the horizontal incision can be placed either buccally or lingually as needed to better cover the grafted site with soft tissue. The papilla is sharply dissected from the underlying bone. The connective tissue within the osseous defect is dissected with a blade and eliminated with curettes and ultrasonic instruments, and the root debrided. The defect is grafted with bone and a resorbable mesh, and the flap is sutured with vertical parallel mattress sutures to obtain primary closure.

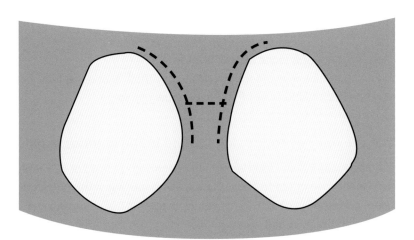

Fig 10-2 Diagram of MIS incision. (Reprinted from Pocket Dentistry.[16])

→

2. Papilla preservation technique, as described by Takei et al,[13] where a palatal incision is made to allow the papilla to move in a buccal direction (Fig 10-3). However, adequate width (> 2 mm) of the papilla is necessary as well as sufficient embrasure space.

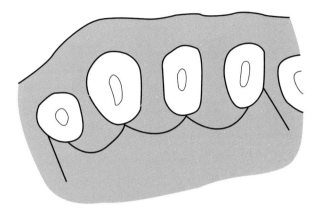

Fig 10-3 A sulcular incision is made along the lingual or palatal aspect of the tooth with a semilunar incision across the interdental papilla (5 mm from gingival margin). This allows the interdental tissue to be dissected from the lingual or palatal aspect so that it can be elevated to the buccal. (Reprinted from Takei et al[13] with permission.)

3. Interdental tissue maintenance[17] (ITM) is a technique used with nonresorbable membranes and grafting material.
4. In the minimally invasive surgical technique (MIST), the defect-associated interdental papilla is accessed either with the simplified papilla preservation flap (SPPF)[18] in narrow (2 mm or narrower) interdental spaces or the modified papilla preservation technique (MPPT)[19] in large (2 mm or wider) interdental spaces (Fig 10-4). The SPPF is a diagonal incision traced as close as possible to the buccal side of the papilla col, whereas the MPPT is a horizontal incision traced on the buccal side of the papilla. Intrasulcular incisions are performed from the interdental side to the buccal and lingual sides of the teeth bordering the defect; tiny buccal and lingual flaps are elevated to expose the residual bone crest. Periosteal incisions are performed only if needed to improve flap reflection. The soft tissue is sharply dissected from the osseous defect, and debridement and root planing are performed with a combination of mini-curettes and power air-driven instruments. It is designed for enamel matrix or growth factors to allow regeneration. →

171

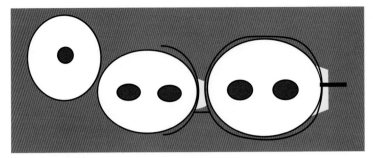

Fig 10-4 MPPT incision. The linear crestal incision performed on the edentulous ridge. Mesial extension of the flap is limited to the mid-buccal and mid-lingual area of the first molar; the distal crestal incision is extended for about 5 to 6 mm. (Reprinted from Cortellini et al[20] with permission.)

5. Modified minimally invasive surgical technique (M-MIST) described by Cortellini and Tonetti[21] consists of a tiny interdental access in which only buccal intrasulcular incisions are made and linked with a buccal horizontal incision of the papilla done as close as possible to the papilla tip (Fig 10-5). Soft tissue filling the osseous defect is "carved" away from under the papilla. Then the root surface is carefully debrided with mini-curettes and power-driven air instruments, avoiding any trauma to the supracrestal fibers of the defect-associated papilla. The palatal tissues are not surgically accessed. The suturing approach is based on the use of a single internal modified mattress suture.[22]

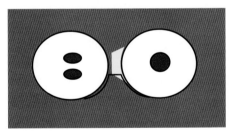

Fig 10-5 The buccal incision to gain access to the defect. (Reprinted from Cortellini et al[20] with permission.)

6. The single-flap approach (SFA)[23] is specifically indicated when the defect extension is prevalent on the buccal. The basic principle of the SFA is the elevation of a limited mucoperiosteal flap to access the defect only on one side (buccal or oral), leaving the opposite side intact. →

7. Figure 10-6 summarizes the minimally invasive surgical techniques.

Buccally positioned incision	Palatally (lingually) positioned incision	Incision can be placed buccal or lingual	Dividing oblique incision
MPPT MIST M-MIST	Papilla preservation technique ITM	MIS	SPPF

Fig 10-6 Summary of minimally invasive surgical techniques.

Q: **What are indications and contraindications for the minimally invasive surgical approaches?**

See Fig 10-7 below.

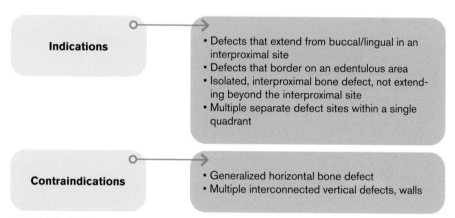

Indications →
- Defects that extend from buccal/lingual in an interproximal site
- Defects that border on an edentulous area
- Isolated, interproximal bone defect, not extending beyond the interproximal site
- Multiple separate defect sites within a single quadrant

Contraindications →
- Generalized horizontal bone defect
- Multiple interconnected vertical defects, walls

Fig 10-7 Indications and contraindications for minimally invasive surgical approaches.[24]

Q: **How should a dentist decide which minimally invasive technique to use?**

The following can affect your flap design[25]:

1. Mesiodistal width of the interdental space
2. Amount of keratinized attached tissue
3. Distance from papilla tip to the bone crest
4. Location of the defect
5. Phenotype of the patient
6. Accessibility of the defect

   Figure 10-8 explains the strategy to decide which flap design is ideal (see next page). →

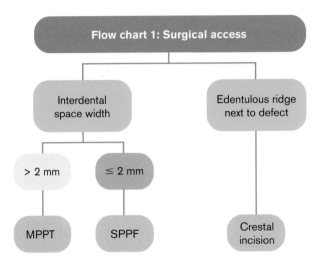

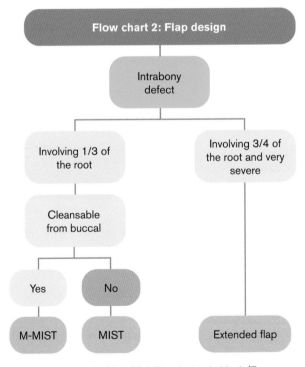

Fig 10-8 How to decide which flap design is ideal. (From Cortellini.[22])

Q: Why are microsurgery techniques advantageous?

Cortellini and Tonetti[26] found that microsurgery can result in the following:

- Improvement of soft tissue healing
- Limited soft tissue damage
- High probability of achieving primary closure
- Limited recession
- Gains in clinical attachment level

Q: Describe how periodontal surgery is performed in your practice.

Note that there can be multiple answers to this question.

1. Scalloped incisions (when there is adequate keratinized tissue) are prepared.
2. The interproximal areas are leveled or ramped (if defect is on the lingual, ramping is performed toward the lingual) first because they will be the highest point (positive architecture). Ramping allows for less bone to be removed from the buccal aspect.
3. A round bur (no. 4) is used to thin the bone on the buccal and lingual aspects.
4. Physiologic architecture is developed, and widow's peaks are removed using hand instruments.
5. A probe is placed interproximally to confirm that no ledges exist.
6. A continuous suture is placed.

Wound Healing

Q: What is the difference between primary, secondary, and tertiary wound healing?

- Primary: The mucosal wound edges are adjacent to one another. They are reapproximated to minimize any scarring (eg, periodontal flaps).
- Secondary: Epithelial cells must migrate (granulate in) to close the wound (eg, gingivectomy).
- Tertiary: Due to necrotic tissue or other impediment, wound closure is not possible until the impediment is removed.

Q: Describe wound healing following osseous surgery.

Table 10-2 presents results from studies of wound healing following osseous surgery.

Table 10-2	Wound healing following osseous surgery	
Study	**Subject**	**Results**
Wood et al[27]	Alveolar crest reduction following full- and partial-thickness flaps	• 0.62-mm crestal bone loss after a full-thickness flap • 0.98-mm crestal bone loss following a partial-thickness flap
Wilderman et al[28]	Histogenesis of repair following osseous surgery	• Osteoblast activity occurs 1 year after surgery • There is 1.2 mm of crestal bone loss but a gain of 0.4 mm for a net loss of 0.8 mm following surgery
Moghaddas and Stahl[29]	Alveolar bone remodeling following osseous surgery	Mean reduction of: • 0.23 mm at the interradicular sites • 0.55 mm at the radicular sites • 0.88 mm at the furcation sites

Q: Describe healing following surgery.

Timeline for healing after surgery[30]:

- 24 hours: Blood clot connects the flap and the tooth or bone surface.
- 1 to 3 days: The space between the flap and the tooth or bone is thinner, and epithelial cells migrate to the site at a rate of 0.5 mm per day.
- 1 week: Epithelial attachment to the root occurs.
- 2 weeks: Collagen fibers form parallel to the tooth surface.
- 1 month: Fully epithelialized gingival crevice.

Q: What are the patient's options when there are unresolved pocket depths?

- No treatment
- Continuous nonsurgical therapy and maintenance →

- Osseous surgery for access to remove the bacteria and/or osseous reshaping for easier maintenance
- Regeneration for deeper pockets

Surgical Versus Nonsurgical Therapy

Q: What has been shown by studies comparing surgical and nonsurgical therapy?

See Table 9-2 in chapter 9 for a synopsis of studies comparing surgical and nonsurgical therapy.

Open Flap Curettage Versus Osseous Recontouring

Q: Compare open flap curettage and osseous recontouring.

In a study comparing open flap curettage and osseous recontouring, Smith et al[31] reported the following:

- Equal reduction of plaque and gingival inflammation for the two techniques
- Improved periodontal health with both techniques
- Pocket recurrence during the 6-month period following open curettage
- Maintenance of pocket reduction during the 6-month period after osseous recontouring
- Lack of bone regeneration with open curettage
- Net loss of attachment with osseous recontouring

Oral Hygiene Following Osseous Surgery

Q: Describe the importance of oral hygiene following surgical therapy.

In a study of 20 patients with advanced periodontal disease, Nyman et al[32] found that treatment was successful in participants in the test group, who $\rightarrow$

received a professional cleaning once every 2 weeks following treatment and were able to maintain a high standard of oral hygiene. Treatment was unsuccessful in patients in the control group, who were recalled for scaling of the teeth once every 6 months and were unable to maintain good oral hygiene.

Root Resection

Q: What are the indications for root resection?

- Severe vertical bone loss on the root not amenable to regeneration
- Furcation invasion not maintainable
- Endodontics impossible on the root
- Vertical/horizontal root fracture

Q: What are the contraindications for root resection?

- Fused roots
- Advanced bone loss with unfavorable crown-to-root ratio
- Inadequate amount of root remaining on the tooth to allow it to serve as an abutment
- Remaining tooth unable to withstand normal occlusal forces
- Inadequate hygiene
- Inability to perform endodontic therapy on the remaining roots
- Remaining furcation involvement between the remaining roots

Q: What is the success rate of root resection?

The most commonly resected root is the distal root of maxillary molars.

Carnevale et al[33] performed osseous recontouring and apically positioned flaps on non–furcation-involved teeth and found a 10-year survival rate of 93% for root-resected teeth and 99% at control sites.

Fuggazzotto[34] reported 96.8% and 97.0% success rates for root-resected molars and molar implants, respectively. The lowest success rate (75%) was reported for resection of the distal root of mandibular molars.

Langer et al[35] found a 62% success rate following root resection. The main reason for failure was root fracture.

Derks et al[36] did a 30-year retrospective study on the retention of molars after root-resective therapy, and they found the cumulative survival rate was

$\rightarrow$

90.6% after 10 years, but then decreased significantly. Molars after root resection had a median survival time of 20 years. The incidence of endodontic complications leading to tooth extraction was only 26.7%, 50% failed due to periodontal problems, and 16.7% because of caries. Mandibular molars had a significantly lower relative risk of loss than molars in the maxilla. Mandibular molars showed a survival probability of almost 80% even 20 years after root resection.

ENAP

Q: What is ENAP?

ENAP stands for *excisional new attachment procedure*, and it was introduced by Yukna et al[37] in 1976. A knife or blade is used to perform subgingival curettage. It is an attempt to gain new attachment in suprabony pockets.

According to a position statement by the American Academy of Periodontology (AAP)[38]:

> Elimination of pocket epithelium by gingival curettage, ENAP or other internal bevel incision designs appears not only nearly impossible but unnecessary for long-term therapeutic goals. In addition, there are no published data that demonstrate that either curettage or ENAP are effective in periodontal regeneration. To the contrary, there is peer reviewed evidence, both in vivo and in vitro, that use of lasers for ENAP procedures and/or gingival curettage may place patients at risk for damage to root surfaces and subjacent alveolar bone that, in turn, could render these tissues incompatible to normal cell attachment and healing.

Surgical Materials

Q: What are the advantages and disadvantages of using surgical dressings?

The advantages and disadvantages of surgical dressings[39,40] are presented in Fig 10-9 (see next page). →

Advantages
- Protects the wound.
- Increases comfort of the patient.
- Stabilizes the flap.
- Retains the graft material.

Disadvantages
- Increases postoperative pain.
- Irritating.
- Plaque retention (increased bacteria): Powell et al[39] found that the use of a postsurgical dressing demonstrated a slightly higher rate of infection (8 infections in 300 procedures, 2.67%) than nonuse of a dressing (14 infections in 753 procedures, 1.86%).
- Jones and Cassingham[40] found that when a dressing was used, patients reported more pain and discomfort and an increased severity of pain and discomfort postoperatively. They concluded that surgical dressings were unnecessary when performing periodontal flap surgery.

Fig 10-9 Advantages and disadvantages of surgical dressings.

Q: What is Surgicel made of? Avitene?

Surgicel (Ethicon) is oxidized cellulose polymer (the unit is polyanhydro-glucuronic acid). It is used to stop postsurgical bleeding. It can be cut in different shapes and placed over the area that is bleeding.

Avitene (Davol) is microfibrillar collagen and another effective hemostatic agent. It is placed on the bleeding site with forceps.

Sutures

Q: What are the ideal properties of sutures?

The ideal properties of sutures are presented in Fig 10-10. →

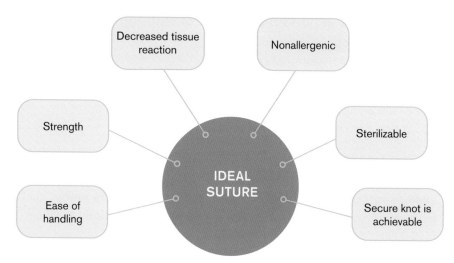

Fig 10-10 Properties of an ideal suture.

Q: What are the different types of sutures?

Figure 10-11 presents the different types of sutures.

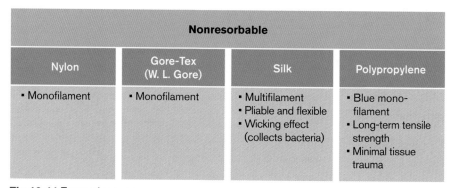

Resorbable		
Plain gut	Chromic gut	Vicryl (Ethicon)
• Harder to tie • 5- to 7-day resorption	• Chromic salt allows greater resistance to resorption	• Multifilament • Absorbed by hydrolysis

Nonresorbable			
Nylon	Gore-Tex (W. L. Gore)	Silk	Polypropylene
• Monofilament	• Monofilament	• Multifilament • Pliable and flexible • Wicking effect (collects bacteria)	• Blue mono-filament • Long-term tensile strength • Minimal tissue trauma

Fig 10-11 Types of sutures.

Q: What are the important principles of suturing?

Dahlberg[41] described the following principles:

- The least reactive material should be used.
- The least amount of suture material should be left beneath the flap.
- The suture should be placed close to the tissue.
- The suture should be removed as soon as possible.

Q: Describe the different techniques for suturing.

- Interrupted: Used when the facial and lingual aspects require similar tension and heights. It is a good choice for a replaced or coronally repositioned flap.
- Sling: The position of the facial or lingual flap is independent of the opposing flap.
- Mattress: Allows for eversion of the edges of the wound and maximum tissue coverage; the vertical mattress suture avoids suture material under the flap, while the horizontal mattress suture can prevent clot destabilization.
- Periosteal: Used to apically displace partial-thickness flaps.
- Figure 8 suture: Helpful in extraction sites when primary closure cannot always be achieved. It looks like a horizontal number 8.

Newell and Brunsvold[42] explained that long, thin papillae should be sutured with a vertical mattress suture, while short, wide papillae should be sutured with a horizontal mattress suture.

Postoperative Period

Q: What instructions should a patient be given following surgery?

Following are instructions to provide to patients following surgery (Sims T, personal communication, 2012):

- Care of your mouth: Immediately after surgery, keep ice-cold water or other cold foods, such as ice cream or frozen yogurt, in your mouth for 6 to 8 hours. Do not brush your teeth in the areas that have dressing or sutures. Perform normal cleaning of all teeth that did not undergo surgery. →

- Activity: Reduce your activity following surgery. No running, weightlifting, or any strenuous aerobic activity or contact sports for 48 hours.
- Discomfort: Following all types of surgery, you can expect some discomfort. Take your pain medication as prescribed. Do not drink alcoholic beverages in combination with pain medication.
- Swelling: In some cases, swelling may be expected, but it will go away in 3 to 4 days.
- Eating: Eat only cold, soft foods on the day of surgery. After the first day, stay on a soft but balanced diet. Do not eat hard, crunchy, or spicy foods.
- Smoking: Do not smoke following surgery. Tobacco smoke is an irritant and delays healing of the tissue. Refrain from smoking for as long as possible.

Miscellaneous

Q: What is the infection rate following periodontal surgery?

In a retrospective study of 395 patients that included 1,053 fully documented surgical procedures, Powell et al[39] reviewed surgical techniques such as osseous resective surgery, flap curettage, distal wedge procedures, gingivectomy, root resection, guided tissue regeneration, dental implant surgery, epithelialized free soft tissue autografts, subepithelial connective tissue autografts, coronally positioned flaps, sinus augmentations, and ridge preservation or augmentation procedures. *Infection*, defined as increasing and progressive swelling with the presence of suppuration, was found at a rate of 2.09% (22/1,053).

Pack and Haber[43] discovered 6/268 (2.2%) surgeries with infection when osseous surgery was performed; whereas 2/336 (0.6%) infections were noted with periodontal surgery without osteoplasty or ostectomy.

Q: How much blood loss occurs in periodontal surgery?

In a study of 26 patients requiring open flap debridement or regeneration, Zigdon et al[44] reported intraoperative blood loss ranging from 6.0 to 145.1 mL, with an overall mean of 59.47 ± 38.2 mL. The volume of blood loss was not related to the amount of local anesthetic, the size of the surgical field, or the duration of the surgery. They concluded that a minimal amount of blood is lost during periodontal surgery. →

Baab et al[45] found that mandibular periodontal surgery caused greater blood loss than maxillary surgery (about a 40-mL difference).

References

1. Rose LF, Mealey BL, Genco RJ, Cohen DW. Periodontics: Medicine, Surgery, and Implants. St Louis: Mosby, 2004:505–506.
2. Serio FG, Hawley C. Manual of Clinical Periodontics. Hudson, OH: Lexi-Comp, 2002.
3. Mörmann W, Ciancio SG. Blood supply of human gingiva following periodontal surgery. A fluorescein angiographic study. J Periodontol 1977;48:681–692.
4. Schluger S. Osseous resection: A basic principle in periodontal surgery. Oral Surg Oral Med Oral Pathol 1949;2:316–325.
5. Friedman N. Periodontal osseous surgery: Osteoplasty and osteoectomy. J Periodontol 1955;26:269.
6. Selipsky H. Osseous surgery—How much need we compromise? Dent Clin North Am 1976;20:79–106.
7. Rose LF, Mealey BL. Periodontics: Medicine, Surgery, and Implants. St Louis: Mosby, 2004:545.
8. Papapanou PN, Wennström JL. The angular bony defect as indicator of further alveolar bone loss. J Clin Periodontol 1991;18:317–322.
9. Ramfjord SP, Nissle RR. The modified Widman flap. J Periodontol 1974;45:601–607.
10. Nabers CL. Repositioning the attached gingiva. J Periodontol 1954;25:38–39.
11. Ochsenbein C, Bohannan HM. The palatal approach to osseous surgery. I. Rationale. J Periodontol 1963;34:60.
12. Tibbetts LS Jr, Ochsenbein C, Loughlin DM. Rationale for the lingual approach to mandibular osseous surgery. Dent Clin North Am 1976;20:61–78.
13. Takei HH, Han TJ, Carranza FA Jr, Kenney EB, Lekovic V. Flap technique for periodontal bone implants. Papilla preservation technique. J Periodontol 1985;56:204–210.
14. Stambaugh RV. A clinician's 3-year experience with perioscopy. Compend Contin Educ Dent 2002;23:1061–1070.
15. Harrel SK, Rees TD. Granulation tissue removal in routine and minimally invasive procedures. Compend Contin Educ Dent 1995;16:960, 962, 964 passim.
16. Pocket Dentistry. The MIS and V-MIS Surgical Procedure. https://pocketdentistry.com/7-the-mis-and-v-mis-surgical-procedure/. Published 20 Jan 2015. Accessed 10 October 2019.
17. Murphy KG. Interproximal tissue maintenance in GTR procedures: Description of a surgical technique and 1-year reentry results. Int J Periodontics Restorative Dent 1996;16:463–477.
18. Cortellini P, Prato GP, Tonetti MS. The simplified papilla preservation flap. A novel surgical approach for the management of soft tissues in regenerative procedures. Int J Periodontics Restorative Dent 1999;19:589–599.
19. Cortellini P, Pini Prato G, Tonetti MS. The modified papilla preservation technique with bioresorbable barrier membranes in the treatment of intrabony defects. Case reports. Int J Periodontics Restorative Dent 1996;16:546–559.
20. Cortellini P, Nieri M, Prato GP, Tonetti MS. Single minimally invasive surgical technique with an enamel matrix derivative to treat multiple adjacent intra-bony defects: Clinical outcomes and patient morbidity. J Clin Periodontol 2008;35:605–613.
21. Cortellini P, Tonetti MS. Improved wound stability with a modified minimally invasive surgical technique in the regenerative treatment of isolated interdental intrabony defects. J Clin Periodontol 2009;36:157–163.
22. Cortellini P. Minimally invasive surgical techniques in periodontal regeneration. J Evid Based Dent Pract 2012;12(3 suppl):89–100.

23. Trombelli L, Farina R, Franceschetti G, Calura G. Single-flap approach with buccal access in periodontal reconstructive procedures. J Periodontol 2009;80:353–360.

24. Nisha S, Shashikumar P, Salini Samyuktha G. Minimally invasive techniques in periodontal regeneration. Int J Oral Health Sci 2017;7:24–29.

25. Mizukama T. Treatment of periodontal diseases and peri-implant diseases. Presented at the 10th Annual Meeting of the American Academy of Periodontology, Vancouver, BC, 30 Oct 2018.

26. Cortellini P, Tonetti MS. Microsurgical approach to periodontal regeneration. Initial evaluation in a case cohort. J Periodontol 2001;72:559–569.

27. Wood DL, Hoag PM, Donnenfeld OW, Rosenfeld LD. Alveolar crest reduction following full and partial thickness flaps. J Periodontol 1972;43:141–144.

28. Wilderman MN, Pennel BM, King K, Barron JM. Histogenesis of repair following osseous surgery. J Periodontol 1970;41:551–565.

29. Moghaddas H, Stahl SS. Alveolar bone remodeling following osseous surgery. A clinical study. J Periodontol 1980;51:376–381.

30. Newman MG, Takei H, Klokkevold PR, Carranza FA. Carranza's Clinical Periodontology, ed 11. St Louis: Elsevier Saunders, 2012:935.

31. Smith DH, Ammons WF Jr, Van Belle G. A longitudinal study of peridontal status comparing osseous recontouring with flap curettage. I. Results after 6 months. J Periodontol 1980;51:367–375.

32. Nyman S, Rosling B, Lindhe J. Effect of professional tooth cleaning on healing after periodontal surgery. J Clin Periodontol 1975;2:80–86.

33. Carnevale G, Pontoriero R, di Febo G. Long-term effects of root-resective therapy in furcation-involved molars. A 10-year longitudinal study. J Clin Periodontol 1998;25:209–214.

34. Fugazzotto PA. A comparison of the success of root resected molars and molar position implants in function in a private practice: Results of up to 15-plus years. J Periodontol 2001;72:1113–1123.

35. Langer B, Stein SD, Wagenberg B. An evaluation of root resections. A ten-year study. J Periodontol 1981;52:719–722.

36. Derks H, Westheide D, Pfefferle T, Eickholz P, Dannewitz B. Retention of molars after root-resective therapy: A retrospective evaluation of up to 30 years. Clin Oral Investig 2018;22:1327–1335.

37. Yukna RA, Bowers GM, Lawrence JJ, Fedi PF Jr. A clinical study of healing in humans following the excisional new attachment procedure. J Periodontol 1976;47:696–700.

38. American Academy of Periodontology. Statement Regarding Use of Dental Lasers for Excisional New Attachment Procedure (ENAP). August 1999.

39. Powell CA, Mealey BL, Deas DE, McDonnell HT, Moritz AJ. Post-surgical infections: Prevalence associated with various periodontal surgical procedures. J Periodontol 2005;76:329–333.

40. Jones TM, Cassingham RJ. Comparison of healing following periodontal surgery with and without dressings in humans. J Periodontol 1979;50:387–393.

41. Dahlberg WH. Incisions and suturing: Some basic considerations about each in periodontal flap surgery. Dent Clin North Am 1969;13:149–159.

42. Newell DH, Brunsvold MA. A modification of the "curtain technique" incorporating an internal mattress suture. J Periodontol 1985;56:484–487.

43. Pack PD, Haber J. The incidence of clinical infection after periodontal surgery. A retrospective study. J Periodontol 1983;54:441–443.

44. Zigdon H, Levin L, Filatov M, Oettinger-Barak O, Machtei EE. Intraoperative bleeding during open flap debridement and regenerative periodontal surgery. J Periodontol 2012;83:55–60.

45. Baab DA, Ammons WF Jr, Selipsky H. Blood loss during periodontal flap surgery. J Periodontol 1977;48:693–698.

Mucogingival Therapy

Background

Q: What is the definition of mucogingival therapy?

A 1996 consensus report by the American Academy of Periodontology defines *mucogingival therapy* as "non-surgical and surgical correction of the defects in morphology, position and/or amount of soft tissue and underlying bone."[1]

In 1988, Miller[2] coined the term *periodontal plastic surgery* to include not only treatment of recession and problems associated with attached gingiva but also "correction of ridge form, exposing unerupted teeth for orthodontic treatment, crown lengthening for esthetic purposes, and frenal surgery."

Q: What is the prevalence of dehiscence and fenestration in the maxilla and the mandible?

Dehiscence refers to when the root area is denuded of bone and extends to the marginal bone.[3] *Fenestration* refers to isolated areas in which the root is denuded of bone (window), and the root surface is covered by periosteum and overlying gingiva. Table 11-1 presents the prevalence of dehiscence and fenestration.[4]

Rupprecht et al[5] found the mean number of either dehiscence or fenestration defects per modern American skull was 3.0. Of the 3,315 individual teeth examined, 4.1% (135) had dehiscences, and 9.0% (298) had fenestrations. Mandibular canines were most often affected by dehiscences (12.9%), while maxillary first molars were most often affected by fenestrations (37.0%).

$\rightarrow$

Table 11-1	Prevalence of dehiscence and fenestration	
	Maxilla	Mandible
Dehiscence (%)	6	14
Fenestration (%)	17	6

Q: What are the endpoints of success with mucogingival therapy?

- Gingival augmentation
- Prevention or cessation of recession
- Facilitation of plaque control
- Elimination of an aberrant frenum
- Increased vestibular depth
- Decreased root sensitivity
- Decreased inflammation
- Improved patient comfort

Q: What circumstances require an increased zone of keratinized tissue (KT)?

According to the World Workshop in Clinical Periodontics, the following are indications for a gingival augmentation procedure[6]:

1. Placement of a restoration with an intracrevicular margin
2. Impingement of major or minor connectors of removable partial dentures
3. Overdenture when there is an absence of gingiva associated with retained teeth

Scheyer et al[7] found a minimum amount of KT is not required to prevent attachment loss when optimal plaque control is present. However, if plaque control is suboptimal, a minimum of 2 mm of KT is essential.

Studies have found a wide band of nonmobile keratinized mucosa, an adequate peri-implant mucosal height, and a thick tissue phenotype might reduce the incidence of tissue inflammation and future complications.[8]

Q: Is there a minimum amount of attached gingiva recommended to reduce the risk of recession?

According to studies by Lang and Löe,[9] a minimum of 2 mm of keratinized gingiva (1 mm attached and 1 mm free gingiva) is needed to maintain gingival health.

According to Maynard and Wilson,[10] if there is good oral hygiene, a lack of attached gingiva does not result in recession.

Q: How does widening the attached gingiva improve esthetics and reduce gingival inflammation?

- Enhances plaque control around the gingival margin
- Reduces inflammation around the restored teeth

Q: What are some of the potential risks associated with mucogingival therapy?

- Increased bleeding
- Bone exposure
- Color discrepancies
- Necrosis of donor site
- Herpetic lesions
- Delayed healing
- Pain
- Swelling
- Difficulty eating
- Speaking
- Graft failure

Gingival Recession

Q: What is gingival recession?

Gingival recession is defined as the apical shift of the gingival margin with respect to the cementoenamel junction (CEJ); it is associated with attachment loss and with exposure of the root surface to the oral environment. It may apply to all surfaces (lingual, buccal, interproximal).[11]

Q: What are causes/risk factors for gingival recession?

- Thin periodontal phenotype: A thin phenotype develops more gingival recession than a thick one.[6]
- Tooth positioned too anterior.
- Underlying bony dehiscence or reduced thickness of the alveolar bone.
- Abrasive and traumatic toothbrushing habits (most important mechanical factor).
- Periodontal inflammation.
- Frenal and muscle attachment encroachment.
- Orthodontic movement (especially in areas with < 2 mm of gingiva).[11]
- Invasion of supracrestal tissue attachment (previously known as *biologic width*; comprised of junctional epithelium and supracrestal connective tissue attachment).
- Absence of attached gingiva.
- Trauma from occlusion; it is controversial as to whether it affects recession (pro[12]; con[13,14]).
- Both lip and tongue piercings are highly correlated with the risk of gingival recession. The incidence of gingival recessions appeared to be 50% in subjects with lip piercings and 44% in subjects with a tongue piercing. Subjects with a lip piercing were 4.14 times more likely to develop gingival recession than those without a lip piercing.[15]

Q: What are the consequences of gingival recession?

Development and progression of gingival recession is not associated with increased tooth mortality.[11] Figure 11-1 presents the consequences of gingival recession.[16]

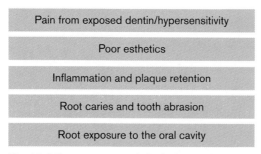

Pain from exposed dentin/hypersensitivity

Poor esthetics

Inflammation and plaque retention

Root caries and tooth abrasion

Root exposure to the oral cavity

Fig 11-1 Consequences of gingival recession.

Q: What is the prevalence of gingival recession?

More than 50% of the population has one or more sites with gingival recession of 1 mm or more. The prevalence of gingival recession was detected in patients with both poor and good oral hygiene. It has been proposed that recession is multifactorial, with one type being associated with anatomical factors and another type with physiologic or pathologic factors. Recession has been found more commonly on buccal surfaces than on other aspects of the teeth.[17]

According to a study by Albandar and Kingman,[18] the prevalence of ≥ 1 mm recession is 58% in individuals 30 years and older and increases with age. The prevalence of recession is 37.8% in those aged 30 to 39 years and increases to 90.4% in persons aged 80 to 90 years.

Q: Once recession is present, can it worsen?

See Fig 11-2 below.

Yes
- Serino et al[19] found a 3-mm recession site worsened 67% of the time. A 4-mm recession site worsened 98% of the time.
- Chambrone and Tatakis[20] found that untreated recession defects in individuals with good oral hygiene have a high probability of progressing during long-term follow-up.
- Agudio et al[21] found that 83% of the 64 treated sites showed recession reduction, whereas 48% of the 64 untreated sites experienced increase in recession.

No
- Kennedy et al[22] reported that the non-grafted sites of 32 patients showed no additional attachment loss or recession over a 6-year observation period on those patients that followed a maintenance routine.

Fig 11-2 Diagram showing studies on whether recessions can worsen.

Classification of Recession

Q: What is the classification system based on interdental CAL measurement?[23]

- Recession Type 1 (RT1): Gingival recession with no loss of interproximal attachment. Interproximal CEJ is clinically not detectable at both mesial and distal aspects of the tooth.
- Recession Type 2 (RT2): Gingival recession associated with loss of interproximal attachment. The amount of interproximal attachment loss (measured from the interproximal CEJ to the depth of the interproximal sulcus/pocket) is less than or equal to the buccal attachment loss (measured from the buccal CEJ to the apical end of the buccal sulcus/pocket).
- Recession Type 3 (RT3): Gingival recession associated with loss of interproximal attachment. The amount of interproximal attachment loss (measured from the interproximal CEJ to the apical end of the sulcus/pocket) is greater than the buccal attachment loss (measured from the buccal CEJ to the apical end of the buccal sulcus/pocket).

With RT1 and RT2 100% root coverage can be achieved, but with RT3 100% root coverage is not achievable. See Fig 11-3.

RT1	RT2	RT3

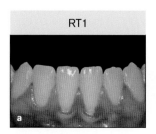 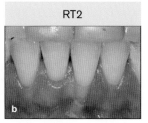 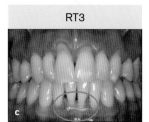

Fig 11-3 Staging.[24]

Q: What is Miller's classification[25] of soft tissue recession?

Miller's classification[25] of soft tissue recession is shown in Fig 11-4 (see next page). →

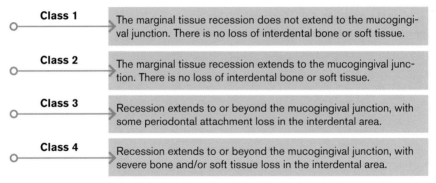

Class 1	The marginal tissue recession does not extend to the mucogingival junction. There is no loss of interdental bone or soft tissue.
Class 2	The marginal tissue recession extends to the mucogingival junction. There is no loss of interdental bone or soft tissue.
Class 3	Recession extends to or beyond the mucogingival junction, with some periodontal attachment loss in the interdental area.
Class 4	Recession extends to or beyond the mucogingival junction, with severe bone and/or soft tissue loss in the interdental area.

Fig 11-4 Miller's classification[25] of soft tissue recession.

Q: What is the expected root coverage for each of Miller's classes?

- Class 1: 100% root coverage.
- Class 2: 100% root coverage.
- Class 3: Partial root coverage is anticipated 50% to 70% of the time.
- Class 4: Root coverage is not anticipated; the success rate is less than 10%.

Q: Describe the Sullivan and Atkins classification[26] of mucogingival defects.

Figure 11-5 presents the Sullivan and Atkins classification[26] of mucogingival defects.

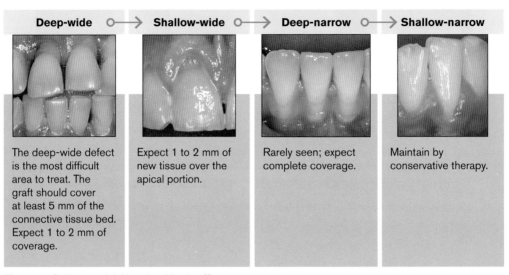

Deep-wide	Shallow-wide	Deep-narrow	Shallow-narrow
The deep-wide defect is the most difficult area to treat. The graft should cover at least 5 mm of the connective tissue bed. Expect 1 to 2 mm of coverage.	Expect 1 to 2 mm of new tissue over the apical portion.	Rarely seen; expect complete coverage.	Maintain by conservative therapy.

Fig 11-5 Sullivan and Atkins classification.[26]

Q: What is the classification system of the four different classes of root concavities?

See Table 11-2 and Fig 11-6 below.

Table 11-2	Classification system of root concavities[27]	
Class	**Step**	**Explanation**
A	–	CEJ detectable without a step
A	+	CEJ detectable with a step
B	–	CEJ undetectable without a step
B	+	CEJ undetectable with step

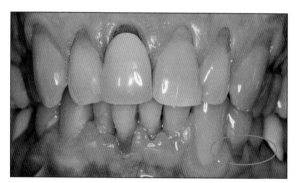

Fig 11-6 Root surface concavities.[24]

Q: How are alveolar ridge defects classified?

Alveolar ridge defects are classified by the Seibert[28] classification:

- Class 1: Buccopalatal loss of tissue with normal apicocoronal ridge height
- Class 2: Apicocoronal loss of tissue with normal buccopalatal ridge width
- Class 3: Combination defect—loss of both width and height of the ridge

Q: How are phenotypes (formerly referred to as *biotypes*) classified?[29]

- *Thin scalloped phenotypes:* Slender triangular crowns, subtle cervical convexity, interproximal contacts close to the incisal edge, and a narrow zone of keratinized tissue, clear and thin tissue, and thin alveolar bone
- *Thick flat phenotypes:* Square-shaped tooth crowns, pronounced cervical convexity, large interproximal contact located apically, keratinized tissue has a broad zone, and thick alveolar bone
- *Thick scalloped phenotypes:* Showing a thick fibrotic gingiva, slender teeth, narrow zone of keratinized tissue, and pronounced gingival scalloping

The mean keratinized tissue width for thick phenotype is 5.72 mm and 4.15 mm for the thin phenotype. The mean buccal bone thickness is 0.343 mm for the thin phenotype and 0.754 mm for thick/average phenotype.[11]

A thin phenotype develops more gingival recession than a thick biotype.[6]

It should be noted that periodontal phenotype, which is the combination of gingival phenotype (3D gingival volume) and the thickness of the buccal bone plate (bone morphotype), should be used as opposed to biotype.[30]

Restorative Considerations and Gingival Recession

Q: How much attached gingiva is required around restorations?

According to studies by Maynard and Wilson,[10] 5 mm of keratinized attached gingiva composed of 2 mm of free gingiva and 3 mm of attached gingiva is needed to meet restorative goals.

Q: Does an intrasulcular restorative margin influence the development of gingival recession?

Teeth with a thin periodontal phenotype restored with intrasulcular restorations may be at greater risk of gingival recession.[30] In such situations, the maintenance of zone of attached keratinized tissue of 3 mm has been suggested, according to Maynard and Wilson.[10]

KT augmentation may prevent the development and progression of gingival recession, especially when restorative margins may interact with the periodontium and/or orthodontic treatment is indicated.[6]

Q: What is the response of periodontal tissues covering a Class V resin?

Martins et al[31] found that the restorative materials (glass ionomer cement and composite resin) used exhibit biocompatibility; however, both materials interfered with the development of new bone and the connective tissue attachment process.

Another study found root coverage improvement without damage to periodontal tissues, supporting the use of a coronally positioned flap for treatment of root surfaces restored with resin-modified glass ionomer or microfilled resin composite as being effective over a 6-month period.[32]

Technique

Q: What are the different technique options for soft tissue augmentation?[33]

1. No treatment with scaling and root planing
2. Apically positioned flap/vestibuloplasty (APF/V)
3. APF/V plus autogenous tissue (eg, connective tissue)
4. APF/V plus allogenic tissue (eg, acellular dermal matrix)
5. APF/V plus tissue-engineered live cell construct (LCC)
6. Xenografts: Extracellular matrix (ECM) or bilayer collagen

Q: What is the technique for placement of a free gingival graft versus a connective tissue graft?

The techniques for placement of free gingival grafts and connective tissue (CT) grafts are presented in Fig 11-7 (see next page). →

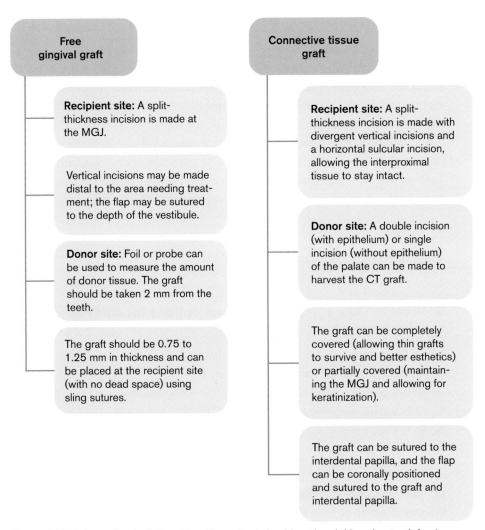

Free gingival graft

Recipient site: A split-thickness incision is made at the MGJ.

Vertical incisions may be made distal to the area needing treatment; the flap may be sutured to the depth of the vestibule.

Donor site: Foil or probe can be used to measure the amount of donor tissue. The graft should be taken 2 mm from the teeth.

The graft should be 0.75 to 1.25 mm in thickness and can be placed at the recipient site (with no dead space) using sling sutures.

Connective tissue graft

Recipient site: A split-thickness incision is made with divergent vertical incisions and a horizontal sulcular incision, allowing the interproximal tissue to stay intact.

Donor site: A double incision (with epithelium) or single incision (without epithelium) of the palate can be made to harvest the CT graft.

The graft can be completely covered (allowing thin grafts to survive and better esthetics) or partially covered (maintaining the MGJ and allowing for keratinization).

The graft can be sutured to the interdental papilla, and the flap can be coronally positioned and sutured to the graft and interdental papilla.

Fig 11-7 Techniques for gingival grafting. The patient should not brush his or her teeth for 4 weeks. MGJ, mucogingival junction.

Q: What are the advantages of a CT graft compared with a free gingival graft?

- Palate can heal by primary intention.
- Patient has less pain. FGG is associated with a greater incidence of donor site pain compared to CT graft at the early postoperative period.[34]
- CT graft is more esthetic (better color match).

Q: **Does the orientation of the CT graft affect root coverage or gingival augmentation?**

Al-Zahrani et al[35] studied 16 pairs of bilateral gingival recessions (Miller class 1 and class 2). For each patient (13 patients), one side received a CT graft with the superficial surface toward the gingival flap, and the other side had the same surface toward the root surface. The study measured Plaque Index, Gingival Index, probing depth, gingival recession, root coverage, and relative clinical attachment level. The study found that neither root coverage nor gingival augmentation were significantly altered by the surface orientation of a CT graft.

Lafzi et al[36] had a similar finding. Their study found that the short-term clinical outcome of a CT graft with a coronally advanced flap (CAF) is not affected by orientation of the CT graft.

Q: **Should CT grafts contain epithelium and/or periosteum?**

The limited available evidence suggests that inclusion of an epithelial collar does not provide additional benefits in terms of root coverage.

There is lack of evidence on the possible effect of periosteum-containing CTGs.[37]

Q: **Are there different outcomes when placing grafts using a microsurgery versus a macrosurgery technique? Using a microscope?**

Burkhardt and Lang[38] found greater vascularization and root coverage immediately, 3 days, and 7 days following microsurgery compared with outcomes at the same time points when the macrosurgery technique was used.

Kang et al[39] found evidence, stemming from two randomized controlled trials, that complete root coverage can be more predictably achieved by subepithelial CT grafts performed with a microscope.

Q: **Which factors may influence the expected outcomes of root coverage procedures?**

See Fig 11-8 on the next page.

Patient-related factors	Site-related factors	Technique-related factors
• Smoking. • Patient expectations. • Patient's systemic health. • Compliance.	• Poor diagnosis (classification). • Noncarious cervical lesions, whether restored or not, may be effectively treated by subepithelial CT graft + CAF and CAF alone. • There is limited evidence that root coverage procedures can be effective in the treatment of previously restored or carious root surfaces. • Defect depth has been demonstrated to negatively correlate with the degree of root coverage attained. • Initial tissue thickness directly correlates with the predictability of root coverage. • Periodontal phenotype. • Presence of aberrant frenal attachment. • Root prominence (surface area, blood supply). • Shallow vestibule. • Palatal anatomy.	• Surgical positioning of the tissue margin coronal to the CEJ improves complete root coverage outcomes. • There is limited evidence that other technical aspects (eg, flap tension and use of vertical releasing incisions) influence outcomes. • Inadequate flap advancement (2.5 mm coronal to CEJ or the graft) increases risk of root coverage failure. • The use of microsurgical techniques results in improved outcomes. • Gingival thickness < 1 mm (root coverage with a CAF without a CT graft) increases risk of root coverage failure.

Fig 11-8 Factors that may influence the expected outcomes of root coverage procedures.[37,40,41]

Q: What are the long- and short-term advantages of root surface biomodification?

Chemical root surface biomodification has not been proven to influence clinical results.[37]

A systematic review and meta-analysis by Barootchi et al[42] found that the adjunct application of ethylenediaminetetraacetic acid (EDTA) may provide benefits when performing a root coverage procedure via CAF and CT graft.

Q: Are live cell therapies effective?

McGuire et al[43] did a randomized controlled study and found living cellular constructs (LCC) regenerated ≥ 2 mm of keratinized gingiva in 95.3% of patients. The free gingival graft (FGG) generated more keratinized gingiva →

than the LCC. The gingiva regenerated with the LCC matched the color and texture of the adjacent gingiva.

In another randomized controlled study McGuire and Nunn[44] found that the FGG group exhibited an average of 1.0 to 1.2 mm more keratinized tissue over time than the LCC group, and the FGG group had about half as much shrinkage as the LCC group over time.

Different Flap Designs

Q: Describe the laterally positioned flap.

Grupe and Warren[45] described the technique in which a split-thickness incision is made one papilla distal or mesial to the affected site beyond the mucogingival junction. The flap is allowed to slide over to the adjacent recipient site. The flap should be made wider than the recipient site. A pedicle flap should have an adequate zone of keratinized tissue in terms of thickness and quantity adjacent to the area of recession. The patient should have an adequate vestibule as well.

Q: Describe the double papilla flap.

The double papilla pedicle flap was first introduced by Cohen and Ross[46] in 1968. According to Cohen and Ross, the procedure is useful for treating recession occurring on the lingual or facial gingiva, and it avoids the need for destruction of the interdental papillae on either side of the area of denudation. The papilla from each tooth is moved over the facial or lingual aspect of the recipient tooth. This technique allows for a dual blood supply. A sling suture is used at the end of the procedure.

Q: Describe the semilunar technique.

Tarnow[47] described a technique that allows the practitioner to make a split-thickness incision parallel to the outline of the gingival margin and 2 mm away from the papilla. This technique is reserved for limited recession. Sutures are not needed for this technique.

Q: When should a coronally positioned flap be used?

The coronally positioned flap was first described by Bernimoulin in 1981.[48] A split-thickness incision is made with vertical incisions that go beyond the mucogingival junction. Some guidelines to perform a coronally positioned flap include:

- Minimum tissue thickness of 0.8 mm (Baldi et al[49])
- Shallow recession of less than 4 mm
- Miller class 1
- Keratinized attached tissue greater than 3 mm
- There should be minimal to no flap tension
- The flap should be placed 2.5 mm coronal to the CEJ

Zucchelli et al[50] found that a coronally positioned flap without vertical incisions (ie, envelope flap) had an increased chance of complete root coverage and decreased postoperative morbidity.

Q: What are some other techniques for treating recession?

Tunnel technique

The tunnel technique (Fig 11-9) is based on what was first introduced as the *envelope technique* by Raetzke in 1985.[51] With the aim to evade any kind of releasing incisions, Raetzke defined this technique, the main distinguishing characteristic of which was the insertion of an autologous CT graft in an envelope that was fashioned in the buccal soft tissues around the exposed root surface by a split-thickness flap preparation.

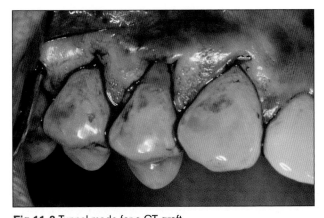

Fig 11-9 Tunnel made for a CT graft.

$\rightarrow$

Vestibular incision subperiosteal tunnel access (VISTA) technique

Placement of the initial incision and a tunnel entrance within the maxillary anterior frenum results in little to no visible scarring, assisting in maximizing the esthetic outcome in this critical restorative area. Next, a subperiosteal tunnel is elevated. VISTA allows for both access as well as a chance to coronally reposition the gingival margins of all affected teeth. Recombinant human platelet-derived growth factor BB saturated onto a matrix of beta-tricalcium phosphate is placed using VISTA over root dehiscences to enhance periodontal healing. The area is sutured via coronally anchored suturing designed to maintain the coronal positioning during healing.[52]

Pinhole surgical technique (PST)

Only one incision (2 to 3 mm) is used, and no releasing incision, no sharp dissection, and no suturing are necessary (when an absorbable membrane is used). Bioresorbable membrane or acellular dermal matrix is used as graft material.[53]

Wound Healing

Q: Describe the wound healing of a free gingival graft.

Following is the timeline for wound healing of a free gingival graft according to Gargiulo and Arrocha[54]:

- 0 to 2 days: Plasmatic circulation
- 2 to 4 days: Vascular invasion
- 4 to 7 days: Connective tissue attachment
- 10 days: Bridge of vascular channels
- 21 days: Connective tissue is well organized

Q: What is the anticipated success and attachment apparatus of root coverage procedures?

There is strong evidence[37] that root coverage procedures result in stable clinical attachment level gains with shallow probing depths. Proof-of-principle human histologic evidence has shown that limited periodontal regeneration can ensue after root coverage procedures. Most of the root coverage techniques result in the formation of a long junctional epithelial attachment.

Q: How much shrinkage can occur after placing the graft?

At 360 days after grafting, Mörmann et al[55] found the percentages of shrinkage to be 45% very thin, 44% thin, and 38% intermediate. Most shrinkage occurs within the first 6 weeks.

Q: Is there a difference between thick and thin grafts in terms of clinical outcome?

Thick grafts do not appear to result in better clinical outcomes than thin grafts. Thick grafts are likely to result in more primary contraction, whereas thin grafts tend to be susceptible to secondary contraction.[6]

Kim and Nevia[6] concluded that a very thin graft (0.5 to 0.6 mm) demonstrates an excellent color blending with that of the neighboring tissues, whereas a thick graft has increased functional resistance. However, a thick graft will result in an unesthetic tissue profile and a deeper donor site wound. Thus, the optimal graft thickness is 1.5 to 2.0 mm (palatal epithelium is 0.34 mm). Thin grafts have been found to revascularize and heal more rapidly than thick ones.

Q: How much creeping attachment can be expected with a free gingival graft?

According to Matter,[56] 0.89 mm of creeping attachment is expected in areas of recession less than 3 mm in width. The mean coverage, obtained principally by creeping attachment, was about 70%.

Q: What is the effect of smoking on mucogingival surgery?

Yadav et al[57] did a systematic study and found that root coverage obtained with a subepithelial CT graft was reduced in smokers. Cyanide, carbon monoxide, and nitrosamines can contribute to poor wound healing in cigarette smokers. Smokers generate less hydroxyproline and collagen—which are crucial for the formation and maintenance of connective tissue—than nonsmokers. Cell death can occur when fibroblasts are subjected to nicotine. This could be the reason for poor periodontal wound healing with CT grafts seen in a cigarette smoker.

Souza et al[58] showed 58.02% and 83.35% of root coverage in smokers and nonsmokers, respectively.

Anatomy for Mucogingival Therapy

Q: When harvesting a CT graft, which area has the greatest soft tissue thickness?

The tuberosity at the mid-distal position has the greatest soft tissue thickness.

Q: What is the average distance from the greater palatine foramen to the CEJ?

Following are the average distances from the greater palatine foramen to the CEJ based on the depth of the palate. According to Reiser et al,[59] these figures are important to consider when taking donor tissue from the palate (Figs 11-10 and 11-11).

- Deep palate: 17 mm
- Average-depth palate: 12 mm
- Shallow palate: 7 mm

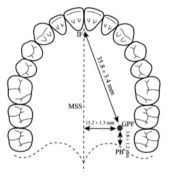

Fig 11-10 Distance to the greater palatine foramen (GPF) from the midsagittal suture (MSS), interincisive foramen (IF), and the posterior border of the hard palate (PB).[60]

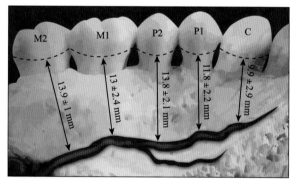

Fig 11-11 Drawing showing the distance from the CEJ to the greater palatine artery.[60]

Q: Is it more effective to place a graft on bone or on periosteum?

- *Bone:* James and McFall[61] believed that there could be 1.5 to 2 times more shrinkage if a graft were placed on periosteum instead of bone. Matter and Cimasoni[62] found that grafts placed on denuded bone shrank 25% and grafts placed on periosteum shrank 50%. Dordick et al[63] found that grafts placed on bone demonstrated less swelling and better hemostasis than did the periosteally placed grafts. A healing lag was observed in the grafts placed on bone, which lasted only for the first two postoperative visits, approximately 2 weeks.
- *Periosteum:* Caffesse and Guinard[64] believed that there is delayed remodeling of grafts placed on bone. Lindhe et al[65] observed greater bone resorption on bone than on periosteum.

Acellular Dermal Matrix (ADM, eg, AlloDerm)

Q: Describe AlloDerm and the technique used to place it.

AlloDerm (BioHorizons) is human dermis made of a matrix of collagen, elastin, vascular channels, and protein that support its revascularization. It has been processed to remove the epidermis and cells that can lead to tissue rejection and graft rejection without damaging the matrix. AlloDerm can be placed in a tunnel as described below:

1. Hydrate the AlloDerm.
2. Scale and root plane the teeth in the affected site.
3. Prepare the tunnel, extending at least one tooth mesial and distal to the site and apical to the mucogingival junction, and the site 3 mm apical to the papilla tip.
4. Trim and place AlloDerm into the tunnel and suture for stability.
5. Place sling sutures (polypropylene sutures are recommended).
6. Suture the gingival tissue detached in the formation of the tunnel to completely cover the acellular dermal matrix.

Q: What is the main contraindication to AlloDerm?

Do not use AlloDerm if the patient is allergic to Gentamicin.

Q: Is an autogenous graft or AlloDerm more effective? Is xenogeneic collagen matrix as effective as an autogenous free gingival graft?

According to studies by Wei et al,[66] AlloDerm is less effective in increasing attached keratinized tissue and can lead to more shrinkage. However, the study found better esthetics with AlloDerm. Henderson et al[67] found that with AlloDerm, there was no creeping attachment and a gain of keratinized attachment of about 1 mm.

A meta-analysis by Gapski et al[68] noted no statistically significant dissimilarities between surgeries using AlloDerm and other mucogingival surgeries.

McGuire and Scheyer[33] found that free gingival graft sites averaged 1.5 mm more width than xenogeneic collagen matrix sites (pure, porcine collagen). However, the amount of new KT generated for both therapies averaged $\geq$ 2 mm. Xenogeneic collagen matrix sites achieved better texture and color matches, and more than two-thirds of patients preferred the appearance of their xenogeneic sites.

The 2015 consensus statement by the American Academy of Periodontology[37] found that for Miller Class 1 and 2 single-tooth recession defects, subepithelial CT graft procedures provide the best outcomes, whereas ADM graft or enamel matrix derivative in conjunction with a coronally advanced flap may be used as an alternative. There is limited evidence that platelet-derived growth factor and xenogeneic collagen matrix may be used as alternatives to autogenous donor tissue.

Q: Compare ADM and a CT graft.

See Table 11-3 below.

Table 11-3	ADM versus CT grafts	
	ADM	**CT**
Handling	Ready to use	Slippery
Availability	Unlimited	Limited
Complications	Necrosis is possible	Minimal

Guided Tissue Regeneration (GTR)

Q: Why would it be beneficial to use GTR as opposed to a soft tissue procedure alone?

- There is not a second surgical site.
- Bone may regenerate.

A challenge is that it is difficult to create enough space for generating tissue between the root surface and membrane.

In a 10-year study comparing CT grafts with GTR, Nickles et al[69] found that CT grafts had a better treatment outcome but caused greater postoperative discomfort compared with GTR.

Oates et al[70] reported greater gains in both root coverage and keratinized tissue width for CT graft procedures compared to GTR.

Q: Is the thickness of the flap a predictor of root coverage?

Table 11-4 presents the percentage of root coverage based on the thickness of the flap according to Harris.[71]

Table 11-4	Thickness of the flap and percentage of root coverage	
Technique	Thin flap (%)	Thick flap (%)
CT with a double pedicle flap	100	95.9
Membrane placement	26.7	96

Q: Based on periodontal informational papers,[72] what is the mean defect coverage for the FGG, pedicle graft, CT graft, coronally positioned graft, GTR, and AlloDerm?

Table 11-5 presents the mean defect coverage for different grafting techniques and AlloDerm. →

Table 11-5	Mean defect coverage using different techniques						
Free gingival graft	Pedicle graft	CT graft	Coronally positioned flap	GTR		AlloDerm
				Resorbable membrane	Nonresorbable membrane	
69%	67%	84%	78%	72%	73%	86%

Enamel Matrix Derivative (EMD)

Q: Has EMD (porcine amelogenin) shown any improvement in mucogingival therapy?

EMD (eg, Emdogain [Straumann]) placed with a coronally placed flap or CT graft seems to accelerate soft tissue healing. According to a position paper,[72] the addition of Emdogain to a flap had a mean defect coverage of 86%.

Subepithelial CT grafts, matrix grafts, and EMD were superior to a coronally advanced flap in achieving complete root coverage, but CT grafts showed the best predictability.[41]

Decision Trees for Treating Recession Defects

Q: Describe the technical factors that enhance root coverage.

See Fig 11-12 below.

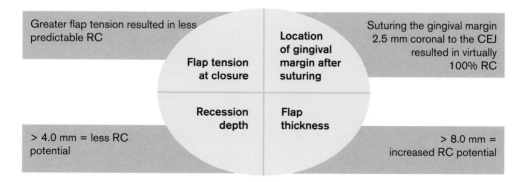

Fig 11-12 Factors that enhance root coverage (RC).[37]

207

Q: Describe the outcome assessment for preoperative hypersensitivity, root surface debridement, growth factor–based procedures, and laser root surface treatment.

See Fig 11-13 below.

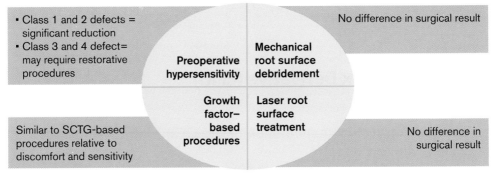

Patient outcomes   **Clinical outcomes**

- Class 1 and 2 defects = significant reduction
- Class 3 and 4 defect= may require restorative procedures

Preoperative hypersensitivity

Mechanical root surface debridement

No difference in surgical result

Growth factor– based procedures

Laser root surface treatment

Similar to SCTG-based procedures relative to discomfort and sensitivity

No difference in surgical result

Fig 11-13 Outcomes assessment.[37] SCTG, subepithelial connective tissue graft.

Q: Describe the decision tree to use when deciding which soft tissue technique to use.

See Fig 11-14 on the next page.

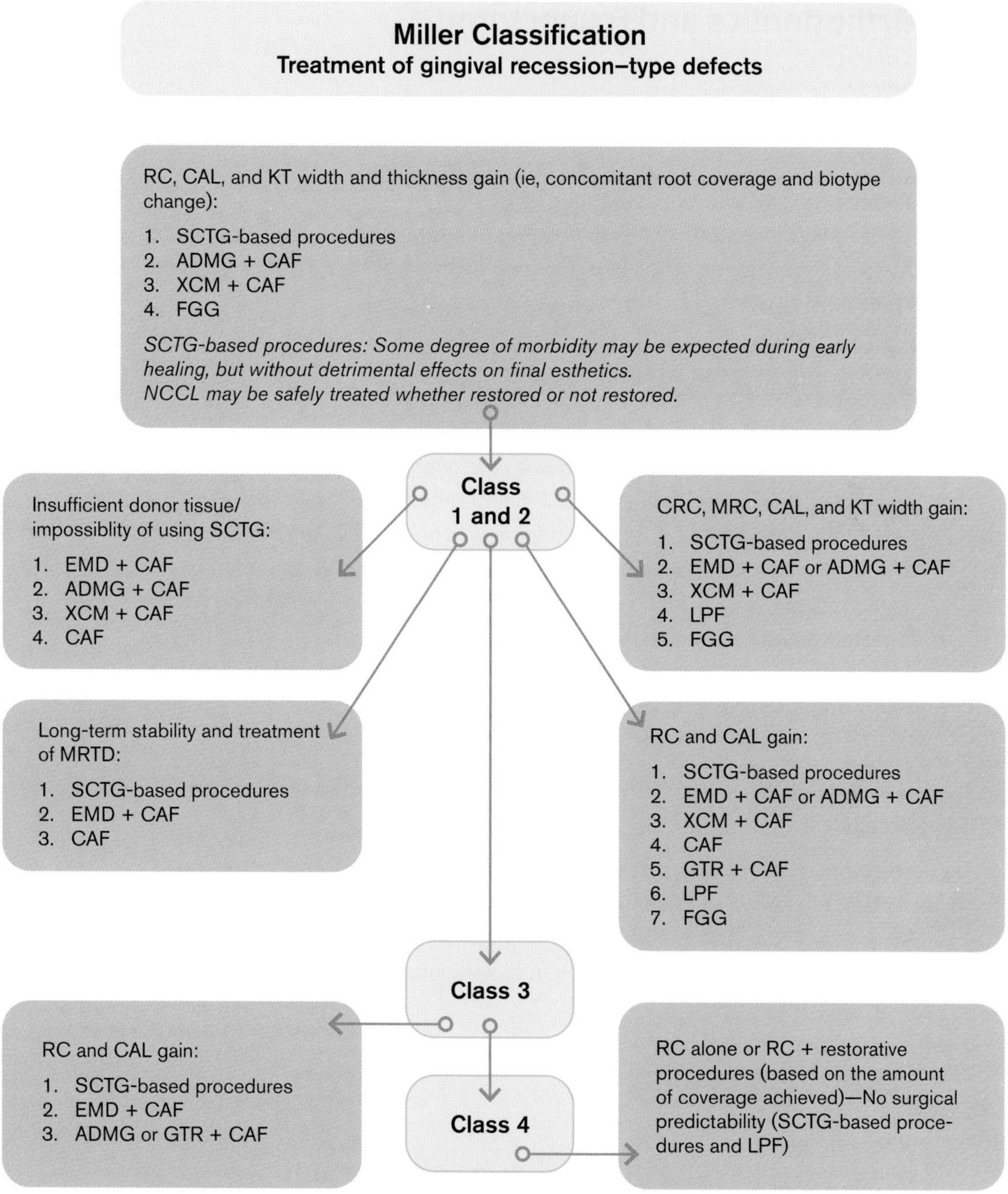

Miller Classification
Treatment of gingival recession–type defects

RC, CAL, and KT width and thickness gain (ie, concomitant root coverage and biotype change):

1. SCTG-based procedures
2. ADMG + CAF
3. XCM + CAF
4. FGG

SCTG-based procedures: Some degree of morbidity may be expected during early healing, but without detrimental effects on final esthetics.
NCCL may be safely treated whether restored or not restored.

Class 1 and 2

Insufficient donor tissue/impossiblity of using SCTG:

1. EMD + CAF
2. ADMG + CAF
3. XCM + CAF
4. CAF

CRC, MRC, CAL, and KT width gain:

1. SCTG-based procedures
2. EMD + CAF or ADMG + CAF
3. XCM + CAF
4. LPF
5. FGG

Long-term stability and treatment of MRTD:

1. SCTG-based procedures
2. EMD + CAF
3. CAF

RC and CAL gain:

1. SCTG-based procedures
2. EMD + CAF or ADMG + CAF
3. XCM + CAF
4. CAF
5. GTR + CAF
6. LPF
7. FGG

Class 3

RC and CAL gain:

1. SCTG-based procedures
2. EMD + CAF
3. ADMG or GTR + CAF

Class 4

RC alone or RC + restorative procedures (based on the amount of coverage achieved)—No surgical predictability (SCTG-based procedures and LPF)

Fig 11-14 Decision tree for treatment of recession.[73] Therapies include free gingival grafts (FGGs); coronally advanced flaps (CAFs) alone or in combination with guided tissue regeneration (GTR), acellular dermal matrix grafts (ADMGs), enamel matrix derivative protein (EMD), xenogenic collagen matrix (XCM) grafts, or other biomaterials (eg, bone substitutes, platelet-rich plasma); and laterally positioned flaps (LPFs). NCCLs, noncarious cervical lesions; RC, root coverage; CAL, clinical attachment level; SCTG, subepithelial connective tissue graft; CRC, complete RC; MRC, mean RC; MRTD, multiple recession-type defects.

Orthodontics and Frenectomy

Q: Is there a need for frenectomy?

According to Ward,[74] a frenectomy and free gingival graft increase the attached gingiva and decrease recession.

According to a study of 1,000 children by Addy et al,[75] frenal attachment had a minor influence on plaque and gingivitis and did not justify mucogingival therapy.

Q: Is there a relationship between orthodontics and recession?

The reported prevalence spans 5% to 12% at the end of treatment.

According to Bollen et al,[76] there is a relationship between orthodontics and recession. The study found 0.03 mm of recession.

Appropriately applied orthodontic forces do not cause permanent damage to a healthy periodontium. The probability of recession during tooth movement in thin biotype is high enough to warrant gingival augmentation when the dimension of gingiva is insufficient (< 2 mm). In addition, cases in which there will be buccal tooth movement outside of the alveolar process need to be considered for a gingival augmentation procedure.[6]

Q: What is periodontally accelerated osteogenic orthodontics (PAOO)?

The procedure combines selective alveolar corticotomy, bone grafting, and orthodontic forces to increase alveolar bone volume, shorten treatment time, reduce root resorption, increase scope of treatment, allow greater post-treatment stability, and increase the height of keratinized gingiva.[77]

Loss of the Papilla

Q: What causes loss of the papilla?

- Loss of periodontal support
- Trauma
- Abnormal tooth shape

Q: What is the classification of loss of papilla height by Nordland and Tarnow?[78]

Following is the classification of loss of papilla height by Nordland and Tarnow[78]:

- Normal: Fills the embrasure space
- Class 1: Tip of the papilla is between the interproximal contact and interproximal CEJ
- Class 2: Tip of the papilla is between the interproximal CEJ and the facial CEJ
- Class 3: Tip of the papilla is apical to the facial CEJ

Q: What occurs when papillae are lost?

- Phonetic problems
- Interproximal food entrapment
- Esthetic impairment

Q: Is it possible for the papillae to be reconstructed?

The success may depend on the distance between the bone crest and the interproximal contact point, as reported by Tarnow et al.[79] According to many studies, predictable reconstruction of lost interproximal papillae is not yet possible.

Gingival Overgrowth and Excessive Gingival Display

Q: What can cause gingival overgrowth?

The following may cause gingival overgrowth[16]:

- Plaque
- Hormones (pregnancy, contraceptives)
- Hereditary gingival fibromatosis
- Scurvy
- Drugs
- Mouth breathing
- Neoplasia
- Granulomatous conditions

Q: What is excessive gingival display and why does it occur?

Excessive gingival display is a condition in which a significant amount of gingiva is visible when the patient smiles. It may be caused by:

- Failure of the gingiva to migrate apically after eruption of the teeth
- Vertical maxillary excess
- Upper lip incompetence/hypermobile upper lip. (Among patients seeking treatment for a gummy smile, hypermobile upper lip is the principal etiology, and it is frequently present in combination with altered passive eruption.[80])

Q: What is Coslet et al's classification[81] of altered passive eruption (gingival margin and sometimes bone located at a more coronal level)? What treatment is recommended for each?

Figure 11-15 presents the classification of altered passive eruption by Coslet et al[81] and the associated treatment approaches.

Mostafa[82] found that botulinum toxin can replace extensive surgical procedures for correction of a gummy smile because it is minimally invasive, quick, and affordable.

*An alternative to surgery ⟶ extrusion of the tooth, but the tooth may still need surgery because the bone moves with the tooth.

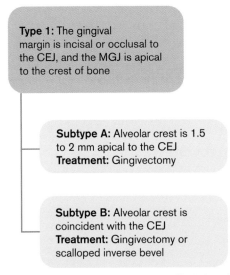
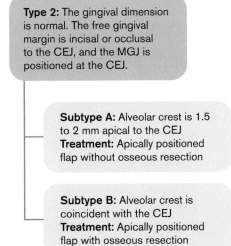

Fig 11-15 Coslet et al classification[39] of altered passive eruption. MGJ, mucogingival junction.

Q: What is active eruption? How is it different from passive eruption?

Active eruption is defined as tooth movement in the occlusal direction as the tooth erupts from its osseous crypt. Altered active eruption (AAE) occurs when teeth achieve the opposite relationship to the occlusal plane prematurely, and the osseous crest is on or very close to the CEJ.

Active eruption is the movement of the teeth in the direction of the occlusal plane, whereas passive eruption is related to the exposure of the teeth by apical migration of the gingiva.

Crown Lengthening

Q: What are the indications for crown lengthening?

- Subgingival fracture/caries
- Endodontic pin/post perforation
- Root resorption
- Inadequate height available for the restoration (Fig 11-16)
- Esthetically short crown
- Altered passive eruption
- Supracrestal tissue attachment would be violated during a restorative procedure. Please note the following dimensions: histologic sulcus (0.69 mm), epithelial attachment (0.97 mm), connective tissue attachment (1.07 mm). Supracrestal tissue attachment is the epithelial attachment plus the connective tissue attachment. (See chapter 2 for a discussion on supracrestal tissue attachment.)

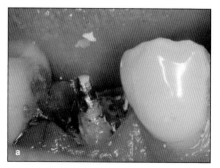 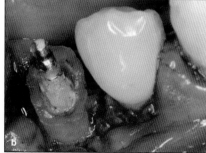

Fig 11-16 *(a)* Before crown lengthening. *(b)* After crown lengthening.

Q: What are contraindications to crown lengthening?

- Stability of the treated dentition may be affected.
- Excessive osseous removal will compromise the crown-to-root ratio.
- Removal of bone in the furcation region associated with the root trunk is a concern.[83]

Q: What are some important considerations when deciding to remove soft tissue or bone during a crown lengthening procedure?

If there is greater than 3 mm of soft tissue between the bone and gingival margin with adequate attached gingiva, crown lengthening by gingivectomy is possible. However, if there is less than 3 mm of soft tissue between the bone and the gingival margin or less than adequate attached gingiva, osseous recontouring is needed.

Q: What are some essential technical factors to consider when performing crown lengthening?

- A full-thickness mucoperiosteal flap should be made.
- A minimum ferrule of 1.5 mm should be allowed for retention.
- A 6-degree preparation taper and a minimum of 3.5 mm (1.5 mm of ferrule and about 2 mm of supracrestal tissue attachment) of circumferential tooth structure are required. However, Wagenberg et al[84] noted that 5 to 5.25 mm of tooth structure above the osseous crest is necessary.
- In the case of caries/fracture, at least 1 mm of sound tooth structure should be provided above the gingival margin for proper restoration.
- Esthetics and the final position of the incisal edge (anterior cases): The average width-to-length ratio of a maxillary central incisor is 75% to 80%.
- The flap should be apically positioned to the new level of the alveolar crest. Deas et al[85] found that the position of the flap in relation to the alveolar crest at suturing seems to be related to tissue rebound. The closer the tissue is sutured to the alveolar crest, the greater the chance of tissue rebound.
- At least 8 weeks should be allowed following surgery before procedures are performed. Brägger et al[86] found 2 to 4 mm of recession of the gingival margin between 6 weeks and 6 months postoperatively in 12% of crown lengthening procedures.

Restorative Considerations for Crown Lengthening

Q: Is it possible to obtain root coverage over caries lesions?

According to Goldstein et al,[87] carious root coverage (92%) is as predictable as coverage of intact roots (97%).

Q: How much tissue healing needs to occur before restorative treatment can be initiated?

Lanning et al[88] reported that coronal advancement of the healing tissues from the osseous crest averages 3 mm by 3 months' time after surgery. They also found that 6 months after surgery, no further significant changes in the vertical position of the free gingival margin were apparent.

Brägger et al[86] found that 12% of the sites with crown lengthening procedure showed 2 to 4 mm recession of the free gingival margin between 6 weeks and 6 months postoperatively.

Q: Which restorative pontic is ideal for gingival tissues?

An ovate pontic is ideal because it tapers to the level of tissue on the palate to allow for hygiene access. It also mimics the natural tooth contour and allows for an esthetic outcome.[89] Spear[90] advocated an ovate pontic because it adapts to the site with a flat or concave outline. However, most restorative dentists prescribe a modified ridge lap because it has better esthetics in areas of reduced bone.

Miscellaneous

Q: What are the indications for soft tissue versus hard tissue grafting?

Soft tissue grafting

- Mild to moderate defects
- Horizontal defects
- Available tissue $\rightarrow$

Hard tissue grafting

- Moderate to severe defects (greater than 4 mm)
- Horizontal and vertical defects
- Inadequate soft tissue quality

Q: What procedures require a vestibule to be successful?

CT grafts, pedicle grafts, and tunnel techniques require the presence of a vestibule.

Q: Is it possible to obtain molar root coverage?

According to a study of 50 cases by Harris,[91] it is possible to achieve 91.1% molar root coverage.

References

1. Prato GP. Advances in mucogingival surgery. J Int Acad Periodontol 2000;2:24–27.
2. Miller PD Jr. Regenerative and reconstructive periodontal plastic surgery. Mucogingival surgery. Dent Clin North Am 1988;32:287–306.
3. Newman MG, Takei H, Klokkevold PR, Carranza FA. Carranza's Clinical Periodontology, ed 11. St Louis: Elsevier Saunders, 2012:84.
4. Elliott JR, Bowers GM. Alveolar dehiscence and fenestration. Periodontics 1963;1:245–248.
5. Rupprecht RD, Horning GM, Nicoll BK, Cohen ME. Prevalence of dehiscences and fenestrations in modern American skulls. J Periodontol 2001;72:722–729.
6. Kim DM, Neiva R. Periodontal soft tissue non-root coverage procedures: A systematic review from the AAP Regeneration Workshop. J Periodontol 2015;86(2 suppl):S56–S72.
7. Scheyer ET, Sanz M, Dibart S, et al. Periodontal soft tissue non-root coverage procedures: A consensus report from the AAP Regeneration Workshop. J Periodontol 2015;86(2 suppl):S73–S76.
8. Lin GH, Madi IM. Soft-tissue conditions around dental implants: A literature review. Implant Dent 2019;28:138–143.
9. Lang NP, Löe H. The relationship between the width of keratinized gingiva and gingival health. J Periodontol 1972;43:623–627.
10. Maynard JG Jr, Wilson RD. Physiologic dimensions of the periodontium significant to the restorative dentist. J Periodontol 1979;50:170–174.
11. Cortellini P, Bissada NF. Mucogingival conditions in the natural dentition: Narrative review, case definitions, and diagnostic considerations. J Periodontol 2018;89(suppl 1):S204–S213.
12. Branschofsky M, Beikler T, Schäfer R, Flemming TF, Lang H. Secondary trauma from occlusion and periodontitis. Quintessence Int 2011;42:515–522.
13. Bernimoulin J, Curilovié Z. Gingival recession and tooth mobility. J Clin Periodontol 1977;4:107–114.
14. Jepsen S, Caton JG, Albandar JM, et al. Periodontal manifestations of systemic diseases and developmental and acquired conditions: Consensus report of workgroup 3 of the 2017 World Workshop on the Classification of Periodontal and Peri-Implant Diseases and Conditions. J Clin Periodontol 2018;45(suppl 20):S219–S229.

15. Hennequin-Hoenderdos NL, Slot DE, Van der Weijden GA. The incidence of complications associated with lip and/or tongue piercings: A systematic review. Int J Dent Hyg 2016;14:62–73.
16. Clerehugh V, Tugnait A, Genco RJ. Periodontology at a Glance. Oxford: Wiley-Blackwell, 2009:64,66.
17. Kassab MM, Cohen RE. The etiology and prevalence of gingival recession. J Am Dent Assoc 2003;134:220–225.
18. Albandar JM, Kingman A. Gingival recession, gingival bleeding, and dental calculus in adults 30 years of age and older in the United States, 1988-1994. J Periodontol 1999;70:30–43.
19. Serino G, Wennström JL, Lindhe J, Eneroth L. The prevalence and distribution of gingival recession in subjects with a high standard of oral hygiene. J Clin Periodontol 1994;21:57–63.
20. Chambrone L, Tatakis DN. Long-term outcomes of untreated buccal gingival recessions: A systematic review and meta-analysis. J Periodontol 2016;87:796–808.
21. Agudio G, Cortellini P, Buti J, Pini Prato G. Periodontal conditions of sites treated with gingival augmentation surgery compared with untreated contralateral homologous sites: An 18- to 35-year long-term study. J Periodontol 2016;87:1371–1378.
22. Kennedy JE, Bird WC, Palcanis KG, Dorfman HS. A longitudinal evaluation of varying widths of attached gingiva. J Clin Periodontol 1985;12:667–675.
23. Cairo F, Nieri M, Cincinelli S, Mervelt J, Pagliaro U. The interproximal clinical attachment level to classify gingival recessions and predict root coverage outcomes: An explorative and reliability study. J Clin Periodontol 2011;38:661–666.
24. Lecture by Dr Greenwell at the American Academy of Periodontology 10/29/18/.
25. Miller PD Jr. A classification of marginal tissue recession. Int J Periodontics Restorative Dent 1985;5(2):8–13.
26. Sullivan HC, Atkins JH. Free autogenous gingival grafts. I. Principles of successful grafting. Periodontics 1968;6:121–129.
27. Pini-Prato G, Franceschi D, Cairo F, Nieri M, Rotundo R. Classification of dental surface defects in areas of gingival recession. J Periodontol 2010;81:885–890.
28. Seibert JS. Reconstruction of deformed, partially edentulous ridges, using full thickness onlay grafts. Part I. Technique and wound healing. Compend Contin Educ Dent 1983;4:437–453.
29. Zweers J, Thomas RZ, Slot DE, Weisgold AS, Van der Weijden FG. Characteristics of periodontal biotype, its dimensions, associations and prevalence: A systematic review. J Clin Periodontol 2014;41:958–971.
30. Jepsen S, Caton JG, Albandar JM, et al. Periodontal manifestations of systemic diseases and developmental and acquired conditions: Consensus report of workgroup 3 of the 2017 World Workshop on the Classification of Periodontal and Peri-Implant Diseases and Conditions. J Periodontol 2018;89(suppl 1):S237–S248.
31. Martins TM, Bosco AF, Nóbrega FJ, Nagata MJ, Garcia VG, Fucini SE. Periodontal tissue response to coverage of root cavities restored with resin materials: A histomorphometric study in dogs. J Periodontol 2007;78:1075–1082.
32. Lucchesi JA, Santos VR, Amaral CM, Peruzzo DC, Duarte PM. Coronally positioned flap for treatment of restored root surfaces: A 6-month clinical evaluation. J Periodontol 2007;78:615–623.
33. McGuire MK, Scheyer ET. Randomized, controlled clinical trial to evaluate a xenogeneic collagen matrix as an alternative to free gingival grafting for oral soft tissue augmentation. J Periodontol 2014;85:1333–1341.
34. Wessel JR, Tatakis DN. Patient outcomes following subepithelial connective tissue graft and free gingival graft procedures. J Periodontol 2008;79:425–430.
35. Al-Zahrani MS, Bissada NF, Ficara AJ, Cole B. Effect of connective tissue graft orientation on root coverage and gingival augmentation. Int J Periodontics Restorative Dent 2004;24:65–69.
36. Lafzi A, Mostofi Zadeh Farahani R, Abolfazli N, Amid R, Safaiyan A. Effect of connective tissue graft orientation on the root coverage outcomes of coronally advanced flap. Clin Oral Investig 2007;11:401–408.
37. Tatakis DN, Chambrone L, Allen EP, et al. Periodontal soft tissue root coverage procedures: A consensus report from the AAP Regeneration Workshop. J Periodontol 2015;86(2 suppl):S52–S55.

38. Burkhardt R, Lang NP. Coverage of localized gingival recessions: Comparison of micro- and macrosurgical techniques. J Clin Periodontol 2005;32:287–293.
39. Kang J, Meng S, Li C, Luo Z, Guo S, Wu Y. Microsurgery for root coverage: A systematic review. Pak J Med Sci 2015;31:1263–1268.
40. Hwang D, Wang HL. Flap thickness as a predictor of root coverage: A systematic review. J Periodontol 2006;77:1625–1634
41. Chambrone L, Pannuti CM, Tu YK, Chambrone LA. Evidence-based periodontal plastic surgery. II. An individual data meta-analysis for evaluating factors in achieving complete root coverage. J Periodontol 2012;83:477–490.
42. Barootchi S, Tavelli L, Ravidà A, Wang CW, Wang HL. Effect of EDTA root conditioning on the outcome of coronally advanced flap with connective tissue graft: A systematic review and meta-analysis. Clin Oral Investig 2018;22:2727–2741.
43. McGuire MK, Scheyer ET, Nevins ML, et al. Living cellular construct for increasing the width of keratinized gingiva: Results from a randomized, within-patient, controlled trial. J Periodontol 2011;82:1414–1423.
44. McGuire MK, Nunn ME. Evaluation of the safety and efficacy of periodontal applications of a living tissue-engineered human fibroblast-derived dermal substitute. I. Comparison to the gingival autograft: A randomized controlled pilot study. J Periodontol 2005;76:867–880.
45. Grupe HE, Warren RF. Repair of gingival defects by a sliding flap operation. J Periodontol 1956;27:92–95.
46. Cohen DW, Ross SE. The double papillae repositioned flap in periodontal therapy. J Periodontol 1968;39:65–70.
47. Tarnow DP. Semilunar coronally repositioned flap. J Clin Periodontol 1986;13:182–185.
48. Bernimoulin JP. Use of a free mucous membrane transplant in mucogingival surgery with special consideration for the treatment of recession [in German]. ZWR 1981;90(12):52–55.
49. Baldi C, Pini-Prato G, Pagliaro U, et al. Coronally advanced flap procedure for root coverage. Is flap thickness a relevant predictor to achieve root coverage? A 19-case series. J Periodontol 1999;70:1077–1084.
50. Zucchelli G, Mele M, Mazzotti C, Marzadori M, Montebugnoli L, De Sanctis M. Coronally advanced flap with and without vertical releasing incisions for the treatment of multiple gingival re-cessions: A comparative controlled randomized clinical trial. J Periodontol 2009;80:1083–1094.
51. Raetzke PB. Covering localized areas of root exposure employing the "envelope" technique. J Periodontol 1985;56:397–402.
52. Zadeh HH. Minimally invasive treatment of maxillary anterior gingival recession defects by vestibular incision subperiosteal tunnel access and platelet-derived growth factor BB. Int J Periodontics Restorative Dent 2011;31:653–660.
53. Chao JC. A novel approach to root coverage: The pinhole surgical technique. Int J Periodontics Restorative Dent 2012;32:521–531.
54. Gargiulo AW, Arrocha R. Histo-clinical evaluation of free gingival grafts. Periodontics 1967;5:285–291.
55. Mörmann W, Schaer F, Firestone AR. The relationship between success of free gingival grafts and transplant thickness. Revascularization and shrinkage—A one year clinical study. J Periodontol 1981;52:74–80.
56. Matter J. Creeping attachment of free gingival grafts. A five-year follow-up study. J Periodontol 1980;51:681–685.
57. Yadav AP, Kulloli A, Shetty S, Ligade SS, Martande SS, Gholkar MJ. Sub-epithelial connective tissue graft for the management of Miller's class I and class II isolated gingival recession defect: A systematic review of the factors influencing the outcome. J Investig Clin Dent 2018;9:e12325.
58. Souza SL, Macedo GO, Tunes RS, et al. Subepithelial connective tissue graft for root coverage in smokers and non-smokers: A clinical and histologic controlled study in humans. J Periodontol 2008;79:1014–1021.
59. Reiser GM, Bruno JF, Mahan PE, Larkin LH. The subepithelial connective tissue graft palatal donor site: Anatomic considerations for surgeons. Int J Periodontics Restorative Dent 1996;16:130–137.

60. Tavelli L, Barootchi S, Ravidà A, Oh TJ, Wang HL. What is the safety zone for palatal soft tissue graft harvesting based on the locations of the greater palatine artery and foramen? A systematic review. J Oral Maxillofac Surg 2019;77:271.e1–271.e9.

61. James WC, McFall WT Jr. Placement of free gingival grafts on denuded alveolar bone. Part I: Clinical evaluations. J Periodontol 1978;49:283–290.

62. Matter J, Cimasoni G. Creeping attachment after free gingival grafts. J Periodontol 1976;47:574–579.

63. Dordick B, Coslet JG, Seibert JS. Clinical evaluation of free autogenous gengival grafts placed on alveolar bone. Part I. Clinical predictability. J Periodontol 1976;47:559–567.

64. Caffesse RG, Guinard EA. Treatment of localized gingival recessions. Part II. Coronally repositioned flap with a free gingival graft. J Periodontol 1978;49:357–361.

65. Lindhe J, Nyman S, Karring T. Connective tissue reattachment as related to presence or absence of alveolar bone. J Clin Periodontol 1984;11:33–40.

66. Wei PC, Laurell L, Geivelis M, Lingen MW, Maddalozzo D. Acellular dermal matrix allografts to achieve increased attached gingiva. Part 1. A clinical study. J Periodontol 2000;71:1297–1305.

67. Henderson RD, Drisko CH, Greenwell H. Root coverage using Alloderm acellular dermal graft material. J Contemp Dent Pract 1999;1:24–30.

68. Gapski R, Parks CA, Wang HL. Acellular dermal matrix for mucogingival surgery: A meta-analysis. J Periodontol 2005;76:1814–1822.

69. Nickles K, Ratka-Krüger P, Neukranz E, Raetzke P, Eickholz P. Ten-year results after connective tissue grafts and guided tissue regeneration for root coverage. J Periodontol 2010;81:827–836.

70. Oates TW, Robinson M, Gunsolley JC. Surgical therapies for the treatment of gingival recession. A systematic review. Ann Periodontol 2003;8:303–320.

71. Harris RJ. A comparative study of root coverage obtained with guided tissue regeneration utilizing a bioabsorbable membrane versus the connective tissue with partial-thickness double pedicle graft. J Periodontol 1997;68:779–790.

72. Greenwell H, Fiorellini J, Giannobile W, et al. Oral reconstructive and corrective considerations in periodontal therapy. J Periodontol 2005;76:1588–1600.

73. Chambrone L, Tatakis DN. Periodontal soft tissue root coverage procedures: A systematic review from the AAP Regeneration Workshop. J Periodontol 2015;86(2 suppl):S8–S51.

74. Ward VJ. A clinical assessment of the use of the free gingival graft for correcting localized recession associated with frenal pull. J Periodontol 1974;45:78–83.

75. Addy M, Dummer PM, Hunter ML, Kingdon A, Shaw WC. A study of the association of fraenal attachment, lip coverage, and vestibular depth with plaque and gingivitis. J Periodontol 1987;58:752–757.

76. Bollen AM, Cunha-Cruz J, Bakko DW, Huang GJ, Hujoel PP. The effects of orthodontic therapy on periodontal health: A systematic review of controlled evidence. J Am Dent Assoc 2008;139:413–422.

77. Soltani L, Loomer PM, Chaar EE. A novel approach in periodontally accelerated osteogenic orthodontics (PAOO): A case report. Clin Adv Periodontics 2019;9:110–114.

78. Nordland WP, Tarnow DP. A classification system for loss of papillary height. J Periodontol 1998;69:1124–1126.

79. Tarnow DP, Magner AW, Fletcher P. The effect of the distance from the contact point to the crest of bone on the presence or absence of the interproximal dental papilla. J Periodontol 1992;63:995–996.

80. Andijani RI, Tatakis DN. Hypermobile upper lip is highly prevalent among patients seeking treatment for gummy smile. J Periodontol 2019;90:256–262.

81. Coslet JG, Vanarsdall R, Weisgold A. Diagnosis and classification of delayed passive eruption of the dentogingival junction in the adult. Alpha Omegan 1977;70(3):24–28.

82. Mostafa D. A successful management of sever gummy smile using gingivectomy and botulinum toxin injection: A case report. Int J Surg Case Rep 2018;42:169–174.

83. Hempton TJ, Dominici JT. Contemporary crown-lengthening therapy: A review. J Am Dent Assoc 2010;141:647–655.

84. Wagenberg BD, Eskow RN, Langer B. Exposing adequate tooth structure for restorative dentistry. Int J Periodontics Restorative Dent 1989;9:322–331.

85. Deas DE, Moritz AJ, McDonnell HT, Powell CA, Mealey BL. Osseous surgery for crown lengthening: A 6-month clinical study. J Periodontol 2004;75:1288–1294.

86. Brägger U, Lauchenauer D, Lang NP. Surgical lengthening of the clinical crown. J Clin Periodontol 1992;19:58–63.

87. Goldstein M, Nasatzky E, Goultschin J, Boyan BD, Schwartz Z. Coverage of previously carious roots is as predictable a procedure as coverage of intact roots. J Periodontol 2002;73:1419–1426.

88. Lanning SK, Waldrop TC, Gunsolley JC, Maynard JG. Surgical crown lengthening: Evaluation of the biological width. J Periodontol. 2003 Apr;74(4):468–474.

89. Orsini G, Murmura G, Artese L, Piattelli A, Piccirilli M, Caputi S. Tissue healing under provisional restorations with ovate pontics: A pilot human histological study. J Prosthet Dent 2006;96:252–257.

90. Spear FM. The use of implants and ovate pontics in the esthetic zone. Compend Contin Educ Dent 2008;29:72–74,76–80.

91. Harris RJ. Root coverage in molar recession: Report of 50 consecutive cases treated with subepithelial connective tissue grafts. J Periodontol 2003;74:703–708.

Regeneration 12

Background

Q: Define periodontal regeneration, reattachment, new attachment, and repair.

- *Periodontal regeneration:* Restoration of the lost periodontium or supporting tissues. It has been defined as the formation of new cementum, alveolar bone, and a functional periodontal ligament on a previously diseased root surface.[1]
- *Reattachment:* Reunion of the epithelium or connective tissue to the root surface or bone.
- *New attachment:* Union of connective tissue or epithelium with the root surface that has been deprived of its original attachment apparatus.
- *Repair:* Healing of the wound by tissue—does not fully restore architecture or function.

  Note that scaling and root planing and most flap surgeries heal by repair.

Q: What are the goals of regeneration?

- Regenerate new bone
- Reduce or eliminate osseous defects
- Stop attachment loss
- Stop or reduce the inflammation
- Increase tooth stability
- Recover esthetics

Q: **Describe the four different cell types that can repopulate the root surface after periodontal surgery.**

Melcher[2] described the four cell types as follows:

1. Long junctional epithelium: If these cells populate first, there will be no bone regeneration.
2. Gingival connective tissue cells: May lead to root resorption.
3. Bone cells: Resorption and ankylosis.
4. Periodontal ligament cells: New cementum forms perpendicular to junctional epithelium.

   Melcher believed that it was important to allow selective repopulation of the wound and exclude epithelium.

Q: **What factors are important for regeneration?**

- Patient factors: The patient should not smoke and must have good oral hygiene.
- Inflammation should be controlled as much as possible before surgery to allow better flap reflection and suturing.
- Defect factors: The deeper, narrower, and greater number of walls, the better (Fig 12-1). Kim et al[3] found that bone regeneration averaged 1.5, 1.7, and 2.3 mm for one-, two-, and three-wall defects, respectively, with the three-wall defects being significantly different from the one-wall defects. They concluded that the number of bone walls is a critical factor determining treatment outcomes in intrabony periodontal defects.

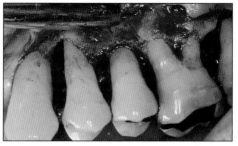

Fig 12-1 Deep and narrow defect between the canine and the premolar.

$\rightarrow$

- Factors associated with technique: Flap design and preservation of the interdental papillae are important. It is also important to perform scaling and root planing of the teeth before regeneration is performed and to minimize trauma to the flap. Lastly, a complete and stable closure of the flaps during healing is necessary to prevent contamination and infection and allow for graft healing. Hence, the buccal and lingual flaps must be sufficiently released to obtain passive closure of the bone grafted area, and it should be stabilized with tension-free sutures.[4]

Q: What is guided tissue regeneration (GTR)?

In GTR, the clinician tries to control the cells repopulating the site by placing a barrier membrane. It is used during wound healing to prevent epithelial and connective tissue growth.

Q: What is guided bone regeneration (GBR)?

GBR is similar to GTR except that a bone graft is generally used in addition to a membrane to successfully augment bone formation.

Q: What is the Misch bone density scale?

- D1: Dense cortical bone found in the anterior mandible
- D2: Thick, dense cortical bone on the crest and coarse trabecular bone within
- D3: Thin, porous cortical bone and fine trabecular bone within
- D4: Fine trabecular bone
- D5: Immature, nonmineralized bone

Q: What is Siebert's classification of ridge deformities?[5]

- Class 1 defects: Buccolingual loss of tissue contour with a normal apico-coronal height
- Class 2 defects: Apicocoronal loss of tissue with normal buccolingual contour
- Class 3 defects: A combination of buccolingual and apicocoronal loss

Bone Grafting

Q: **What is the difference between osteogenic, osteoinductive, and osteoconductive bone material?**

- *Osteogenic:* New bone formation occurs as a result of bone-forming cells contained in the graft.
- *Osteoinductive:* Bone formation is induced in the surrounding soft tissue immediately adjacent to the grafted material. An example is demineralized freeze-dried bone allograft (DFDBA).
- *Osteoconductive:* Graft material does not directly contribute to new bone formation but serves as a scaffold for bone formation by adjacent host bone. An example is freeze-dried bone allograft (FDBA).

Q: **Describe the different types of graft material.**

- *Autogenous graft:* Graft is transferred from one position to another within the same individual. A second surgical site is needed (eg, retromolar pad, maxillary tuberosity).
- *Allogeneic bone graft:* A graft between genetically dissimilar members of the same species.
- *Xenograft:* A graft from a donor of another species.
- *Alloplast:* Synthetic or inorganic implant material used as a substitute for a bone graft.

Q: **What are the advantages and disadvantages of autogenous bone grafts?**

See Fig 12-2 below.

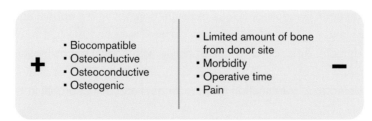

Fig 12-2 Advantages and disadvantages of autogenous bone grafts.

Q: Are allogeneic bone grafts safe?

Most bone banks adhere to the guidelines of the American Association of Tissue Banks (AATB).[6] The AATB excludes collection in the following circumstances:

- Donor is from a high-risk group
- Donor tests positive for HIV
- Autopsy of the donor reveals occult disease
- Donor tests positive for bacterial contamination
- Donor and bone test positive for hepatitis B or C
- Donor tests positive for syphilis

Mellonig et al[7] found that spiked and infected bone treated with a virucidal agent inactivates HIV.

Q: Do cortical or cancellous bone grafts resorb faster?

Cancellous onlay bone grafts resorb faster than cortical grafts.[8]

Q: What are the different applications for onlay, veneer block, and saddle grafts?

- Onlay graft: Vertical or horizontal reconstruction of bone
- Veneer block graft: Horizontal augmentation of bone
- Saddle graft: Horizontal and vertical augmentation of bone—could use a J- or L-shaped graft

Q: What is the success rate for allogeneic bone block augmentation?

In a multicenter evaluation, Keith et al[9] found the following success rates for allogeneic bone block grafts by region:

- Anterior maxilla: 94% (2/35 block grafts lost)
- Maxillary molar region: 100% (0 lost)
- Anterior mandible: 67% (1/3 lost)
- Mandibular molar region: 87% (5/38 lost)

Q: What is the resorption rate for block grafts?

Nissan et al[10] evaluated the outcome of ridge augmentation with cancellous freeze-dried block allogeneic bone grafts in the posterior atrophic mandible

→

followed by placement of dental implants. Horizontal augmentation was 5.6 mm, and vertical augmentation was 4.3 mm. Resorption of the buccal bone averaged 0.5 mm at the time of implant placement and 0.2 mm at stage-two surgery.

McAllister and Haghighat[11] noted that augmentation with autogenous bone grafts resulted in resorption rates of 0% to 25% at implant placement and up to 60% at the time of abutment placement. The study found that barrier membranes placed with block grafts optimized ridge augmentation (in regard to graft resorption).

Q: Describe some studies that show that bone grafting is effective.

- In 1991, Mellonig[12] conducted a study in which 327 sites were treated with FDBA only and 176 sites were treated with FDBA and autogenous bone. The study found complete or greater than 50% bone fill in 67% of sites treated with FDBA alone and 78% of sites treated with FDBA and autogenous bone.
- The results of a 2003 meta-analysis by Reynolds et al[13] supported the following statements regarding the treatment of intrabony defects: *(1)* Bone grafts increase bone level, reduce crestal bone loss, increase clinical attachment level, and reduce probing depth compared with open-flap debridement (OFD) procedures. *(2)* Randomized controlled studies provide evidence that DFDBA supports the formation of a new attachment apparatus in intrabony defects, whereas OFD results in periodontal repair characterized primarily by the formation of a long junctional epithelial attachment.
- In a 1989 histologic evaluation of new attachment apparatus formation by Bowers et al,[14] data from 12 patients with 32 DFDBA-grafted and 25 non-grafted defects were studied. A long junctional epithelium formed along the entire length of exposed root in nongrafted sites. In contrast, grafted sites gained new attachment apparatus, new cementum, new connective tissue, and new bone.
- In 2000, Mellonig[15] conducted a human histologic evaluation of a bovine-derived bone xenograft (Bio-Oss, Geistlich) in the treatment of periodontal osseous defects. In three of the four specimens, histologic observations demonstrated new bone, new cementum, and new periodontal ligament. Grafting with a bovine-derived xenograft allows for periodontal regeneration.
- In a 1970 study of iliac transplants in periodontal therapy, Schallhorn et al[16] found that iliac grafts are effective, but they can cause external resorption, infection, and sequestra. →

- Buser et al[17] carried out lateral ridge augmentation using autografts and barrier membranes in a 1996 clinical study with 40 partially edentulous patients, demonstrating that the combined application of autografts and expanded polytetrafluoroethylene (ePTFE) membranes is a predictable surgical procedure for lateral ridge augmentation that results in a 4-mm increase of bone width.

Although there is significant evidence acclaiming the effectiveness of bone grafting, Cortellini and Tonetti[18] did a study without regenerative materials and obtained results similar to those of studies that did use regenerative materials. A group of 45 patients received either a modified minimally invasive surgery technique (M-MIST) alone, with enamel matrix protein, or with enamel matrix protein and xenograft. Significant clinical and radiographic improvements were found when M-MIST was used with or without regenerative materials. The human body can induce regeneration of its own tissue.

Q: Is there a difference between bone graft materials (FDBA, DFDBA, and xenografts)?

Wood and Mealey[19] found that FDBA had a significantly decreased percentage of vital bone at 24.63% versus DFDBA at 38.42%. FDBA also had a significantly greater mean percentage of residual graft particles at 25.42% compared with DFDBA at 8.88%. Yukna and Vastardis,[20] on the other hand, found that FDBA stimulates faster and more substantial new bone formation than DFDBA in a monkey jaw defect model system.

A 2005 American Academy of Periodontology (AAP) position paper[21] found bone fill ranging from 1.3 to 2.6 mm when FDBA was used to treat defects. Human trials using DFDBA have demonstrated bone fill similar to that achieved with FDBA, ranging from 1.7 to 2.9 mm. Rummelhart et al[22] studied 22 defects in nine patients using DFDBA and FDBA and found no significant differences between the treatment groups.

The 2015 consensus from the AAP[1] concluded that DFDBA had the largest body of evidence to support it as a predictable material for periodontal regeneration of intrabony defects.

Q: Discuss the variability in the ability of DFDBA to induce new bone formation.

The following are possible reasons for the variability in new bone formation induced by DFDBA[6]:

- Bone induction proteins are not present in sufficient quantity to produce detectable bone formation.
- Bone-inductive components of DFDBA are present but are in an inactive form.
- Some DFDBA batches are more active than others (based on content of bone-inductive factors in donor).
- Sterilization processing may be an important contributor to variability of DFDBA.
- Wide variations in commercial bone bank preparations of DFDBA exist.
- Donor age, but not sex, may also play a role.
- Particle size also appears to be an important variable in the success of DFDBA as a bone-inductive material. Particles in the range of 125 to 1,000 μm possess a higher osteogenic potential than do particles below 125 μm.

Q: Is the alloplast calcium sulfate effective?

Choi et al[23] found bone regeneration with the synthetic biomaterials amorphous calcium phosphate (ACP) and micro-macroporous biphasic calcium phosphate (MBCP) similar to that with FDBA in surgically generated three-wall intrabony defects adjacent to implants. The study concluded that FDBA is as effective as ACP and MBCP at osteoconduction.

Aimetti et al[24] evaluated whether the placement of medical-grade calcium sulfate hemihydrate in fresh extraction sockets might affect the quality of newly formed bone and influence crestal bone changes. The study found that from the crestal to the apical region of specimens treated with the alloplast, the mean percentage of lamellar bone increased from 16.4% to 43.6%, compared with 11.1% to 22.2% in unfilled specimens.

Q: Does particle size make a difference in the success of the bone graft material?

Shapoff et al[25] indicated that there was significantly decreased new bone formation associated with large-particle (1,000- to 2,000-μm) FDBA plus autogenous marrow than with small-particle (100- to 300-μm) FDBA plus →

autogenous marrow. In addition, large-particle FDBA plus autogenous marrow tended to display less resorption than small-particle FDBA plus autogenous marrow.

In a study by Fucini et al,[26] after reentry average bony defect fill was 1.32 mm for the small-particle (250- to 500-µm) group and 1.66 mm for the large-particle (850- to 1,000-µm) group. Different particle sizes of DFDBA showed no statistically significant difference in bony fill.

Q: Does adding tetracycline to the bone graft make it more effective?

Figure 12-3 shows a site grafted with particulate bone plus tetracycline.

Drury and Yukna[27] mixed tetracycline and FDBA in experimental defects in baboons. The study found that FDBA in combination with tetracycline improves new bone formation in experimental alveolar bone defects.

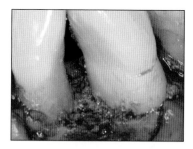

Fig 12-3 Particulate bone mixed with tetracycline in a grafted site.

A study by Masters et al[28] found only a slight difference in bone fill between a DFDBA and tetracycline group (2.27 mm) and a DFDBA only group (2.20 mm) and reported no statistically significant differences between the groups in any clinical parameters. The authors concluded that the addition of 50 mg/mL of tetracycline hydrochloride to the allograft did not result in any significant benefits.

Q: Is decortication of the bone important?

Rompen et al[29] demonstrated greater regeneration in skulls perforated with nine 0.8-mm-diameter holes (172.8%) compared with skulls with an intact osseous surface (141%). De novo bone formation occurs by stimulation of the blood supply and access of bone-forming cells by cortical perforations.

Adeyemo et al[30] found no difference in terms of healing and integration of the bone graft between perforated and nonperforated recipient cortical beds.

Greenstein et al[31] did a review of the literature and found that there is inconsistent literature and inadequate clinical research to make any conclusions as to the benefits of bone decortication preceding GBR procedures.

Membranes

Q: What are some important properties of membranes?

Figure 12-4 presents properties that membranes should possess to be clinically effective.

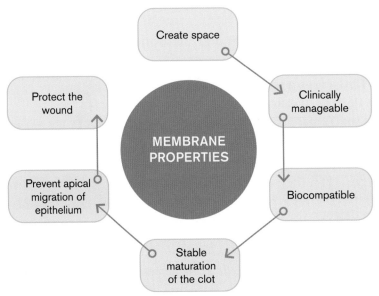

Fig 12-4 Properties of membranes.

Q: What are the two types of membranes?

Figure 12-5 presents characteristics of the two types of membranes: resorbable and nonresorbable.

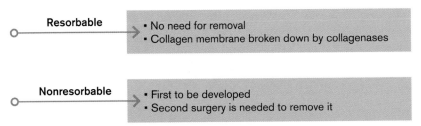

Fig 12-5 Characteristics of resorbable and nonresorbable membranes.

Q: Is there a difference in treatment outcome between resorbable and nonresorbable membranes?

In a 2010 study, Merli et al[32] randomly allocated patients into two treatment groups—resorbable and titanium-reinforced membranes. Each group had 11 patients needing vertical bone augmentation. The study noted no statistically significant difference in bone loss between the two groups at either 1 or 3 years. At the 3-year mark, the resorbable membrane group lost an average of 0.55 mm of bone, while patients in the nonresorbable barrier group had an average of 0.53 mm of bone loss.

In a 1997 study, Caffesse et al[33] randomly placed patients in resorbable and nonresorbable membrane groups. In the nonresorbable group, the membrane was removed at 6 weeks. The study found no differences between the groups. The study concluded that, in terms of treating grade II furcations and intrabony defects, the resorbable membrane and the nonresorbable ePTFE membrane were equally effective.

In a 1998 study, Laurell et al[34] concluded that there is no difference between resorbable and nonresorbable membranes. The study came to this conclusion by evaluating studies presented during the previous 20 years on the surgical treatment of intrabony defects. The authors examined treatment outcomes of OFD, bone replacement grafts, and GTR.

Due to the proven effectiveness of resorbable membranes, ePTFE membranes are limited to specific indications, such as three-dimensional reconstruction.[35]

Q: What is the effect of membrane exposure?

Figure 12-6 shows an exposed resorbable membrane during a socket grafting procedure.

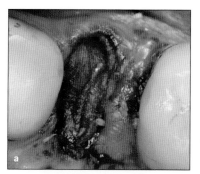 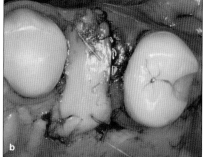

Fig 12-6 *(a)* Exposed resorbable membrane after socket grafting. *(b)* The exposed resorbable membrane covered with a free gingival graft.

$\rightarrow$

Machtei[36] found that nonresorbable and resorbable membrane exposure during healing had a minimal effect on GTR around natural teeth. However, it had a significant negative impact on GBR around dental implants; exposed membranes had 0.56 mm and submerged membranes had 3.01 mm of bone regeneration around implants.

An analysis by De Sanctis et al[37] found that exposed areas of membranes had bacterial colonization in all the microscopic fields. Although no bacteria-positive field was observed in the most apical portion of the membranes, the middle portion of many of the membranes (16 of 39 [41%]) demonstrated microbial colonization.

Q: How is membrane exposure managed postoperatively?

Figure 12-7 presents the steps involved in postoperative management of membrane exposure. Note that if a nonresorbable membrane is exposed, it should be removed in 4 to 6 weeks to prevent a negative effect on bone regeneration.

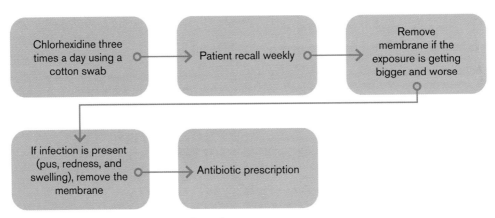

Fig 12-7 Postoperative management of membrane exposure.

Q: Should antibiotics be given to patients when a membrane is placed?

The patient should take antibiotics for 1 week and rinse with 12% chlorhexidine for 12 weeks after GBR to reduce postoperative infection and ensure optimal clinical results.[38]

In a study by Nowzari et al,[39] the experimental group received Augmentin (GlaxoSmithKline) and GTR (nonresorbable membrane), while the control →

group only had GTR (nonresorbable membrane). A significantly higher gain in mean probing attachment was found at 6 months in the test group (36.5% of potential gain) compared with the control group (22.4% of potential gain). When the membranes were removed, significantly fewer organisms were found in the test group (52.2 × 10⁶) compared with the control group (488.6 × 10⁶).

Q: Is there a difference between cross-linked and non–cross-linked membranes?

Tal et al[40] found that although both cross-linked and non–cross-linked membranes degraded when exposed to the oral environment, both membranes were resistant to tissue degradation and preserved continuity throughout the study.

When membranes were prematurely exposed, Moses et al[41] found bony defect healing to be significantly higher in the cross-linked Ossix (OraPharma) group than in the other two groups (non–cross-linked Bio-Gide [Geistlich] and Gore-Tex [W. L. Gore]). They also found statistically similar defect reduction in the patients with prematurely exposed Ossix membranes and those with unexposed membranes.

Bornstein et al[42] found that the cross-linked membrane placed in dog mandibles for bone regeneration had a limited beneficial effect when healing was uneventful. They compared the cross-linked membrane to a collagen membrane.

Q: What is the difference between Bio-Gide and BioMend membranes?

Figure 12-8 presents the characteristics of Bio-Gide and BioMend (Zimmer) membranes.

Bio-Gide
- Non–cross-linked, porcine-derived collagen (type I and type III).
- Resorption time varies depending on a number of factors, including but not limited to the surgical site, occurrence of dehiscence, loading, type of fixation, and the patient.

BioMend
- Bovine achilles tendon collagen (type I).
- BioMend collagen membrane is absorbed in approximately 8 weeks.
- BioMend Extend collagen membrane is absorbed in approximately 18 weeks.

Fig 12-8 Bio-Gide versus BioMend.

Q: What is the technique for membrane placement?

1. Slightly divergent vertical incisions are initiated at proximal line angles one tooth anterior and one tooth posterior to the treated tooth/area. They should extend apical to the mucogingival junction.
2. A horizontal incision is made, and a full-thickness flap is carried out to expose the entire perimeter of the dehiscence.
3. Degranulation is performed.
4. The membrane should cover 3 mm of bone beyond the defect margins, and the apical margin of the membrane should be 2 to 3 mm apical to the flap margin.

Q: What are tacks and screws used for?

Tacks are used to stabilize the membrane.[43] Screws are used for bone stabilization. It is important to place at least two screws to prevent rotation.

Technique

Q: Describe management of deficiencies in the esthetic zone.

See Fig 12-9 below.

	Protocol 1	Protocol 2	Protocol 3
Description	Partially edentulous patients having less than 6.0 mm and more than 4.0 mm of residual horizontal bone width[44]	Thin ridge that needs lateral ridge augmentation[45,46]	Vertical loss
Technique	2 mm autogenous bone covered with 2 mm xenograft, then a resorbable membrane can be placed	• Fixation of the bone graft; autogenous bone and xenograft placed with a resorbable membrane • Must be very stable	• Titanium-reinforced membrane fixated on the buccal and lingual • May need to do it in stages • Use screws and tacks

Fig 12-9 Management of deficiencies in the esthetic zone.[47]

Q: Describe a guided bone regeneration technique.[47]

1. Establish periodontal health in natural dentition.
2. Full-thickness flap elevation.
3. Clean and perforate bone surface.
4. Release the periosteum to loosen the flap.
5. Trim the membrane.
6. Use a bone scraper to get autogenous bone and place in saline.
7. Prepare xenograft (with growth factor/blood/saline).
8. Mix the graft 1:1.
9. Apply and fix membrane with suture/tacks.
10. Apply bone graft.
11. Adapt and fix the membrane to cover the bone graft.
12. Advance the flap and suture with PTFE material.
13. Temporize the site with no tissue contact.

Considerations for Regeneration

Q: What are some ideal anatomical considerations when regenerating bone?

Tonetti et al[48] found greater linear gains in deeper pockets. The study also found that, at an angle of 25 degrees or less (bony wall to long axis of the tooth), there was 1.6 mm more attachment than in defects with an angle of 37 degrees or more.

Laurell et al[34] compared OFD alone and OFD plus DFDBA, FDBA, or autogenous GTR. The study found that the intrabony defect has to be at least 4 mm deep to benefit from GTR procedures.

Q: How does GTR compare to OFD?

Figure 12-10 presents studies comparing GTR and OFD (see next page). →

Laurell et al[34] (1998)	Murphy and Gunsolley[49] (2003)	Needleman et al[50] (2006)
• This article reviews studies presented during the last 20 years on the surgical treatment of intrabony defects. Treatments include OFD; OFD plus DFDBA, FDBA, or autogenous bone; and GTR. • GTR resulted in significant pocket reduction, clinical attachment gain of 4.2 mm, and bone fill averaging 3.2 mm versus OFD with clinical attachment gain of 1.5 mm and bone fill of 1.1 mm.	• This review's aim was to compare GTR in control patients and patients with periodontal osseous defects. • Patients who received GTR had a gain of clinical attachment and a reduction in probing depth compared with those receiving OFD. • Physical barriers and bone replacement grafts placed together have been shown to enhance clinical outcome in furcation defects. • Coverage of the barrier with a coronally advanced flap is associated with a better outcome.	• The study compared GTR and OFD in the treatment of periodontal infrabony defects using the Cochrane Oral Health Group Trials Register, MEDLINE, and EMBASE up to April 2004. • Although there is a marked variability between studies, improved attachment gain, less increase in gingival recession, more gain in hard tissue, and reduced pocket depth were observed with GTR compared with OFD at reentry surgery.

Fig 12-10 Studies comparing GTR and OFD.

Q: Does grafting a site with a membrane and bone differ in effectiveness compared to using just a membrane?

A systematic review found that the combination of barrier membranes and grafting materials resulted in histologic evidence of periodontal regeneration, chiefly bone repair. In supra-alveolar and two-wall intrabony (missing buccal wall) defect models of periodontal regeneration, the added use of a grafting material gave superior histologic results of bone repair to barrier membranes alone. In one study, combined graft and barrier membrane gave a better result than graft alone.[51]

Q: What is distraction osteogenesis?

Distraction osteogenesis is based on the concept that new bone fills a gap created when two pieces of bone are separated slowly under tension. It is important to have a minimum of 6 to 7 mm of bone height above vital structures. The ridge defect should be greater than 3 to 4 mm, and the edentulous

$\rightarrow$

ridge span should be three or more missing teeth.[11] Figure 12-11 presents the phases of distraction osteogenesis.

Latency	Distraction	Consolidation
7 days for soft tissue healing	Two pieces of bone undergo separation at a rate of 1 mm per day	Allows bone regeneration in the created space

Fig 12-11 Distraction osteogenesis phases.

Q: What are the options for horizontal ridge augmentation?

▪ Bone and membrane (Fig 12-12): Fuggazotto[52] completed 289 ridge augmentation surgeries. Various configurations of Gore-Tex membranes were used in addition to various nonautogenous particulate materials. Of the 289 augmented ridges, 279 had adequate regenerated hard tissues for implant placement in ideal prosthetic positions. The horizontally augmented ridges had a success rate of 97%.

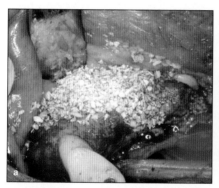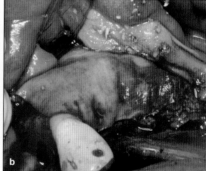

Fig 12-12 *(a)* Allograft material placed for horizontal augmentation. *(b)* Membrane placed over the allograft for horizontal augmentation.

▪ Autogenous block graft (eg, tuberosity, chin, and lateral ramus).
▪ Ridge splitting (Fig 12-13): When doing the procedure, it is important to prevent fracture of the buccal plate. Sethi and Kaus[53] performed a 5-year study evaluating 449 implants placed in maxillary ridges expanded by the ridge-split technique. The study revealed a survival rate of 97%. According to McAllister and Haghighat,[11] the avoidance of a separate donor site with the ridge-split technique, whether it uses particulate, block graft, or GBR, and its associated reduced treatment time and morbidity represent its primary advantage compared with other lateral augmentation techniques.

→

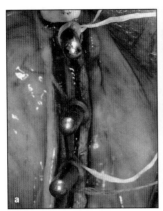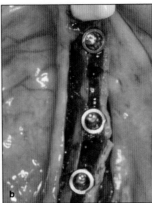

Fig 12-13 *(a)* Ridge split with direction indicators. *(b)* Ridge split with implants placed.

- Distraction osteogenesis: Laster et al[54] treated nine patients with distraction osteogenesis, increasing the alveolar width from 4 to 6 mm. Of the 21 implants placed, 20 implants successfully osseointegrated. After 12 months' follow-up, no marginal bone resorption was observed. They listed soft tissue expansion, high dimensional stability, reduced treatment time, and the avoidance of a graft as the advantages of horizontal distraction compared with block grafting.
- Block allograft: Because allograft is not living bone, it must be hydrated, and air bubbles must be removed. Nissan et al[55] did a study on 40 patients (83 implants) with 60 cancellous freeze-dried bone block allografts. The study had an average percentage of newly formed bone of 33% and implant survival of 98.8%. In a two-stage implant placement procedure, cancellous bone block allograft is osteoconductive and biocompatible, allowing new bone formation following augmentation of extremely atrophic anterior maxillae.

Esposito et al[56] conducted a systematic review and observed no statistically significant differences when comparing various horizontal augmentation techniques.

Q: What are the options for vertical ridge augmentation?

- Bone and membrane (GBR with the possibility of using pins): Simion et al[57] performed a study in which vertical augmentation was performed in six

$\longrightarrow$

different surgical sites. Five patients received 15 conical Brånemark-type implants that protruded 4 to 7 mm from the bone crest, and miniscrews were placed distally to the implants. The miniscrews and implants were enclosed with a titanium-reinforced membrane. There was vertical augmentation of 3 to 4 mm, and the retrieved miniscrews were in contact with bone based on histology. Vertical augmentation with GBR is more technique sensitive than horizontal augmentation.

- Lateral window sinus elevation (discussed in chapter 13).
- Osteotome sinus elevation (discussed in chapter 13).
- Onlay graft: Barone and Covani[58] found that the success rate of block grafts was very good. They found a very low rate of resorption both clinically and radiographically following bone graft and implant placement and concluded that grafts from the anterosuperior edge of the iliac wing are a "promising treatment" in cases of severe maxillary atrophy.
- Distraction osteogenesis: Esposito et al[56] found that distraction osteogenesis (more than any other technique) permits simultaneous horizontal and vertical augmentation.
- Amato et al[59] found orthodontic extrusion was a viable treatment for hopeless teeth to regenerate hard and soft tissues. Its efficacy was about 70% for bone regeneration and 60% for gingival augmentation.

Esposito et al[56] found in a systematic review that there can be many complications associated with vertical augmentation, and as a result, short implants may be a better option in patients with resorbed mandibles.

Vertical augmentation is difficult because it is challenging to achieve fixation, and there is a high resorption rate.

Another option is to place zygomatic implants if the ridge cannot be grafted and/or the patient does not want grafting done.[60]

Q: What is the decision tree when deciding the best treatment for an intrabony periodontal defect?

See Fig 12-14 on next page. →

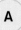

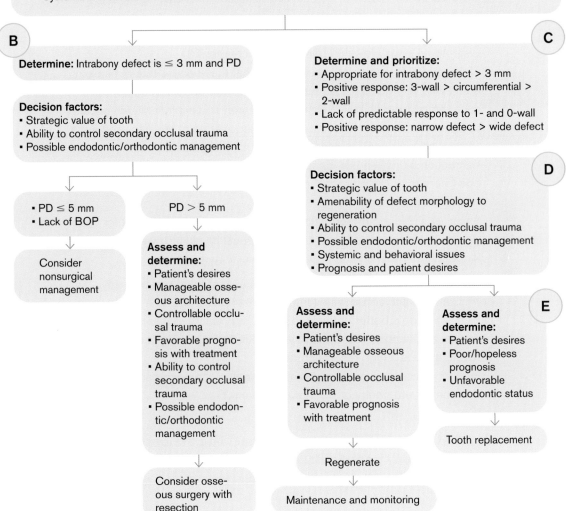

A   **Assess intrabony periodontal defect (after initial therapy and occlusal adjustment as needed)**
- Probing depth (PD) and clinical attachment level
- Bleeding on probing (BOP)
- Mobility
- Radiographic and clinical assessment of osseous architecture
- Concurrent endodontic/orthodontic needs/treatment
- Systemic and behavioral issues

B

Determine: Intrabony defect is ≤ 3 mm and PD

Decision factors:
- Strategic value of tooth
- Ability to control secondary occlusal trauma
- Possible endodontic/orthodontic management

- PD ≤ 5 mm
- Lack of BOP

Consider nonsurgical management

PD > 5 mm

Assess and determine:
- Patient's desires
- Manageable osseous architecture
- Controllable occlusal trauma
- Favorable prognosis with treatment
- Ability to control secondary occlusal trauma
- Possible endodontic/orthodontic management

Consider osseous surgery with resection

C

Determine and prioritize:
- Appropriate for intrabony defect > 3 mm
- Positive response: 3-wall > circumferential > 2-wall
- Lack of predictable response to 1- and 0-wall
- Positive response: narrow defect > wide defect

D

Decision factors:
- Strategic value of tooth
- Amenability of defect morphology to regeneration
- Ability to control secondary occlusal trauma
- Possible endodontic/orthodontic management
- Systemic and behavioral issues
- Prognosis and patient desires

Assess and determine:
- Patient's desires
- Manageable osseous architecture
- Controllable occlusal trauma
- Favorable prognosis with treatment

Regenerate

Maintenance and monitoring

E

Assess and determine:
- Patient's desires
- Poor/hopeless prognosis
- Unfavorable endodontic status

Tooth replacement

Fig 12-14 Decision tree.[61]

Socket Grafting

Q: What is socket grafting or ridge preservation?

After extraction of the tooth, it is important to maintain the dimensions of the ridge. Placing a bone graft into the socket (Fig 12-15) allows for this preservation, especially in the esthetic zone.

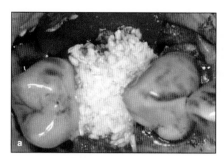 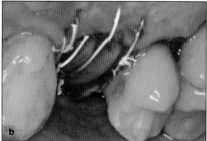

Fig 12-15 (a) Socket preservation with allogeneic bone graft and resorbable membrane. (b) Membrane sutured over the graft.

Q: What is the rationale for socket grafting?[62]

1. To enable installation and stability of a dental implant
2. To reduce loss of alveolar bone volume
3. To reduce need for additional bone grafting procedures
4. To enable the generated tissues to provide implant osseointegration
5. To improve the esthetic outcome of the final prosthesis
6. To regenerate bone faster, allowing earlier implantation and restoration

Q: Describe the healing that occurs after tooth extraction.

Amler et al[63] found that after extraction, a blood clot filled the socket. After 7 days, granulation tissue filled the socket. Collagen replaced the granulation tissue, and bone formation began at the base and around the extraction socket after 20 days. Bone filled about two-thirds of the socket at 5 weeks. It took 24 to 35 days for the epithelium, which grew progressively as it enveloped granulation, debris, and bone particles, to completely cover the extraction socket. At all stages, bone regeneration began at the apex and outside of the socket, progressing gradually toward its center and the crest of bone.[64] $\rightarrow$

After socket grafting, first a blood clot forms, then a few days after grafting, the first phase of the graft material dissolves. Nutrient canals and osteoblasts invade the graft, and maturation occurs.

Q: Is socket grafting effective?

In a meta-analysis, Vignoletti et al[65] found vertical and horizontal contraction of the alveolar bone crest to be less in patients who had received socket preservation. Test and control sites had a difference of 1.47 mm in bone height. The meta-analysis concluded that socket preservation limits vertical and horizontal dimensional changes after a tooth has been extracted.

McAllister and Haghighat[11] noted that bone regeneration could occur without socket grafting in extraction sockets with intact bony walls, and therefore socket grafting at the time of extraction may not always be beneficial. They cited studies in which the healing processes of socket grafts were altered when various bone grafting materials were used to preserve the alveolar ridge and socket dimensions.

A randomized clinical trial[66] found that implants placed into grafted sites displayed a clinical performance comparable to that of implants positioned in non-grafted sites with respect to implant survival and marginal bone loss. Yet grafted sites allowed for fewer augmentation surgeries and placement of larger implants.

Tan et al[67] did a systematic review and found horizontal bone loss of 29% to 63% and vertical bone loss of 11% to 22% after 6 months following tooth extraction. There were rapid reductions in the first 3 to 6 months, followed by gradual reductions in dimensions thereafter.

Q: Does the thickness of the buccal bone plate matter when grafting the socket?

Cardaropoli[68] found that the thinner the bone plate was at baseline, the greater the alveolar bone loss after 4 months, while a thicker buccal plate at baseline had less alveolar bone loss after 4 months, confirming that the thickness of the buccal bony wall in the extraction site influences hard tissue changes during healing.

Avila-Ortiz[69] found sites presenting a buccal bone thickness greater than 1.0 mm exhibited more favorable ridge preservation outcomes, as compared to sites with a thinner buccal wall.

Q: When should implants be placed after socket preservation?

Beck and Mealey[70] found no significant differences in the amount of new bone growth of the grafted allograft bone at 3 versus 6 months following extraction and ridge preservation. Therefore, the study did not support waiting longer periods of time following extraction and ridge preservation to permit bone regeneration.

Cardaropoli et al[71] did a 12-month postloading study and reported the success rate as 95.83% in the patients with ridge preservation and 91.66% in the group with no ridge preservation. No statistically significant differences in the marginal bone level were detected between the two groups.

Note that it may be prudent to look at other factors (eg, number of bony walls, angle of the defect, and age of the patient) to determine the amount of time to wait before implant placement.

Growth Factors

Q: What are some bioactive agents used in regeneration?

1. Platelet-derived growth factor
2. Insulin-like growth factor
3. Fibroblast growth factor
4. Bone morphogenetic proteins
5. Enamel matrix derivative

Q: What are the benefits and drawbacks of using growth factors for bone regeneration?[72]

The advantages and disadvantages of using growth factors for bone regeneration are shown in Fig 12-16.

+	−
• Excellent wound healing • Bone induction and chemotactic effect • Decreased need for autogenous bone • Decreased surgical time and thus less trauma to the patient • Better tissue regeneration	• Higher cost • New technologic advancement that needs to be developed over time • Greater swelling

Fig 12-16 Advantages and disadvantages of using growth factors for bone regeneration.

Q: What is enamel matrix derivative (EMD), and is it effective?

EMD is derived from porcine teeth, and it has a protein that mimics the matrix proteins that induce cementogenesis. It is a tissue-healing modulator that mimics events that occur during root development and helps stimulate peri-odontal regeneration.

Studies on EMD include the following:

- Froum et al[73] found that EMD use resulted in statistically larger gains in clinical attachment level and decreased probing depth.
- In a meta-analysis, Koop et al[74] found that EMD is as effective as resorb-able membranes in the treatment of intrabony defects. EMD and a coronally advanced flap is as effective as a connective tissue graft.
- Esposito et al[75] found that EMD significantly improved probing attachment levels by 1.1 mm and pocket depth reduction by 0.9 mm when compared with a control, although they stated that the actual clinical advantages of using EMD were not certain. There were no findings of differences between GTR and EMD with the exception of significantly more postoper-ative complications in the GTR group.
- Rösing et al[76] treated 16 patients with chronic periodontitis who had greater than 6-mm defects using a split-mouth design. The control sites received a placebo, and the test sites received the EMD solution. EMD did not impact or improve clinical and radiographic parameters compared with the placebo.
- Giannobile and Somerman[77] found that clinical attachment level gain and reduction of pocket depth have been promoted with the use of EMD in osseous defects. Compared with control procedures (usually OFD), EMD has shown superior results with great consistency.

Q: Describe the importance of bone morphogenetic proteins (BMPs).

BMP-2 and BMP-7 (osteogenic protein 1), which are glycoproteins and osteoinductive, start a cycle of cellular events resulting in differentiation of cells into phenotypes involved in periodontal regeneration. They enhance bone and cementum formation. In a 1994 study, Ripamonti et al[78] made acute defects in baboons and applied BMP to the experimental group. They found that the experimental group had 2.5 times more bone and cemen-tum height than the controls. A review by King and Cochran[79] found that a number of studies have demonstrated the potential for BMPs to increase $\rightarrow$

periodontal regeneration. The effects of BMPs are influenced by root surface conditioning, occlusal loading, dosage, and carrier systems.

Q: What is platelet-derived growth factor (PDGF) and what does it do?

PDGF is derived from platelets, macrophages, and osteoblasts. It stimulates DNA and protein synthesis and regulates cell growth and division. Kaigler et al[80] suggest that PDGF in combination with osteoconductive matrices, based on clinical results of its use in various periodontal and peri-implant applications, could potentially come into routine use.

Fagan et al[81] noted that when FDBA, recombinant human PDGF (rhPDGF), and a titanium-reinforced membrane were placed for implant site augmentation, hard tissue augmentation was histologically apparent. Soft tissue was also augmented after pediculated connective tissue was rinsed with rhPDGF.

Q: What is growth factor–enhanced matrix?

Growth factor–enhanced matrix (GEM 21S, Lynch Biologics) combines rhPDGF and β-tricalcium phosphate (β-TCP), which mix and are released into the surrounding environment after implantation. rhPDGF then binds to specific cell surface receptors on the target cells, initiating a cascade of intracellular signaling pathways. rhPDGF-induced intracellular events lead to directed cell migration or chemotaxis and cell proliferation or mitogenesis of osteoblasts, periodontal ligament fibroblasts, and cementoblasts.[82]

In 11 clinical centers, Nevins et al[83] performed surgical treatment on 180 patients with a 4-mm or greater intrabony periodontal defect. Patients were randomly placed into one of three treatment groups: *(1)* β-TCP + 0.3 mg/mL rhPDGF-BB in buffer, *(2)* β-TCP + 1.0 mg/mL rhPDGF-BB in buffer; and *(3)* β-TCP + buffer (active control). At 3 months, clinical attachment gain was significantly greater for group 1 (3.8 mm) compared with group 3 (3.3 mm). Group 1 had greater defect fill (57% versus 18%) and greater linear bone gain (2.6 versus 0.9 mm) than group 3 at 6 months.

Q: Are biologics effective in the treatment of intrabony defects?

A Consensus Report from the AAP Regeneration Workshop[1] found EMD and rhPDGF-BB with B-TCP were shown to be efficacious in regenerating intrabony defects. The level of evidence is supported by multiple studies →

documenting effectiveness. The clinical application of biologics supports improvements in clinical parameters comparable with selected bone replacement grafts and GTR. Smoking and excessive tooth mobility negatively affect regeneration.

Miscellaneous

Q: Does tooth vitality affect regenerative outcomes in intrabony defects?

Cortellini and Tonetti[84] demonstrated that deep intrabony defects do not negatively influence tooth vitality. They also found that the healing response of deep intrabony defects treated with GTR therapy is not negatively affected by root canal therapy.

Q: How does hypermobility affect regeneration?

Cortellini et al[85] found that severe hypermobility can negatively impact the clinical outcome of regeneration.

Q: Does demineralization of the root surface improve regeneration?

It was believed that exposure of the collagen in the dentinal matrix would facilitate adhesion of the blood clot to the root. However, in five out of six citric acid–treated specimens, Stahl and Froum[86] found no evidence suggesting that citric acid applications either initiated or accelerated cementogenesis or functional connective tissue attachment at root surfaces previously exposed to periodontal pockets. Moreover, a meta-analysis performed by Mariotti[87] on 28 clinical trials did not show any significant effects of acid root treatment on attachment level gains or probing depth. Evidence to date suggests that the use of citric acid, tetracycline, or ethylenediaminetetraacetic acid (EDTA) to modify the root surface provides no clinically significant benefit to regeneration in patients with chronic periodontitis.

Q: How does smoking affect regeneration?

Tonetti et al[88] performed a retrospective study investigating the influence of cigarette smoking on the healing response after GTR in deep defects. Nonsmokers gained significantly more probing attachment level (5.2 mm) than smokers (2.1 mm).

Rosen et al[89] conducted a study on DFDBA in intrabony defects. At 1 year posttreatment, significant reductions in mean probing depth were observed for nonsmokers (3.8 mm) and smokers (3.0 mm). However, when relative improvements in clinical measures were compared at the 1- and 2- to 5-year follow-ups, nonsmokers were found to exhibit significantly better treatment effects. Compared to pretreatment findings, there were changes in progress detected for the clinical attachment level at the 1-year evaluation (29.2% for smokers and 42.5% for nonsmokers).

Stavropoulos et al[90] examined 47 intrabony defects in 32 patients treated by means of polylactic acid/citric acid ester copolymer resorbable membranes. Smokers had less pocket reduction than nonsmokers (4.5 ± 0.7 versus 5.5 ± 0.7 mm, respectively), which resulted in greater residual pocket depth in smokers compared with nonsmokers (3.6 ± 1.0 versus 3.4 ± 1.1 mm).

The 2015 Consensus Report from the AAP Regeneration Workshop found regeneration in intrabony defects are negatively affected by smoking and poor oral hygiene.[1]

Q: How can researchers measure regeneration?

- Histology (many believe this is the only way)
- Radiographic analysis
- Probing

References

1. Reynolds MA, Kao RT, Camargo PM, et al. Periodontal regeneration—Intrabony defects: A consensus report from the AAP Regeneration Workshop. J Periodontol 2015;86(2 suppl):S105–S107.
2. Melcher AH. On the repair potential of periodontal tissues. J Periodontol 1976;47:256–260.
3. Kim CS, Choi SH, Chai JK, et al. Periodontal repair in surgically created intrabony defects in dogs: Influence of the number of bone walls on healing response. J Periodontol 2004;75:229–235.
4. Ronda M, Stacchi C. A novel approach for the coronal advancement of the buccal flap. Int J Periodontics Restorative Dent 2015;35:795–801.
5. Seibert JS. Reconstruction of deformed, partially edentulous ridges, using full thickness onlay grafts. Part I. Technique and wound healing. Compend Contin Educ Dent 1983;4:437–453.

6. Committee on Research, Science and Therapy of the American Academy of Periodontology. Tissue banking of bone allografts used in periodontal regeneration. J Periodontol 2001;72:834–838.

7. Mellonig JT, Prewett AB, Moyer MP. HIV inactivation in a bone allograft. J Periodontol 1992;63:979–983.

8. Buchman SR, Ozaki W. The ultrastructure and resorptive pattern of cancellous onlay bone grafts in the craniofacial skeleton. Ann Plast Surg 1999;43:49–56.

9. Keith JD Jr, Petrungaro P, Leonetti JA, et al. Clinical and histologic evaluation of a mineralized block allograft: Results from the developmental period (2001–2004). Int J Periodontics Restorative Dent 2006;26:321–327.

10. Nissan J, Ghelfan O, Mardinger O, Calderon S, Chaushu G. Efficacy of cancellous block allograft augmentation prior to implant placement in the posterior atrophic mandible. Clin Implant Dent Relat Res 2011;13:279–285.

11. McAllister BS, Haghighat K. Bone augmentation techniques. J Periodontol 2007;78:377–396.

12. Mellonig JT. Freeze-dried bone allografts in periodontal reconstructive surgery. Dent Clin North Am 1991;35:505–520.

13. Reynolds MA, Aichelmann-Reidy ME, Branch-Mays GL, Gunsolley JC. The efficacy of bone replacement grafts in the treatment of periodontal osseous defects. A systematic review. Ann Periodontol 2003;8:227–265.

14. Bowers GM, Chadroff B, Carnevale R, et al. Histologic evaluation of new attachment apparatus formation in humans. Part III. J Periodontol 1989;60:683–693.

15. Mellonig JT. Human histologic evaluation of a bovine-derived bone xenograft in the treatment of periodontal osseous defects. Int J Periodontics Restorative Dent 2000;20:19–29.

16. Schallhorn RG, Hiatt WH, Boyce W. Iliac transplants in periodontal therapy. J Periodontol 1970;41:566–580.

17. Buser D, Dula K, Hirt HP, Schenk RK. Lateral ridge augmentation using autografts and barrier membranes: A clinical study with 40 partially edentulous patients. J Oral Maxillofac Surg 1996;54:420–433.

18. Cortellini P, Tonetti MS. Clinical and radiographic outcomes of the modified minimally invasive surgical technique with and without regenerative materials: A randomized-controlled trial in intra-bony defects. J Clin Periodontol 2011;38:365–373.

19. Wood RA, Mealey BL. Histologic comparison of healing after tooth extraction with ridge preservation using mineralized versus demineralized freeze-dried bone allograft. J Periodontol 2012;83:329–336.

20. Yukna RA, Vastardis S. Comparative evaluation of decalcified and non-decalcified freeze-dried bone allografts in rhesus monkeys. I. Histologic findings. J Periodontol 2005;76:57–65.

21. Wang HL, Greenwell H, Fiorellini J, et al; Research, Science and Therapy Committee of the American Academy of Periodontology. Position paper: Periodontal regeneration. J Periodontol 2005;76:1601–1622.

22. Rummelhart JM, Mellonig JT, Gray JL, Towle HJ. A comparison of freeze-dried bone allograft and demineralized freeze-dried bone allograft in human periodontal osseous defects. J Periodontol 1989;60:655–663.

23. Choi JY, Jung UW, Lee IS, Kim CS, Lee YK, Choi SH. Resolution of surgically created three-wall intrabony defects in implants using three different biomaterials: An in vivo study. Clin Oral Implants Res 2011;22:343–348.

24. Aimetti M, Romano F, Griga FB, Godio L. Clinical and histologic healing of human extraction sockets filled with calcium sulfate. Int J Oral Maxillofac Implants 2009;24:902–909.

25. Shapoff CA, Bowers GM, Levy B, Mellonig JT, Yukna RA. The effect of particle size on the osteogenic activity of composite grafts of allogeneic freeze-dried bone and autogenous marrow. J Periodontol 1980;51:625–630.

26. Fucini SE, Quintero G, Gher ME, Black BS, Richardson AC. Small versus large particles of demineralized freeze-dried bone allografts in human intrabony periodontal defects. J Periodontol 1993;64:844–847.

27. Drury GI, Yukna RA. Histologic evaluation of combining tetracycline and allogeneic freeze-dried bone on bone regeneration in experimental defects in baboons. J Periodontol 1991;62:652–658.
28. Masters LB, Mellonig JT, Brunsvold MA, Nummikoski PV. A clinical evaluation of demineralized freeze-dried bone allograft in combination with tetracycline in the treatment of periodontal osseous defects. J Periodontol 1996;67:770–781.
29. Rompen EH, Biewer R, Vanheusden A, Zahedi S, Nusgens B. The influence of cortical perforations and of space filling with peripheral blood on the kinetics of guided bone generation. A comparative histometric study in the rat. Clin Oral Implants Res 1999;10:85–94.
30. Adeyemo WL, Reuther T, Bloch W, et al. Influence of host periosteum and recipient bed perforation on the healing of onlay mandibular bone graft: An experimental pilot study in the sheep. Oral Maxillofac Surg 2008;12:19–28.
31. Greenstein G, Greenstein B, Cavallaro J, Tarnow D. The role of bone decortication in enhancing the results of guided bone regeneration: A literature review. J Periodontol 2009;80:175–189.
32. Merli M, Lombardini F, Esposito M. Vertical ridge augmentation with autogenous bone grafts 3 years after loading: Resorbable barriers versus titanium-reinforced barriers. A randomized controlled clinical trial. Int J Oral Maxillofac Implants 2010;25:801–807.
33. Caffesse RG, Mota LF, Quiñones CR, Morrison EC. Clinical comparison of resorbable and non-resorbable barriers for guided periodontal tissue regeneration. J Clin Periodontol 1997;24:747–752.
34. Laurell L, Gottlow J, Zybutz M, Persson R. Treatment of intrabony defects by different surgical procedures. A literature review. J Periodontol 1998;69:303–313.
35. Fontana F, Maschera E, Rocchietta I, Simion M. Clinical classification of complications in guided bone regeneration procedures by means of a nonresorbable membrane. Int J Periodontics Restorative Dent 2011;31:265–273.
36. Machtei EE. The effect of membrane exposure on the outcome of regenerative procedures in humans: A meta-analysis. J Periodontol 2001;72:512–516.
37. De Sanctis M, Zucchelli G, Clauser C. Bacterial colonization of bioabsorbable barrier material and periodontal regeneration. J Periodontol 1996;67:1193–1200.
38. Villar CC, Cochran DL. Regeneration of periodontal tissues: Guided tissue regeneration. Dent Clin North Am 2010;54:73–92.
39. Nowzari H, Matian F, Slots J. Periodontal pathogens on polytetrafluoroethylene membrane for guided tissue regeneration inhibit healing. J Clin Periodontol 1995;22:469–474.
40. Tal H, Kozlovsky A, Artzi Z, Nemcovsky CE, Moses O. Cross-linked and non-cross-linked collagen barrier membranes disintegrate following surgical exposure to the oral environment: A histological study in the cat. Clin Oral Implants Res 2008;19:760–766.
41. Moses O, Pitaru S, Artzi Z, Nemcovsky CE. Healing of dehiscence-type defects in implants placed together with different barrier membranes: A comparative clinical study. Clin Oral Implants Res 2005;16:210–219.
42. Bornstein MM, Bosshardt D, Buser D. Effect of two different bioabsorbable collagen membranes on guided bone regeneration: A comparative histomorphometric study in the dog mandible. J Periodontol 2007;78:1943–1953.
43. Block MS. Preserving alveolar ridge anatomy following tooth removal in conjunction with delayed implant placement. Atlas Oral Maxillofac Surg Clin North Am 1999;7:61–77.
44. Meloni SM, Jovanovic SA, Pisano M, De Riu G, Baldoni E, Tallarico M. One-stage horizontal guided bone regeneration with autologous bone, anorganic bovine bone and collagen membranes: Follow-up of a prospective study 30 months after loading. Eur J Oral Implantol 2018;11:89–95.
45. Urban IA, Nagursky H, Lozada JL. Horizontal ridge augmentation with a resorbable membrane and particulated autogenous bone with or without anorganic bovine bone-derived mineral: A prospective case series in 22 patients. Int J Oral Maxillofac Implants 2011;26:404–414.
46. Urban IA, Nagursky H, Lozada JL, Nagy K. Horizontal ridge augmentation with a collagen membrane and a combination of particulated autogenous bone and anorganic bovine bone-derived mineral: A prospective case series in 25 patients. Int J Periodontics Restorative Dent 2013;33:299–307.
47. Sascha Jovanovic lecture at the AAP. Tissue Engineering and Hard Tissue Reconstruction. Tuesday 10/30/2018.

48. Tonetti MS, Pini-Prato G, Cortellini P. Periodontal regeneration of human intrabony defects. IV. Determinants of healing response. J Periodontol 1993;64:934–940.

49. Murphy KG, Gunsolley JC. Guided tissue regeneration for the treatment of periodontal intrabony and furcation defects. A systematic review. Ann Periodontol 2003;8:266–302.

50. Needleman IG, Worthington HV, Giedrys-Leeper E, Tucker RJ. Guided tissue regeneration for periodontal infra-bony defects. Cochrane Database Syst Rev 2006;(2):CD001724.

51. Sculean A, Nikolidakis D, Schwarz F. Regeneration of periodontal tissues: Combinations of barrier membranes and grafting materials—Biological foundation and preclinical evidence: A systematic review. J Clin Periodontol 2008;35(8 suppl):106–116.

52. Fugazzotto PA. Report of 302 consecutive ridge augmentation procedures: Technical considerations and clinical results. Int J Oral Maxillofac Implants 1998;13:358–368.

53. Sethi A, Kaus T. Maxillary ridge expansion with simultaneous implant placement: 5-year results of an ongoing clinical study. Int J Oral Maxillofac Implants 2000;15:491–499.

54. Laster Z, Rachmiel A, Jensen OT. Alveolar width distraction osteogenesis for early implant placement. J Oral Maxillofac Surg 2005;63:1724–1730.

55. Nissan J, Marilena V, Gross O, Mardinger O, Chaushu G. Histomorphometric analysis following augmentation of the anterior atrophic maxilla with cancellous bone block allograft. Int J Oral Maxillofac Implants 2012;27:84–89.

56. Esposito M, Grusovin MG, Felice P, Karatzopoulos G, Worthington HV, Coulthard P. The efficacy of horizontal and vertical bone augmentation procedures for dental implants—A Cochrane systematic review. Eur J Oral Implantol 2009;2:167–184.

57. Simion M, Trisi P, Piattelli A. Vertical ridge augmentation using a membrane technique associated with osseointegrated implants. Int J Periodontics Restorative Dent 1994;14:496–511.

58. Barone A, Covani U. Maxillary alveolar ridge reconstruction with nonvascularized autogenous block bone: Clinical results. J Oral Maxillofac Surg 2007;65:2039–2046.

59. Amato F, Mirabella AD, Macca U, Tarnow DP. Implant site development by orthodontic forced extraction: A preliminary study. Int J Oral Maxillofac Implants 2012;27:411–420.

60. Tuminelli FJ, Walter LR, Neugarten J, Bedrossian E. Immediate loading of zygomatic implants: A systematic review of implant survival, prosthesis survival and potential complications. Eur J Oral Implantol 2017;10(suppl 1):79–87.

61. Kao RT, Nares S, Reynolds MA. Periodontal regeneration—Intrabony defects: A systematic review from the AAP Regeneration Workshop. J Periodontol 2015;86(2 suppl):S77–S104.

62. Pagni G, Pellegrini G, Giannobile WV, Rasperini G. Postextraction alveolar ridge preservation: Biological basis and treatments. Int J Dent 2012;2012:151030.

63. Amler MH, Johnson PL, Salman I. Histological and histochemical investigation of human alveolar socket healing in undisturbed extraction wounds. J Am Dent Assoc 1960;61:32–44.

64. Steiner GG, Francis W, Burrell R, Kallet MP, Steiner DM, Macias R. The healing socket and socket regeneration. Compend Contin Educ Dent 2008;29:114–116,118,120–124.

65. Vignoletti F, Matesanz P, Rodrigo D, Figuero E, Martin C, Sanz M. Surgical protocols for ridge preservation after tooth extraction. A systematic review. Clin Oral Implants Res 2012;23(suppl 5):22–38.

66. Barone A, Orlando B, Cingano L, Marconcini S, Derchi G, Covani U. A randomized clinical trial to evaluate and compare implants placed in augmented versus non-augmented extraction sockets: 3-year results. J Periodontol 2012;83:836–846.

67. Tan WL, Wong TL, Wong MC, Lang NP. A systematic review of post-extractional alveolar hard and soft tissue dimensional changes in humans. Clin Oral Implants Res 2012;23(suppl 5):1–21.

68. Cardaropoli D, Tamagnone L, Roffredo A, Gaveglio L. Relationship between the buccal bone plate thickness and the healing of postextraction sockets with/without ridge preservation. Int J Periodontics Restorative Dent 2014;34:211–217.

69. Avila-Ortiz G, Chambrone L, Vignoletti F. Effect of alveolar ridge preservation interventions following tooth extraction: A systematic review and meta-analysis. J Clin Periodontol 2019;46(suppl 21):195–223.

70. Beck TM, Mealey BL. Histologic analysis of healing after tooth extraction with ridge preservation using mineralized human bone allograft. J Periodontol 2010;81:1765–1772.

71. Cardaropoli D, Tamagnone L, Roffredo A, Gaveglio L. Evaluation of dental implants placed in preserved and nonpreserved postextraction ridges: A 12-month postloading study. Int J Periodontics Restorative Dent 2015;35:677–685.

72. Jovanovic SA. Out of the vein or out of the bottle? Presented at the 98th Annual Meeting of the American Academy of Periodontology, Los Angeles, 2 Oct 2012.

73. Froum S, Lemler J, Horowitz R, Davidson B. The use of enamel matrix derivative in the treatment of periodontal osseous defects: A clinical decision tree based on biologic principles of regeneration. Int J Periodontics Restorative Dent 2001;21:437–449.

74. Koop R, Merheb J, Quirynen M. Periodontal regeneration with enamel matrix derivative in reconstructive periodontal therapy: A systematic review. J Periodontol 2012;83:707–720.

75. Esposito M, Grusovin MG, Papanikolaou N, Coulthard P, Worthington HV. Enamel matrix derivative (Emdogain[R]) for periodontal tissue regeneration in intrabony defects. Cochrane Database Syst Rev 2009;(4):CD003875.

76. Rösing CK, Aass AM, Mavropoulos A, Gjermo P. Clinical and radiographic effects of enamel matrix derivative in the treatment of intrabony periodontal defects: A 12-month longitudinal placebo-controlled clinical trial in adult periodontitis patients. J Periodontol 2005;76:129–133.

77. Giannobile WV, Somerman MJ. Growth and amelogenin-like factors in periodontal wound healing. A systematic review. Ann Periodontol 2003;8:193–204.

78. Ripamonti U, Heliotis M, van den Heever B, Reddi AH. Bone morphogenetic proteins induce periodontal regeneration in the baboon (Papio ursinus). J Periodontal Res 1994;29:439–445 [erratum 1995;30:149–151].

79. King GN, Cochran DL. Factors that modulate the effects of bone morphogenetic protein-induced periodontal regeneration: A critical review. J Periodontol 2002;73:925–936.

80. Kaigler D, Avila G, Wisner-Lynch L, et al. Platelet-derived growth factor applications in periodontal and peri-implant bone regeneration. Expert Opin Biol Ther 2011;11:375–385.

81. Fagan MC, Miller RE, Lynch SE, Kao RT. Simultaneous augmentation of hard and soft tissues for implant site preparation using recombinant human platelet-derived growth factor: A human case report. Int J Periodontics Restorative Dent 2008;28:37–43.

82. The Science of rhPDGF-BB: Scientifically Proven Mechanism of Action. Osteohealth website. http://www.osteohealth.com/TheScienceofrhPDGFBB.aspx. Accessed 16 October 2012.

83. Nevins M, Giannobile WV, McGuire MK, et al. Platelet-derived growth factor stimulates bone fill and rate of attachment level gain: Results of a large multicenter randomized controlled trial. J Periodontol 2005;76:2205–2215.

84. Cortellini P, Tonetti MS. Evaluation of the effect of tooth vitality on regenerative outcomes in infrabony defects. J Clin Periodontol 2001;28:672–679.

85. Cortellini P, Labriola A, Tonetti MS. Regenerative periodontal therapy in intrabony defects: State of the art. Minerva Stomatol 2007;56:519–539.

86. Stahl SS, Froum SJ. Human clinical and histologic repair responses following the use of citric acid in periodontal therapy. J Periodontol 1977;48:261–266.

87. Mariotti A. Efficacy of chemical root surface modifiers in the treatment of periodontal disease. A systematic review. Ann Periodontol 2003;8:205–226.

88. Tonetti MS, Pini-Prato G, Cortellini P. Effect of cigarette smoking on periodontal healing following GTR in infrabony defects. A preliminary retrospective study. J Clin Periodontol 1995;22:229–234.

89. Rosen PS, Marks MH, Reynolds MA. Influence of smoking on long-term clinical results of intrabony defects treated with regenerative therapy. J Periodontol 1996;67:1159–1163.

90. Stavropoulos A, Mardas N, Herrero F, Karring T. Smoking affects the outcome of guided tissue regeneration with bioresorbable membranes: A retrospective analysis of intrabony defects. J Clin Periodontol 2004;31:945–950.

Implants

Background

Q: **Which classification is important to take into account before placing implants?**

Lekholm and Zarb[1] classified the jaws according to bone quantity and quality (Fig 13-1).

Bone quantity	Bone quality
A: The alveolar ridge is intact B: Moderate ridge resorption has occurred C: Advanced residual ridge resorption has occurred D: Some resorption of the basal bone has begun E: Extreme resorption of the basal bone has transpired	1: Entire jaw is cortical bone 2: Thick cortical bone surrounds a core of dense trabecular bone 3: Thin layer of cortical bone surrounds a core of dense trabecular bone 4: Thin layer of cortical bone surrounds low-density trabecular bone

Fig 13-1 Lekholm and Zarb classification[1] of bone quantity and quality.

Q: What are the criteria for successful dental implants?

Following are criteria for a successful outcome with implant placement[2,3]:

- The implant is immobile (less than 1-mm mobility in any direction) and functioning.
- No radiographic evidence of radiolucency.
- Vertical bone loss is less than 0.2 mm annually following the implant's first year of service.
- Implant has an absence of persistent and/or irreversible signs.
- Patient and clinician satisfaction.
- The hard and soft tissues are healthy.
- A trained and experienced surgeon.
- Maintenance and oral hygiene.
- Management of the soft tissues.
- A well-designed restoration.

Q: What is the mean success rate of implants? What is the mean survival rate?

Moraschini et al[4] did a systematic study and found a cumulative mean success value (using Albrektsson criteria)[2] of 89.7% with a mean follow-up of 15.7 years. The study found a mean survival rate of 94.6% with a mean follow-up of 13.4 years.

Q: How much remodeling can be expected after an implant is placed?

Adell et al[5] found an average of 1.5 mm of marginal bone loss during healing and the first year after connection of the partial denture. Subsequently, an average of 0.1 mm was lost annually.

After the initial period of healing, 75% of implants experience no additional bone loss, but osseointegration occurs.[6]

Q: What are some factors that affect soft and hard tissue deficiencies at dental implants?

See Table 13-1 on the next page. →

Table 13-1	Factors affecting soft and hard tissue deficiencies.[7]		
Soft tissue deficiencies prior to implant placement	Soft tissue deficiencies after implant placement	Hard tissue deficiencies prior to implant placement	Hard tissue deficiencies after implant placement
• Tooth loss • Periodontal disease • Systemic diseases	• Lack of buccal bone • Papilla height (height determined by the bone crest between the implants) • Keratinized tissue • Migration of teeth and lifelong skeletal changes	• Tooth loss • Trauma from tooth extraction • Periodontitis • Endodontic infections • Longitudinal root fractures • General trauma • Bone height in the posterior maxilla (due to sinus floor) • Systemic diseases (eg, ectodermal dysplasia)	• Defects in healthy situations (eg, mandibular under-cuts, fenestrations) • Malpositioning of implants • Peri-implantitis • Mechanical overload • Soft tissue thickness • Systemic diseases

Q: What are some factors that affect implant success?

- Bone quantity and quality
- Surgical technique (eg, overheating of the bone and torque forces)
- Implant length and width
- Smoking
- Amount of plaque
- Occlusion (avoiding nonaxial forces, cantilevers, and lateral excursive movements)
- Lack of keratinized attached gingiva
- Anatomy (lingual concavity, mental nerve, sinus location)
- Surface texture

Q: What factors may lead to implant failure?

- Infection (bacterial contamination and increased inflammation)
- Fracture
- Impaired healing $\rightarrow$

- Improper implant preparation (eg, overheating or overpreparation; Fig 13-2)
- Improper mechanical stability following insertion of the implant (mobility)
- Premature loading of the implant
- Pain

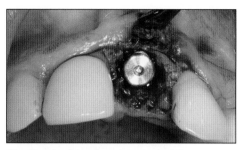

Fig 13-2 Implant placed too buccal (improper implant preparation).

Q: What factors are associated with recession of the peri-implant mucosa?

The principal reason for recession of the peri-implant mucosa is malpositioning of the implants, lack of keratinized tissue, lack of buccal bone, thin soft tissue, surgical trauma, and the status of the attachment of the adjacent teeth.[8] Contour of the abutment and/or crown overcontour can cause recession, and undercontour can allow tissue to move coronally.

Evans and Chen[9] reported implants with a buccal shoulder position showed three times more recession than implants with a lingual shoulder position, with the difference being highly statistically significant.

Q: Should peri-implant tissues be probed?

Using a light probing force (probing depth and bleeding on probing [BOP]) is an important and safe aspect of the oral exam. The dentist can ascertain the therapeutic needs of the patient by following the change in the probing depths between visits.

Q: Does location of the implant in the maxilla or mandible have an impact on implant success?

Cochran[3] found that mandibular implants have superior outcomes compared with maxillary implants. One reason for this variability is the difference in the quality of the bone. Areas with cortical bone (anterior mandible) have greater success rates compared with areas with reduced bone quality (posterior maxilla).

Q: What are contraindications to implant therapy?

Figure 13-3 presents contraindications to implant therapy.

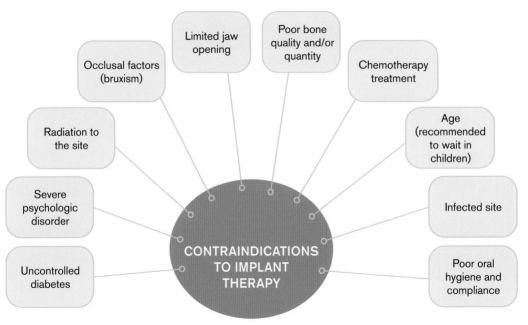

Fig 13-3 Contraindications to implant therapy.

Q: What is the definition of osseointegration?

Osseointegration is the formation of a direct attachment between an implant and bone, without any intervening soft tissue on a light microscope level.

Q: Should preoperative antibiotics be given to patients receiving implants?

Laskin et al[10] noted the benefits of prophylactic antibiotics in a study of 2,973 implants. The study demonstrated that patients who receive preoperative antibiotics have a significantly higher survival rate at each phase of treatment.

A Cochrane review by Esposito et al[11] found some evidence suggesting that 2 g amoxicillin given orally 1 hour preoperatively significantly reduces failures of dental implants placed under ordinary conditions. No significant adverse events were reported. The paper states that although it is not certain that postoperative antibiotics are beneficial or which antibiotics are most effective, it might make sense to prescribe a single dose of 2 g amoxicillin prior to implant placement for prophylactic purposes.

Q: Describe some differences between natural teeth and implants.

Table 11-2 details some of the differences (see next page):

- Host response: Schierano et al[12] found no significant differences between implants and teeth in terms of both pro- and anti-inflammatory cytokines. Lang et al[13] reported that while plasma cells and lymphocytes dominated in both types of lesions, neutrophil granulocytes and macrophages occurred in larger proportions in peri-implantitis than in periodontitis. The condition is self-limiting around teeth but not around implants.
- Conversion of mucositis to peri-implantitis versus that of gingivitis to periodontitis: Lang et al[14] assumed, based on data, that mucositis lesions may progress to peri-implantitis earlier than gingivitis converts to periodontitis. The paper also found that the apical extension of the lesion was more pronounced in peri-implantitis than in periodontitis. →

Table 13-2 Comparison between periodontal tissue and peri-implant tissue

	Periodontal tissues	Peri-implant tissues	Notes
Bacteria	No significant difference	No significant difference	Leonhardt et al[14] found no significant microbiologic difference between titanium implants and teeth in healthy conditions and in gingivitis and periodontitis. According to Lang et al,[13] because a host response is a reaction to a bacterial challenge, there is no reason to assume that it will be different in the peri-implant mucosa when compared with the gingiva.
Anatomy	• Have a periodontal ligament, bundle bone, dento-alveolar and dentogingival fiber bundles, and root cementum • Fiber orientation: Perpendicular	• Implants lack bundle bone, fiber bundles, root cementum, and a periodontal ligament, but they do have sulcular and junctional epithelium. They have a more limited vascular supply than those of teeth. • Peri-implant epithelium is longer and the connective tissue zone has no inserting fibers into the implant. • Fiber orientation: Parallel	• Hämmerle et al[15] showed that the natural teeth had an 8.75 times higher mean threshold for tactile sensibility than implants. • While a tooth may adapt to movement through intrusion or slight rotation, the dental implant-bone interface may absorb all the forces. Although forces are evenly distributed along the natural tooth, the forces are concentrated at the crestal bone level surrounding the implant.[16]
Peri-implant mucositis vs gingivitis	Reversible	Reversible	Peri-implant mucositis versus gingivitis: At the onset of mucositis/gingivitis, there is no evidence that the host response to the bacterial challenge is different at tooth and implant sites. Both mucositis and gingivitis are reversible.

Table 13-2 (cont)	Comparison between periodontal tissue and peri-implant tissue		
	Periodontal tissues	Peri-implant tissues	Notes
Margin of the gingiva	Follows the CEJ (health)	Follows the contour of the crestal bone or the connective tissue adhesion[6]	"Epithelial sealing" around implants is considered to be identical to that of teeth.[13]
Fulcrum to lateral forces	Apical third of the root	Crestal bone level	
Mobile or anchored in relation to the surrounding bone under occlusal forces[16]	Mobile Axial mobility: 25–100 μm Horizontal mobility: 56–150 μm	Rigidly anchored Axial mobility: 3–5 μm Horizontal mobility: 10–50 μm	
Histopathology at peri-implantitis site vs periodontitis site	Similar to peri-implantitis sites, dominated by plasma cells and lymphocytes	• Characterized by larger proportions of plasma cells, polymorphonuclear leukocytes and macrophages than periodontitis • Size of lesion twice as large as those found in periodontitis sites • IL-1α is a dominant osteoclast activating cytokine at peri-implantitis sites[17]	

Q: What are some of the surface modifications used to create a rough surface of a dental implant?

Surface modifications of implants include[18]:

- Grit-blasted or grit-blasted and acid-etched
- Microgrooved or plasma-sprayed titanium
- Plasma-sprayed hydroxyapatite coatings
- Thickened oxide layer (Nobel Biocare) (crystalline and phosphate enriched)

Q: Are rough surface implants more successful than smooth surface implants?

According to Cochran,[3] rough surfaces have a superior success rate for all implants, regardless of location, compared with smooth surfaces (Fig 13-4).

Khang et al[19] found that 36 (12 dual acid-etched and 24 machined surface) implants failed out of 432 implants (247 dual acid-etched, 185 machined surface). The collective success rates were 86.7% for the machined surface implants and 95% for the dual acid-etched implants at 36 months.

Nasatzky et al[20] showed that osteoblasts are sensitive to surface roughness, displaying decreased proliferation and a more differentiated phenotype on rougher surfaces. Instead of the usual 12 weeks, roughened titanium implants require a shorter healing period before loading (6 to 8 weeks), which can be advantageous. Shorter (6- to 8-mm) roughened implants can also be employed.

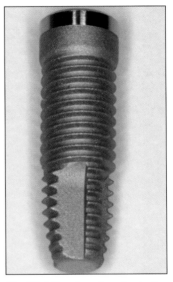

Fig 13-4 Rough surface implant.

Lang et al[13] found that peri-implantitis is more likely to develop with titanium plasma-sprayed than with minimally rough implants following exposure to the oral environment. Two animal studies further showed that susceptibility to disease progression may be higher for some moderately rough implant surfaces than others.

Q: Is keratinized attached tissue around an implant important?

Bouri et al[21] found significantly increased mean Gingival Index and Plaque Index scores, radiographic bone loss, and BOP for implants with less than 2 mm of keratinized mucosa. They found reduced mean alveolar bone loss and better soft tissue health with greater width of keratinized mucosa around implants.

Chung et al[22] suggested that the lack of adequate keratinized mucosa or attached mucosa around implants, regardless of the surface type, is not associated with increased bone loss, but it was associated with higher plaque accumulation and gingival inflammation.

Souza et al[23] reported that brushing at implant sites with a band of less than 2 mm of keratinized mucosa was shown to be considerably more uncomfortable and prone to plaque accumulation and peri-implant soft tissue inflammation when compared to implant sites with at least 2 mm of keratinized mucosa.

Lin et al[24] in a systematic review found a lack of adequate keratinized mucosa around implants is associated with more inflammation, mucosal recession, attachment loss, and plaque accumulation.

However, the 2017 World Workshop[17] concluded that although the absence or reduced width of keratinized mucosa may negatively impact oral hygiene measures, there is limited evidence that these factors constitute a risk for peri-implantitis.

Q: Are implants placed in patients with periodontal disease successful?

Baelum and Ellegaard[25] found the 5-year survival rate of implants placed in patients with a history of periodontitis to be similar to that observed with implants placed in patients without periodontitis. The authors recommended implant treatment as a good therapeutic option for periodontally compromised patients despite the fact that the 10-year survival rate of one-stage implants was somewhat lower in this population than in individuals without periodontal disease.

Karoussis et al[26] found that a history of chronic periodontitis was associated with significantly greater long-term probing depth, peri-implant marginal bone loss, and peri-implantitis. Ong et al[27] conducted a literature review and found that of the five studies presenting data on implant survival, four reported higher implant survival for non-periodontitis patients in comparison with treated periodontitis patients. The authors also point to evidence of →

increased implant loss and complications in patients previously treated for periodontitis compared with those with no history of periodontal disease.

Swierkot et al[28] found in their prospective long-term study that patients who were treated for generalized aggressive periodontitis had a 3-fold greater risk of mucositis, a 5-fold greater risk of implant failure, and a 14-fold greater risk of peri-implantitis.

Roccuzzo et al[29] conducted a 10-year study following 101 patients and found patients with a history of periodontitis presented a statistically significantly higher number of sites that required additional treatment. The study concluded that patients with a history of periodontitis should be notified that they are at a greater risk for peri-implant disease.

Q: Compare crestal bone changes at teeth and implants in periodontally healthy and periodontally compromised patients.

Rasperini et al[30] found that:

> ...natural teeth yielded better long-term results with respect to survival rate and marginal bone level changes compared with dental implants. Moreover, these findings also extend to teeth with an initial reduced periodontal attachment level, provided adequate periodontal treatment and maintenance are performed. As a consequence, the decision of tooth extraction attributable to periodontal reasons in favor of a dental implant should be carefully considered in partially edentulous patients.

Q: Where is the greatest force on an implant located?

The greatest force occurs at the neck of the implant.

Implant Placement

Q: What presurgical steps need to be taken before implant placement?

- Restorative requirements, the interarch space and jaw relationships, the location of edentulous areas, and the quantity and quality of available bone should be evaluated before implants are selected as a treatment option. It is also a good idea to get study casts and photographs to be able to perform case analysis when the patient is not present.[18] →

▪ Radiographs and cone beam images are necessary to determine the height of available bone in three dimensions and for selection of the dimensions of the implants. They also may be needed to determine the location of anatomical structures (eg, nerves and vessels).
▪ Written informed consent must be obtained from the patient.

Q: Describe the basic technique for implant placement.

The basic implant placement technique is outlined in Fig 13-5.

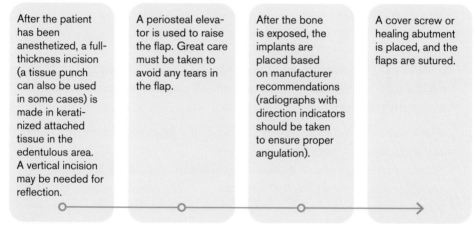

| After the patient has been anesthetized, a full-thickness incision (a tissue punch can also be used in some cases) is made in kerati-nized attached tissue in the edentulous area. A vertical incision may be needed for reflection. | A periosteal eleva-tor is used to raise the flap. Great care must be taken to avoid any tears in the flap. | After the bone is exposed, the implants are placed based on manufacturer recommendations (radiographs with direction indicators should be taken to ensure proper angulation). | A cover screw or healing abutment is placed, and the flaps are sutured. |

Fig 13-5 Implant placement technique.

There are three principles that must be followed when placing implants[12] (Fig 13-6):

1. The surgical procedure must minimize thermal trauma to the bone. Copious irrigation should be used to avoid overheating of the bone.
2. A primary healing period of variable duration must be allowed to permit osseointegration to be achieved (some studies are starting to question this principle).
3. There should be no micromotion greater than 100 µm during the healing period.

If multiple implants are to be placed, it has been found that arranging implants in a nonlinear manner creates a more stable base that is more resistant to torquing forces. →

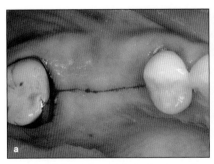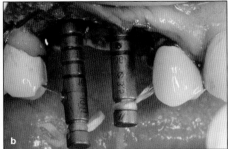

Fig 13-6 *(a)* Incision made for implant placement in keratinized attached tissue. *(b)* Direction indicators placed.

Q: How much anterior-posterior (A-P) spread is needed in the maxilla and mandible when an implant-supported prosthesis is treatment planned?

A-P spread is the distance from the center of the most anterior implant to the distal surface of the most posterior implant.
- Maxilla: An A-P spread of 2 cm with six implants. The cantilever length should not exceed half the A-P spread.
- Mandible: An A-P spread of 1 cm with four implants. The cantilever length should not exceed twice the A-P spread.

Q: What is the difference between a single-stage technique and a two-stage technique?

- Single-stage technique: The implant is exposed, and a healing abutment or restoration (most likely provisional) is placed but not loaded.
- Two-stage technique: The implant is placed and covered with a cover screw and gingiva. After 2 to 6 months, the implant is exposed, and a healing abutment and subsequently the restoration are placed.

Q: When would you perform two-stage surgery?[31]

- Situations where simultaneous bone grafting is necessary at the same time as implant placement because membranes are covered (less chance of exposure).
- Poor initial stability.
- Gingival tissues need to be augmented at the stage-two surgery. $\rightarrow$

- With dense cortical bone and good initial stability 2 to 4 months are needed for healing.
- In areas of loose trabecular bone and poor initial stability 4 to 6 months or more is needed.

Q: How much space is needed between the apex of an implant and the mental nerve?

A minimum of 2 mm is needed between the apex of an implant and the mental nerve.

Q: What are other options if a standard implant cannot be placed?

- Short implants
- Zygoma implants—cumulative survival rate is 96.7%[32]

Q: Is there a difference in peri-implantitis rate between specialists and general dentists?

Patients with periodontitis and with four or more implants, as well as implants of certain brands and prosthetic therapy delivered by general practitioners, exhibited higher odds ratios for moderate/severe peri-implantitis.[33]

Implants and Esthetics

Q: What does the distance from the interproximal contact point to the crest of bone have to be to have the papilla present 100% of the time?

Tarnow et al[34] found that the papilla was present 100% of the time when the measurement from the interproximal contact point to the crest of bone was 5 mm or less. The papilla was present 56% of the time when the distance was 6 mm, and the papilla was present 27% of the time or less when the distance was 7 mm or more.

Tarnow et al[35] also found that between two neighboring implants, the average height of papillary tissue was 3.4 mm, with a range of 1 to 7 mm. The most frequently probed heights were 2 mm (16.9%), 3 mm (35.3%), and 4 mm (37.5%).

Q: What does the distance between two implants and between an implant and a tooth have to be to preserve interdental bone?

According to Tarnow et al,[35] the distance between two implants should be at least 3 mm in order to preserve interdental bone (Fig 13-7). Vela et al[36] recommended 1.5 mm between the implant and the tooth to maintain bone adjacent to the teeth and 1 mm between the implant and the tooth when using platform-switched implants.

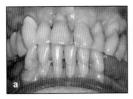 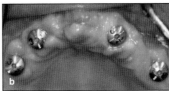 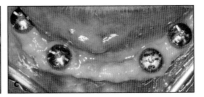

Fig 13-7 (a) Intraoral view before extractions. (b) Maxillary implants placed. (c) Mandibular implants placed.

Q: What appears to be the primary variable for success in peri-implant papilla reconstruction in terms of the abutment junction?

The subcrestal formation of the implant biologic width (which relates to the implant-abutment junction) is the primary variable for success. The flat design of the coronal portion of some implants, which results in flat interdental bone, is a serious hindrance in achieving an esthetically pleasing implant-supported restoration. A scalloped implant-abutment junction may enhance treatment success.[37]

Q: What should be evaluated when placing an anterior implant?

The following should be included in the evaluation prior to placing an anterior implant[38]:

- Mesiodistal dimension of the edentulous area
- 3D radiographs of the site
- Neighboring teeth (tooth dimensions, form, position, and orientation; periodontal/endodontic status; length of roots; crown-to-root ratio)
- Interarch relationships (vertical dimension of occlusion, interocclusal space)
- Esthetic parameters (height of upper smile line, lower lip line, occlusal plane orientation, dental and facial symmetry) →

- Patient expectations
- Plaque control
- Primary stability of the implant

Q: **What are the relative possible contraindications for immediate implant placement in the esthetic zone?**

- Heavy smoker
- Patient with very high expectations
- Immunocompromised patient
- Highly scalloped and thin biotype
- Triangular crowns
- Soft tissue defects
- High lip line

Q: **What surgical guidelines need to be followed for placement of an esthetic implant?**

Figure 13-8 presents the surgical guidelines for placing esthetic implants.

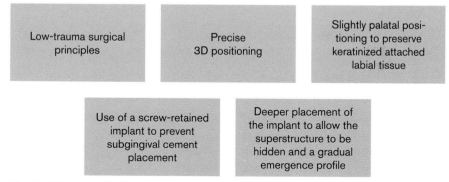

Fig 13-8 Surgical guidelines for esthetic implant placement.

Q: **How thick is the buccal wall in the esthetic area? Vertical mucosal thickness?**

Huynh-Ba et al[39] suggested that thin ($\leq$ 1 mm) buccal walls were found in most extraction sites in the anterior maxilla. As a result, augmentation $\rightarrow$

procedures are necessary to attain sufficient bony contours around the implant in most clinical situations.

The vertical peri-implant mucosal thickness measured 3.6 mm overall in healthy volunteers, with a big variation from 1.6 to 7 mm.[42]

Q: Does soft tissue grafting of the maxillary anterior area after immediate implant placement result in a gain of volume?

Grunder[41] did a study on 24 patients, with 12 in the grafted group (a subepithelial connective tissue graft was placed using the tunnel technique at the time of tooth extraction and implant placement) and 12 in the non-grafted group. Measurements of the labial volume were taken before treatment and 6 months after implant placement. The non-grafted group lost a mean of 1.063 mm of volume, as opposed to the grafted group, which gained 0.34 mm. At the time of immediate implant placement in the esthetic zone, insertion of a soft tissue graft can be advantageous.

Q: What is the survival rate of a single anterior implant placed immediately after extraction?

The mean survival rate based on many studies[42] is 97%.

Q: What is the best abutment to prevent soft tissue recession?

Rompen et al[43] found that with implants placed in the esthetic zone with concave, gingivally converging abutments, 87% of the sites showed facial soft tissue stability or gain, while recession (13% of the sites) was never greater than 0.5 mm. This is contrary to existing data from the literature, which demonstrate that 0.5 to 1.5 mm of recession may be expected with a majority of implants.

Patil et al[44] found angled abutments elicit more labial recession.

Q: What is the best abutment height to prevent marginal bone loss?

Galindo-Moreno et al[45] reported marginal bone loss rates were higher for prosthetic abutment heights less than 2 mm versus 2 mm or greater, for periodontal versus non-periodontal patients, for grafted versus pristine bone, and for a heavier smoking habit.

Implant Shape and Length

Q: When can short implants be used?

Figure 13-9 presents the indications for placing short implants.

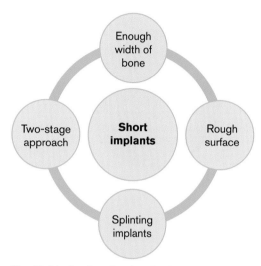

Fig 13-9 Indications for short implants.

Q: Are short implants successful?

Fugazzotto[46] performed a retrospective analysis on 1,774 patients and placed 2,073 implants of 6, 7, 8, or 9 mm in length. The implants were either supporting short-span fixed prostheses or single crowns. The survival rates for the implants were 98.1% to 99.7%. The study concluded that survival rates for implants 6 to 9 mm in length are comparable to those of longer implants.

Camps-Font et al[47] found placement of short implants (5 to 8 mm) appears to be the best option for treating atrophic posterior areas of the mandible, since this option is less invasive and has a significantly lower complication rate when compared with more challenging grafting procedures. Furthermore, survival rates and marginal bone level changes after 1 year of loading seem similar.

Q: What are the main implant shapes?

Tapered and straight are the main implant shapes[48] (Fig 13-10). $\rightarrow$

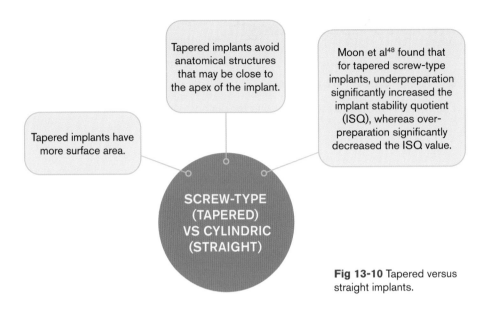

Tapered implants avoid anatomical structures that may be close to the apex of the implant.

Moon et al[48] found that for tapered screw-type implants, underpreparation significantly increased the implant stability quotient (ISQ), whereas over-preparation significantly decreased the ISQ value.

Tapered implants have more surface area.

SCREW-TYPE (TAPERED) VS CYLINDRIC (STRAIGHT)

Fig 13-10 Tapered versus straight implants.

Immediate Implants

Q: When can an immediate implant be useful?

If there is potential for postextraction bone resorption and ridge deformation, an immediate implant can be effective provided that stability is achieved.[18]

However, Araújo et al[49] discovered that implant placement in the extraction site did not stop the remodeling that occurred in the walls of the socket. At 3 months, they found that the buccal and lingual wall heights were similar in implant and edentulous sites.

Q: Can an immediate implant achieve osseointegration?

Wilson et al[50] conducted a histologic study of implants placed in immediate extraction sites and noted that titanium plasma-sprayed implants can achieve osseointegration when placed immediately into extraction sockets. They also found that the most critical aspect relating to the ultimate extent of bone-implant contact is the horizontal component of the peri-implant defect.

If there is a distance of more than 2 mm from the socket to the implant, bone graft materials are required to ensure success. Kahnberg[51] demon-strated a submerged surgical technique that had satisfactory clinical and →

radiographic outcomes over a 2-year period in 26 patients. The study noted that using autologous bone graft material to fill the gap between implant and labial bone resulted in implants being placed effectively in fresh extraction sockets.

Artzi et al[52] demonstrated that both delayed and immediate placement of implants are clinically effective, but immediate placement of implants leads to greater bone resorption around the implant neck and as a result decreases implant stability.

Q: What is the success rate for immediate implants?

In a prospective clinical trial of 134 implants in 81 patients, Becker et al[53] placed implants at the time of tooth extraction without barrier membranes or graft materials. The cumulative success rate for the 47 implants with 4- to 5-year follow-up was 93.3%.

Al-Shabeeb et al[54] suggested that multiple immediate implants placed in contiguous extraction sites are associated with significantly greater buccal bone remodeling than that seen with a single immediate implant placed in an extraction site.

Covani et al[55] conducted a prospective clinical study that found that immediate implants have a 91.8% success rate after 10 years. Guided bone regeneration made no difference in the success or survival of implants. During the 10-year evaluation, the clinical attachment level, marginal bone loss, and soft tissue measurements were stable.

Q: Is preservation of pink esthetics possible after immediate implant placement?

One study found that preservation of pink esthetics is feasible following immediate implant placement; however, to accomplish that, a connective tissue graft may be needed in about one-third of patients. Major alveolar process remodeling is the key cause for additional treatment.[56]

Q: Is there recession after immediate implant placement?

Chen et al[57] reported significant recession of the mesial papilla (-6.2% +/− 6.8%), distal papilla (-7.4% +/− 7.5%), and facial mucosa (-4.6% +/− 6.6%) between surgical placement (immediate placement without a flap) and 1 year postoperative.

Q: What is platform switching?

Platform switching is the use of an abutment that is smaller than the implant. The theory is that the microgap is moved away from the adjacent crestal bone, and there is a buffer zone to prevent bone loss since the shoulder of the platform has an extra zone of connective tissue.

Q: Has platform switching been shown to be effective?

Cappiello et al[58] found that the vertical bone loss for patients who did not receive a platform-switched abutment was between 1.3 and 2.1 mm. Patients who received an abutment 1 mm narrower than the platform had vertical bone loss between 0.6 and 1.2 mm. These figures validate the significant role of the microgap between the abutment and the implant in the remodeling of the peri-implant crestal bone. Not only does platform switching increase the long-term predictability of implant therapy, but it also reduces peri-implant crestal bone resorption.

Canullo et al[59] found that the group that received a narrower abutment had a bone reduction level of 0.30 mm, whereas the control had a bone reduction level of 1.19 mm. The study did not find differences between the two groups in bleeding on probing and pocket probing depth.

Effect of Smoking on Implants

Q: What is the failure rate of implants in smokers?

Strietzel et al[60] conducted a meta-analysis and found that smokers had a greater risk of implant failure (implant-related odds ratio [OR] of 2.25) compared with nonsmokers. The OR for implant placement with augmentation was 3.61 in smokers. Overall, the review suggested that the risk of biologic complications is significantly higher for smokers than for nonsmokers.

Moy et al[61] found that smokers had a relative risk ratio of 1.56 for implant failure. They noted that implant failure significantly increased among patients who were 60 years or older, smoked, had a history of diabetes or head and neck radiation, or were postmenopausal and taking hormone replacement therapy.

However, Aguirre-Zorzano et al[62] found no association between smoking and peri-implant disease. →

The 2017 World Workshop concluded that there is no conclusive evidence that smoking constitutes a risk factor for peri-implantitis.[17]

Q: Why can implants fail in smokers?

The reasons behind the high failure rate of implants in smokers include the following[63]:

- Carbon monoxide reduces oxygenation of the healing tissues.
- Nicotine is vasoconstrictive, increasing platelet aggregation and adhesiveness and reducing blood flow.
- Cytotoxic effects on fibroblasts and polymorphonuclear cells disrupt cell repair and defense.
- Wound healing is impaired, leading to a higher complication rate.

Peri-implant Mucositis and Peri-implantitis

Q: What is peri-implant mucositis?

An inflammatory lesion of the mucosa surrounding an endosseous implant without loss of supporting peri-implant bone. It occurs following accumulation of bacterial biofilms around osseointegrated dental implants.[64]

Q: What is peri-implantitis?

Peri-implantitis is defined as an inflammatory process affecting the tissue around an implant in function that has resulted in loss of supporting bone. Anaerobic bacteria are the primary factor for bone loss and have been observed in the sulcus of implants, especially when probing depths are greater than 5 mm.[65]

Q: Describe the difference between health, peri-implant mucositis, and peri-implantitis.

See Table 13-3 on the next page.

Table 13-3   Difference between health, peri-implant mucositis, and peri-implantitis[8,66]

	Peri-implant health	Peri-implant mucositis	Peri-implantitis

Clinical signs	• No erythema.
	• No BOP.
	• No inflammation, suppuration, or swelling.
	• The probing depth is less than 5 mm (probing depths at implant sites are usually greater than tooth sites).[8]
	• No changes ≥ 2 mm during or after the first year.
	• The mucosa forms a tight seal around the implant.
		• Swelling.
		• Redness.
		• Soreness.
		• Any BOP with inflammatory changes. Note that a local dot of blood could be from trauma and may not be mucositis.
		• The key parameter for the diagnosis of peri-implant mucositis is bleeding on gentle probing (0.25 N).[13]
		• Suppuration.
		• No bone loss.
		• An increase in probing depth is often observed due to swelling or decrease in probing resistance.
			• Soft tissue inflammation.
			• BOP.
			• Redness.
			• Edema.
			• Mucosal enlargement.
			• Suppuration is a common finding in peri-implantitis sites.[13]
			• Gradual bone loss is detected on radiographs.[17]
			• Same clinical signs of inflammation as peri-implant mucositis.[66]
			• Increasing probing depths compared to measurements obtained at placement.
			• Progression appears to be non-linear and faster than periodontitis.
			• In the absence of previous examination:
			  • Presence of bleeding and/or suppuration with gentle probing
			  • Probing depth ≥ 6 mm
			  • Bone levels ≥ 3 mm apical of the most coronal portion of the intraosseous part of the implant

Radiographic bone loss	No changes ≥ 2 mm at any point during or after the first year.	Changes ≥ 2 mm at any point during or after the first year should be considered pathologic.	• ≥ 2 mm of bone loss during or after the first year • Surgical entry at peri-implantitis sites often reveals a circumferential pattern of bone loss.[17]

Table 13-3 (cont)	Difference between health, peri-implant mucositis, and peri-implantitis[8,66]		
	Peri-implant health	Peri-implant mucositis	Peri-implantitis
Histologic characteristics	• The peri-implant mucosa is 3 to 4 mm high with an epithelium that is 2 mm long. • The buccal aspect is 3 to 4 mm high from crest of bone to the mucosal margin. • It contains a core of connective tissue, mainly comprised of collagen fibers and matrix elements (85%), few fibroblasts (3%), and vascular units (5%). Outer aspect of connective tissue is covered with orthokeratinized epithelium. • Mucosa facing the implant: Comprised of a coronal (thin barrier epithelium) and sulcular epithelium, and a more apical part in which the connective tissue seems to be in direct contact with the implant.[6] As in the natural dentition, the junctional epithelium is attached to the implant surface via a basal lamina and hemidesmosomes.[67] • Intrabony part of the implant is in contact with the bone.	• Inflammatory lesion lateral to the junctional/pocket epithelium with an infiltrate of vascular structures, lymphocytes, and plasma cells. • The infiltrate does not go apical to the junctional/pocket epithelium.	• Lesions extend apical of the junctional/pocket epithelium and contain macrophages, plasma cells, and neutrophils. • Lesions are larger than those at peri-implant mucositis sites.
Etiology		• Bacteria and plaque • Smoking, diabetes, and radiation therapy may modify the condition • Reversible	• Gram-negative bacteria and *Staphylococcus aureus* may be an important bacterium in initiation of peri-implantitis. A 2012 study[68] found colonization by bacteria at the implant sulcus was influenced by microorganisms in the gingival crevice of adjacent teeth as opposed to those on contralateral and occluding teeth. • Patients without regular maintenance therapy are at a higher risk of developing peri-implantitis.

Q: Describe the similarities and differences between gingivitis and peri-implant mucositis.

See Table 13-4 below.

Table 13-4	Comparison of biofilm-induced gingivitis and peri-implant mucositis[64]			
	Definition	**Symptoms**	**Can it be reversed?**	**Histology**
Gingivitis	Gingival inflammation without periodontal attachment loss	Swelling, redness, and bleeding on gentle probing	After biofilm control, experimental gingivitis can be reversed.	Increased proportions of inflammatory cells in connective tissue
Peri-implant mucositis	Peri-implant mucosal inflammation in absence of continuous marginal peri-implant bone loss	Swelling, suppuration, redness, and bleeding on gentle probing	It may take 3 weeks for reversal of experimental peri-implant mucositis.[69] Another study by Salvi et al[70] found that although experimental gingivitis and peri-implant mucositis were reversible at the biomarker level, 3 weeks of continued plaque control did not yield pre-experimental levels of gingival and peri-implant mucosal health, signifying that longer healing periods are needed.	Increased proportions of inflammatory cells in connective tissue

Q: Describe the similarities and differences between periodontitis and peri-implantitis.

See Fig 13-11 below.

Apical lesion	Histology	Self-limiting?	Biofilm formation
• The apical extension of the lesion was more pronounced in peri-implantitis than in periodontitis. • Peri-implantitis lesions are circumferential in nature.	• While plasma cells and lymphocytes dominated in both types of lesions, neutrophil granulocytes and macrophages occurred in larger proportions in peri-implantitis than in periodontitis. • Peri-implantitis lesions, in contrast to periodontitis lesions, exhibit signs of acute inflammation and large amounts of osteoclasts that line the surface of the crestal bone.	• A "self-limiting" process existed in the tissues around teeth that resulted in a protective connective tissue capsule that separated the lesion from the alveolar bone. • Such a "self-limiting" process did not occur in peri-implant tissues, and the lesion can extend to the bony crest.	The basic principles of biofilm formation are similar.

Fig 13-11 Similarities and differences between periodontitis and peri-implantitis.

Wong et al[71] found that peri-implantitis does not respond as well to insult removal as periodontitis.

Q: What can cause/be associated with peri-implantitis? Peri-implant mucositis?

- Cement trapped below the gingiva.[72]
- Risk indicator for peri-implant mucositis.[73]
- Foreign bodies primarily consisting of titanium and dental cement were found to be associated with an inflammatory infiltrate.[74]
- Inadequate seating of the restoration on the abutment.
- Overcontouring the restoration.
- Implant malpositioning—Canullo et al[75] found that malpositioning was the most important factor with an odds ratio of 48 for signs and symptoms of peri-implantitis.
- Submucosal restoration margins.[76]
- IL-1RN gene polymorphism.[77]
- Endodontic pathology—In a retrospective study, Quirynen et al[78] noted that endodontic pathology of an extracted tooth (scar tissue–impacted tooth),

$\rightarrow$

residual granulomatous tissue at the recipient site, or potential endodontic pathology from a neighboring tooth can trigger retrograde peri-implantitis.
- Radiation.

Heitz-Mayfield[79] found substantial evidence that the following factors are associated with peri-implantitis:

- Poor oral hygiene.
- History of periodontitis.[17]
- Cigarette smoking—risk indicator for peri-implant mucositis.[73]
- Thin soft tissues lead to increased marginal bone loss compared to thick soft tissues at implants.[7]

There is limited evidence that the following factors are associated with peri-implantitis:

- Poorly controlled diabetes (see below question)
- Alcohol consumption
- Metal and titanium particles detected in peri-implant supporting tissues[80]

Monje et al[81] found (in a cross-sectional study) that compliance with maintenance therapy was associated with 86% fewer conditions of peri-implantitis. Koldsland et al[82] found a strong association between the presence of plaque and inflammation, but no association was found between the presence of plaque and detectible bone loss. Thus the 2017 World Workshop[17] concluded that there is evidence that poor control and lack of regular maintenance therapy constitutes risk factors/indicators for peri-implantitis. However, the workshop found no evidence that occlusal overload constitutes a risk factor for the onset or progression of peri-implantitis.

Berglundh et al[83] proposed that the development of peri-implantitis, if untreated, is less distinct at implants with a polished surface than at implants with a moderately rough surface (sandblasted acid-etched surfaces).

Q: When do you know an implant has failed?

Implant failure is defined as the state where the implant is no longer integrated after placement. Failure may occur early (ie, before osseointegration and usually during the first year) or late (ie, during and after the restorative treatment).[84] Primary stability at the time of implant placement is necessary to ensure successful osseointegration. One meta-analysis found the failure rate at 7.7% over a 5-year period (bone graft excluded).[85] Another study[86] found implant failure of 2% to 3% when the implant was in function and for implants supporting fixed reconstructions. Patients with overdentures had a 5% failure

$\rightarrow$

rate during a 5-year period. No evident differences in implant survival were found between the different implant systems.[87]

Q: **If an implant is mobile, what would be the reason?**

1. Infection
2. Host factors (smoking, autoimmune disorders)
3. Occlusion and loading
4. Poor bone quality
5. Poor prosthetic design[84]
6. Inability of the surgeon to achieve primary stability
7. Trauma to the tissue (pressure necrosis and overheating of the bone[84])
8. Prior history of periodontitis

Q: **Is diabetes associated with peri-implant mucositis?**

Ferreira et al[88] did a cross-sectional study with 193 patients and found peri-implant mucositis was more associated with the participants over 57 years of age, with systemic disease, and with their prostheses in function for more than 5 years. Ferreira et al[89] also found that subjects with uncontrolled diabetes presented higher risks of developing peri-implantitis (OR: 1.9; 95% confidence interval: 1.0–2.2).

However, Costa et al[90] found diabetes was not associated with the occurrence of peri-implant disease in subjects with preexisting peri-implant mucositis. Similarly, Shi et al[91] did a meta-analysis that failed to show a difference in the failure rates for dental implants between patients with well-controlled diabetes and patients with diabetes that was not well controlled. Thus the 2017 World Workshop found that the available evidence is inconclusive as to whether diabetes is a risk factor/indicator for peri-implantitis. They also found that evidence suggesting other systemic disease to be a risk factor for peri-implantitis is limited.[17]

Q: **Does progressive crestal bone loss around implants transpire without soft tissue inflammation?**

Progressive crestal bone loss around implants without soft tissue inflammation is a rare finding.[17]

Q: In what percentage of patients do peri-implant mucositis and peri-implantitis occur?

Jepsen[73] found prevalence for peri-implant mucositis of 43% and for peri-implantitis of 22%. See Fig 13-12.

Lindhe et al[93] noted that peri-implantitis occurs in between 28% and 56% of patients treated with implants and peri-implant mucositis occurs in about 80% of patients.

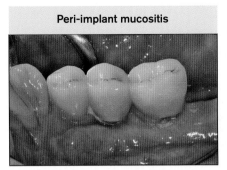
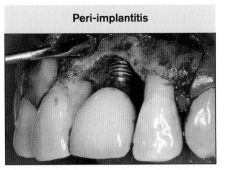

Peri-implant mucositis

Peri-implantitis

Fig 13-12 Clinical example of peri-implant mucositis and peri-implantitis.[92]

Q: What is the incidence of peri-implantitis in individuals with peri-implant mucositis?

Costa et al[90] did a longitudinal study and found the incidence of peri-implantitis as 31.2% in individuals with mucositis in a 5-year follow-up study. The study found 18% of the patients complying with supportive therapy presented with peri-implantitis, while the corresponding proportion in patients who did not adhere to supportive therapy was 43.9%. The study also found that the absence of preventive maintenance in individuals with preexisting peri-implant mucositis was related with a high incidence of peri-implantitis. Clinical parameters, such as bleeding on peri-implant probing, periodontal probing depth, and the presence of periodontitis were related with an elevated risk of developing peri-implantitis at 5 years.

Q: Describe the pattern and severity of peri-implantitis.

Fransson et al[94] found that the average bone loss after the first year of function was 1.68 mm and 32% of the implants exhibited bone loss 2 mm or greater. The multilevel model showed that the bone loss presented a non-linear pattern and that the rate of bone loss increased over time. →

Surgical entry at peri-implantitis sites shows a circumferential pattern of bone loss.[17]

Q: How effective is chlorhexidine in treating peri-implant mucositis?

Menezes et al[95] found 0.12% chlorhexidine was not more effective than placebo in treatment of peri-implant mucositis.

Heitz-Mayfield et al[76] found adjunctive chlorhexidine gel application did not show improvements compared with mechanical cleansing alone in patients with peri-implant mucositis.

Q: Does the addition of adjunctive methods (antiseptics, systemic antibiotics, and air abrasive device) improve peri-implant mucositis?

A systematic study[96] found adjunctive therapy may not improve the efficacy of professionally administered plaque removal in reducing bleeding on probing, Gingival Index, and pocket depth scores at mucositis sites.

Q: How should peri-implantitis be treated?

Byrne[97] noted that the evidence is inconclusive regarding the most effective method of treating peri-implantitis. In most cases, simple mechanical debridement seemed to achieve results that were similar to those of more complex therapies.

See Fig 13-13 on the next page on the management of peri-implantitis (cumulative interceptive supportive therapy).[98]

A novel surgical approach is the circumferential occlusal access procedure (COAP),[99] a minimally invasive, flapless surgical technique designed to access and detoxify a contaminated implant surface and facilitate bone repair or regeneration while reducing the potential for membrane exposure and recession. A curette is used around the implant with no restoration. Granulation tissue is removed, and the area is detoxified.

A study comparing CO_2 laser and hydrogen peroxide versus saline on a cotton pellet found re-osseointegration of 21% and 82% at laser-treated turned-surface implants and sand-blasted large-grit acid-etched (SLA) implants, respectively, and 22% and 84% at saline-treated turned-surface implants and SLA implants, respectively.[100] Another study[101] comparing the Er:YAG laser (ERL) versus plastic curettes + cotton pellets + sterile saline →

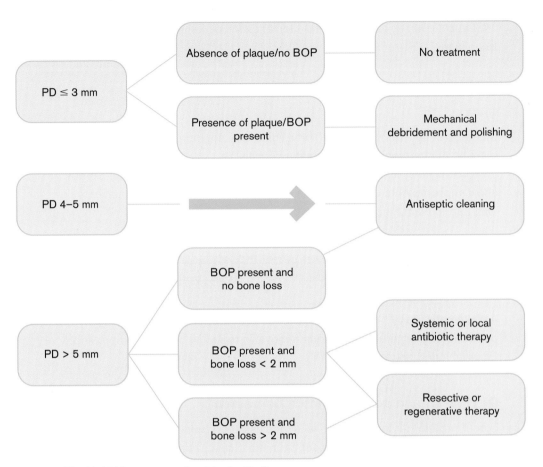

Fig 13-13 Management of peri-implantitis.[98]

(CPS) found that the CPS-treated sites tended to reveal higher reductions in mean BOP (CPS: 85.2% ± 16.4% versus ERL: 71.6% ± 24.9%) and clinical attachment level values (CPS: 1.5 ± 2.0 mm versus ERL: 1.2 ± 2.0 mm).

Implant Hygiene

Q: What instruments can be used on implant surfaces?

Mengel et al[102] studied the effect of the DenSonic sonic scaler (Senova) with universal tips, the Cavitron Jet ultrasonic unit (Dentsply), rubber cups, a plastic curette, a titanium curette, and a Gracey curette on the implant surface. All instruments except the rubber cup and Cavitron Jet air polishing system

$\rightarrow$

left marked traces at the transition of the implant head to the titanium plasma coating of the full-screw implants. The study found that the plastic curette, Cavitron Jet air polishing system, DenSonic sonic scaler (in some situations), and rubber cup are appropriate for cleaning the implant surface.

Fox et al[103] found that metal instruments considerably changed the titanium surface, as opposed to plastic instruments, which produced an insignificant alteration of the implant surface.

Q: What is the impact of regular maintenance on implant survival?

Gay et al[104] performed a retrospective study and found that subjects with no maintenance had the lowest cumulative survival rate as compared to subjects with regular maintenance. Regular maintenance patients had the dental implant failure rate reduced by 90% as compared to no maintenance.

Sinus Elevation

Q: What is the function of the maxillary sinus?

1. Reduce skull weight
2. Produce mucus
3. Resonance of a person's voice
4. Warming of air

Q: What percentage of sinuses have septa?

According to Ulm et al,[105] 30% of sinuses have septa (usually in the middle) between the second premolar and first molar.

Q: Describe the shape and dimensions of the maxillary sinus.

The maxillary sinus is pyramidal in shape (Fig 13-14; see next page). It averages 3.75 cm in height and 2.5 cm in width. Its anteroposterior depth averages 3 cm.

Q: What is the blood supply to the sinus?

Blood is supplied to the sinus through the posterior superior alveolar artery, infraorbital artery, and posterior superior nasal artery.

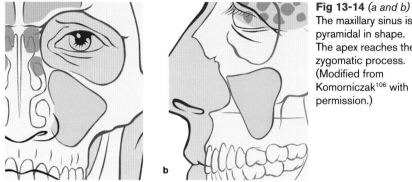

Fig 13-14 *(a and b)* The maxillary sinus is pyramidal in shape. The apex reaches the zygomatic process. (Modified from Komorniczak[106] with permission.)

Q: What is the innervation to the sinus?

The superior alveolar nerves (anterior, medial, and posterior) and infraorbital nerve innervate the sinus.

Q: Describe how to perform a sinus elevation.

Boyne and James[107] and Tatum[108] first described the procedure. The lateral window procedure is described in Fig 13-15.

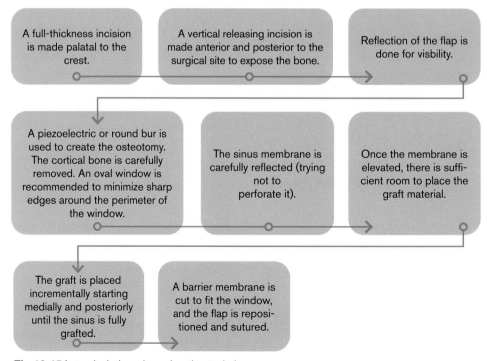

A full-thickness incision is made palatal to the crest.

A vertical releasing incision is made anterior and posterior to the surgical site to expose the bone.

Reflection of the flap is done for visbility.

A piezoelectric or round bur is used to create the osteotomy. The cortical bone is carefully removed. An oval window is recommended to minimize sharp edges around the perimeter of the window.

The sinus membrane is carefully reflected (trying not to perforate it).

Once the membrane is elevated, there is sufficient room to place the graft material.

The graft is placed incrementally starting medially and posteriorly until the sinus is fully grafted.

A barrier membrane is cut to fit the window, and the flap is repositioned and sutured.

Fig 13-15 Lateral window sinus elevation technique.

Q: What is the average rate of sinus membrane perforation?

Tan et al[109] performed a meta-analysis on the osteotome technique and found that membrane perforation varied between 0% and 21.4%, with a mean of 3.8%.

Malet et al[110] state that perforation of the sinus membrane is the most frequent complication, occurring in about 20% of procedures.

Q: Is there a difference in the rate of sinus membrane perforation when using a round bur versus a piezoelectric instrument?

Wallace et al[111] found that employing the piezoelectric technique reduced the membrane perforation rate (in 100 cases) from the mean reported rate of 30% with rotary instrumentation to 7%. Additionally, all perforations with the piezoelectric technique did not happen with the piezoelectric inserts but during hand instrumentation.

Toscano et al[112] noted that during 56 sinus elevation procedures using the piezoelectric technique, no perforations of the sinus membrane occurred. However, using the hand instrumentation technique, two perforations were noted. The overall sinus perforation rate was 3.6%.

Q: In general, what is the infection rate when a sinus elevation is performed?

Tan et al[109] found that infection was the most common postoperative complication associated with sinus elevation. Of the 19 reviewed studies, with 884 implants, only six reported on postoperative infection. The mean postoperative infection rate was 0.8% (range, 0% to 2.5%).

Malet et al[110] reported an infection rate of grafted sinuses of approximately 3% and graft loss from severe complications at a rate of approximately 2%.

Q: What steps should be taken if a patient develops an infection following a sinus elevation procedure?

Rosen[113] recommends taking the steps presented in Fig 13-16 in cases of postoperative infection following sinus elevation. →

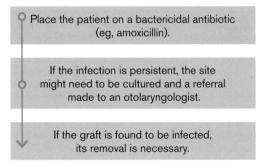

Place the patient on a bactericidal antibiotic (eg, amoxicillin).

If the infection is persistent, the site might need to be cultured and a referral made to an otolaryngologist.

If the graft is found to be infected, its removal is necessary.

Fig 13-16 Steps to be taken to treat an infection following sinus elevation.

Q: Which bone material has been found to be the most beneficial for sinus augmentation?

A systematic review by Wallace and Froum[114] found that block grafting of the sinus resulted in a statistically significantly lower implant survival rate (83.3%) than particulate grafts (92.3%). The review found no difference in implant survival between particulate autogenous bone and particulate bone replacement grafts.

Froum et al[115] found anorganic bovine bone to be an effective graft material with 98.2% implant survival.

Piero et al[116] performed a study in which 28 implants were placed in 15 patients (with an average residual bone height of 6.2 mm) with sinus membrane elevation without biomaterials. At the 1-year follow-up, all 28 implants had survived.

Al Nawas and Schiegnitz[117] did a systematic review and found no difference between autogenous bone and bone substitute materials when used in maxillary sinus floor augmentation and vertical and/or lateral alveolar ridge augmentation.

Q: Has platelet-rich plasma (PRP) been shown to be beneficial when placed in the sinus?

A review by Wallace and Froum[114] found insufficient data to recommend PRP for sinus graft surgery.

Sánchez et al[117] did not find sufficient dental implant literature regarding the use of PRP. Of the six human studies using PRP, five were case series or reports. The study could not recommend the use of PRP mixed with bone graft material during regeneration procedures due to a lack of scientific $\rightarrow$

evidence. Well-designed, controlled studies are needed to provide evidence for the use of PRP.

Q: What is the success rate of dental implants in a staged sinus elevation procedure?

Bornstein et al[118] found that titanium screw-type implants with a titanium plasma-sprayed or SLA surface inserted in a two-stage sinus elevation procedure in the posterior maxilla had a 98% 5-year success rate.

Q: Is it necessary to place a membrane over the window?

Tarnow et al[119] studied 12 patients who received sinus elevations with and without placement of a nonresorbable membrane. They found that place-ment of the barrier membrane tends to increase vital bone formation. It also has a positive effect on implant survival. Those who received a membrane had an implant survival of 100% versus 92.6% for those who did not have a membrane placed.

Tawil and Mawla[120] reported a survival rate of 93.1% for the membrane group and 78.1% for the no-membrane group in their controlled study.

McAllister and Haghighat[121] found that the placement of graft material and a resorbable or nonresorbable barrier membrane over the lateral sinus window aided in graft containment, prevented soft tissue encleftation, and enhanced the implant success rate.

Q: Does the implant surface affect the survival of the implant in the sinus?

Wallace and Froum[114] found that the survival rates of rough surface implants and machined surface implants were 94.6% and 90%, respectively, in the sinus.

Q: Can implants be placed simultaneously with sinus elevation?

The sinus elevation should be performed 4 to 6 months before implant placement if there is 4 to 6 mm of vertical bone between the antral floor and the crest of the ridge. However, if there is greater than 4 to 6 mm of bone, implants can be placed simultaneously as long as they are stable[122] (Fig 13-17). →

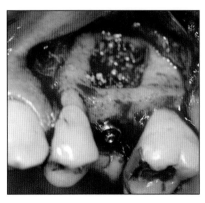

Fig 13-17 Implant placement and sinus augmentation performed simultaneously.

Osteotome

Q: What is the osteotome technique?

Summers1[123] introduced the bone-added osteotome sinus floor elevation procedure in 1994. The sinus floor is elevated by inward collapse of the residual crestal floor with specially designed osteotomes. Bone graft material can be introduced through the prepared osteotomy, if needed, with or without simultaneous implant placement. The amount of augmentation achieved by the osteotome technique was 3 to 5 mm.[121]

Q: Describe the osteotome technique.

During the procedure, radiographs should be taken.

- A 2-mm twist drill is used to drill within 1 mm of the sinus floor.
- An osteotome is used to elevate the sinus floor.
- Bone is pushed into the area of the osteotomy before implant placement.

Q: What is the minimum bone height needed to perform the osteotome technique?

Rosen et al[124] treated 101 patients with 174 implants. Screw-type and cylindric implants with machined, titanium plasma-sprayed, and hydroxyapatite surfaces from different manufacturers were used. When pretreatment bone height was 5 mm or more, the survival rate was 96% or higher; however, when pretreatment bone height was 4 mm or less, the survival rate fell to $\rightarrow$

85.7%. Preexisting bone height between the sinus floor and the crest was the most important factor influencing implant survival.

Toffler[125] found that the osteotome technique has a survival rate of 93.5%. The survival rate fell to 73.3% when only sites with a residual bone height of 4 mm or less were considered. The height of the residual alveolar ridge was the chief determinant. Graft material, implant design, and the method of sinus floor infracture (direct or bone-cushioned) exerted minimal influence on survival outcome; conversely, issues such as an overdenture prosthesis, edentulism, and osteoporosis were shown to negatively impact postloading survival of implants placed in regions of limited residual bone height.

Q: Is there a difference in implant survival between implants placed conventionally and implants placed at the time of osteotomy?

The survival rate of implants placed with the osteotome technique is high and does not differ with respect to implant placement with the conventional technique.[126]

Shi et al[127] did a review and found cumulative survival rates were significantly higher in the group that did the osteotome technique and did not graft than in the graft group. Early failures (< 1 year functional loading) accounted for most of the implant failures. The cumulative survival rates in the graft group were considerably lower when the residual bone height was < 5 mm, while the cumulative survival rates in the non-graft group exhibited no statistically signif-icant difference based on residual bone height. Shorter (< 8-mm) implants demonstrated significantly lower cumulative survival rates than longer implants.

Q: Describe the advantages and disadvantages of a lateral window versus a crestal sinus elevation.

See Fig 13-18 on the next page.[128]

Q: What is the success rate for implants placed using the osteotome method compared with implants placed with a sinus elevation?

Pal et al[129] reported that the gain in bone height was significantly greater in a direct procedure through lateral antrostomy (mean, 8.5 mm) than through a crestal approach by osteotome technique (mean, 4.4 mm). Both sinus eleva-tion techniques did not seem to affect the implant success rate.

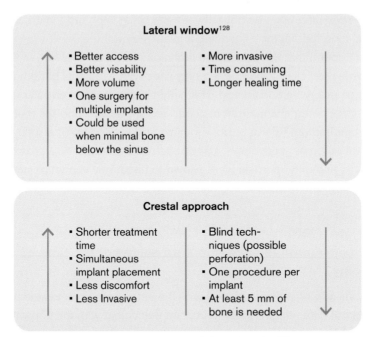

Fig 13-18 Lateral window versus crestal sinus elevation.[128]

Alternatives to Implants

Q: Are fixed partial dentures a better option than an implant-supported single implant? How does root canal therapy compare with both options?

Torabinejad et al[130] found success rates for root canal therapy and fixed partial dentures to be lower than those for an implant-supported single implant, yet success criteria differed greatly among the various treatments, which makes comparisons challenging. A stand-alone implant and root canal therapy had survival rates comparable and superior to that of fixed partial dentures.

Salinas and Eckert[131] performed a systematic review and found that fixed partial dentures of all designs at 60 months exhibited an 84.0% success rate, while single-implant restorations at 60 months demonstrated a 95.1% success rate.

Iqbal and Kim[132] found no substantial dissimilarities in survival between single-tooth implants and restored root canal–treated teeth.

Q: What are the alternatives to implants?

Figure 13-19 presents the alternatives to implant placement.

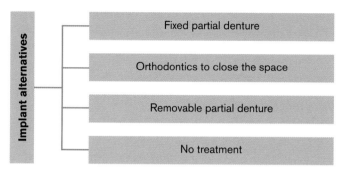

Fig 13-19 Alternatives to implant placement.

Miscellaneous

Q: Is there a difference in success rate with placement of an implant in a clean versus a sterile condition?

Scharf and Tarnow[133] found implant success rates of 98.9% under sterile conditions and 98.2% under clean conditions (not statistically significant). In order to attain a similar high rate of osseointegration, implant surgery can be performed under both sterile and clean conditions.

Q: Describe the interface between an implant and the epithelium.

The interface between an implant and the epithelium consists of hemidesmosomes and basal lamina. The biologic width is 3 to 4 mm with 2 mm of epithelial attachment and 1 mm of connective tissue attachment. Collagen fibers are parallel to the implant.

Q: What is the survival rate of implants placed in irradiated bone?

Buddula et al[134] did a retrospective study and found that implants placed in patients with head and neck cancer who had received radiation treatment had a greater risk of failure compared with those placed in nonirradiated $\rightarrow$

bone. The survival of the implants at 1 year was 98.9%, at 5 years 89.9%, and at 10 years 72.3%. The study also found that implants placed in the maxilla had a greater chance of failure than those placed in the mandible. Lastly, implants placed in the posterior region had a greater likelihood of failure than those placed anteriorly.

Q: Can an implant be placed in sclerotic bone?

A CBCT scan, preferably with high resolution and a small field of view, should be ordered to assess how sclerotic the bone is and the extent of the changes. The problem with sclerotic bone is the decreased vascularity, which may compromise healing and osseointegration.

References

1. Brånemark PI, Zarb GA, Albrektsson T (eds). Tissue-Integrated Prostheses. Chicago: Quintessence, 1985.
2. Zarb GA, Albrektsson T. Criteria for determining clinical success with osseointegrated dental implants [in French]. Cah Prothese 1990;(71):19–26.
3. Cochran DL. A comparison of endosseous dental implant surfaces. J Periodontol 1999;70:1523–1539.
4. Moraschini V, Poubel LA, Ferreira VF, Barboza Edos S. Evaluation of survival and success rates of dental implants reported in longitudinal studies with a follow-up period of at least 10 years: A systematic review. Int J Oral Maxillofac Surg 2015;44:377–388.
5. Adell R, Lekholm U, Rockler B, Brånemark PI. A 15-year study of osseointegrated implants in the treatment of the edentulous jaw. Int J Oral Surg 1981;10:387–416.
6. Araujo MG, Lindhe J. Peri-implant health. J Periodontol 2018;89(suppl 1):S249–S256.
7. Hämmerle CHF, Tarnow D. The etiology of hard- and soft-tissue deficiencies at dental implants: A narrative review. J Periodontol 2018;89(suppl 1):S291–S303.
8. Berglundh T, Armitage G, Araujo MG, et al. Peri-implant diseases and conditions: Consensus report of workgroup 4 of the 2017 World Workshop on the Classification of Periodontal and Peri-Implant Diseases and Conditions. J Periodontol 2018;89(suppl 1):S313–S318.
9. Evans CD, Chen ST. Esthetic outcomes of immediate implant placements. Clin Oral Implants Res 2008;19:73–80.
10. Laskin DM, Dent CD, Morris HF, Ochi S, Olson JW. The influence of preoperative antibiotics on success of endosseous implants at 36 months. Ann Periodontol 2000;5:166–174.
11. Esposito M, Grusovin MG, Loli V, Coulthard P, Worthington HV. Does antibiotic prophylaxis at implant placement decrease early implant failures? A Cochrane systematic review. Eur J Oral Implantol 2010;3:101–110.
12. Schierano G, Pejrone G, Roana J, et al. A split-mouth study on microbiological profile in clinical healthy teeth and implants related to key inflammatory mediators. Int J Immunopathol Pharmacol 2010;23:279–288.
13. Lang NP, Berglundh T; Working Group 4 of Seventh European Workshop on Periodontology. Periimplant diseases: Where are we now?—Consensus of the Seventh European Workshop on Periodontology. J Clin Periodontol 2011;38(suppl 11):178–181.

14. Leonhardt A, Berglundh T, Ericsson I, Dahlén G. Putative periodontal pathogens on titanium implants and teeth in experimental gingivitis and periodontitis in beagle dogs. Clin Oral Implants Res 1992;3:112–119.
15. Hämmerle CH, Wagner D, Brägger U, et al. Threshold of tactile sensitivity perceived with dental endosseous implants and natural teeth. Clin Oral Implants Res 1995;6:83–90.
16. Sheridan RA, Decker AM, Plonka AB, Wang HL. The role of occlusion in implant therapy: A comprehensive updated review. Implant Dent 2016;25:829–838.
17. Schwarz F, Derks J, Monje A, Wang HL. Peri-implantitis. J Periodontol 2018;89(suppl 1):S267–S290.
18. The Research, Science and Therapy Committee of the American Academy of Periodontology. Position paper: Dental implants in periodontal therapy. J Periodontol 2000;71:1934–1942.
19. Khang W, Feldman S, Hawley CE, Gunsolley J. A multi-center study comparing dual acid-etched and machined-surfaced implants in various bone qualities. J Periodontol 2001;72:1384–1390.
20. Nasatzky E, Gultchin J, Schwartz Z. The role of surface roughness in promoting osteointegration [in Hebrew]. Refuat Hapeh Vehashinayim 2003;20:8–19,98.
21. Bouri A Jr, Bissada N, Al-Zahrani MS, Faddoul F, Nouneh I. Width of keratinized gingiva and the health status of the supporting tissues around dental implants. Int J Oral Maxillofac Implants 2008;23:323–326.
22. Chung DM, Oh TJ, Shotwell JL, Misch CE, Wang HL. Significance of keratinized mucosa in maintenance of dental implants with different surfaces. J Periodontol 2006;77:1410–1420.
23. Souza AB, Tormena M, Matarazzo F, Araújo MG. The influence of peri-implant keratinized mucosa on brushing discomfort and peri-implant tissue health. Clin Oral Implants Res 2016;27:650–655.
24. Lin GH, Chan HL, Wang HL. The significance of keratinized mucosa on implant health: A systematic review. J Periodontol 2013;84:1755–1767.
25. Baelum V, Ellegaard B. Implant survival in periodontally compromised patients. J Periodontol 2004;75:1404–1412.
26. Karoussis IK, Kotsovilis S, Fourmousis I. A comprehensive and critical review of dental implant prognosis in periodontally compromised partially edentulous patients. Clin Oral Implants Res 2007;18:669–679.
27. Ong CT, Ivanovski S, Needleman IG, et al. Systematic review of implant outcomes in treated periodontitis subjects. J Clin Periodontol 2008;35:438–462.
28. Swierkot K, Lottholz P, Flores-de-Jacoby L, Mengel R. Mucositis, peri-implantitis, implant success, and survival of implants in patients with treated generalized aggressive periodontitis: 3- to 16-year results of a prospective long-term cohort study. J Periodontol 2012;83:1213–1225.
29. Roccuzzo M, Bonino F, Aglietta M, Dalmasso P. Ten-year results of a three arms prospective cohort study on implants in periodontally compromised patients. Part 2: Clinical results. Clin Oral Implants Res 2012;23:389–395.
30. Rasperini G, Siciliano VI, Cafiero C, Salvi GE, Blasi A, Aglietta M. Crestal bone changes at teeth and implants in periodontally healthy and periodontally compromised patients. A 10-year comparative case-series study. J Periodontol 2014;85:e152–e159.
31. Newman MG, Takei HH, Klokkevold PR, Carranza FA. Newman and Carranza's Clinical Periodontology, ed 13. Philadelphia: Elsevier, 2019:785.
32. Chrcanovic BR, Abreu MH. Survival and complications of zygomatic implants: A systematic review. Oral Maxillofac Surg 2013;17:81–93.
33. Derks J, Schaller D, Håkansson J, Wennström JL, Tomasi C, Berglundh T. Effectiveness of implant therapy analyzed in a swedish population: Prevalence of peri-implantitis. J Dent Res 2016;95:43–49.
34. Tarnow DP, Magner AW, Fletcher P. The effect of the distance from the contact point to the crest of bone on the presence or absence of the interproximal dental papilla. J Periodontol 1992;63:995–996.
35. Tarnow D, Elian N, Fletcher P, et al. Vertical distance from the crest of bone to the height of the interproximal papilla between adjacent implants. J Periodontol 2003;74:1785–1788.

36. Vela X, Méndez V, Rodríguez X, Segalá M, Tarnow DP. Crestal bone changes on platform-switched implants and adjacent teeth when the tooth-implant distance is less than 1.5 mm. Int J Periodontics Restorative Dent 2012;32:149–155.

37. Pradeep AR, Karthikeyan BV. Peri-implant papilla reconstruction: realities and limitations. J Periodontol 2006;77:534–544.

38. Besler U, Vernard JP, Buser D. Implant placement in the esthetic zone: In: Lindhe J, Karring T, Lang NP (eds). Clinical Periodontology and Implant Dentistry, ed 4. Oxford, UK: Blackwell Munksgaard, 2003:918.

39. Huynh-Ba G, Pjetursson BE, Sanz M, et al. Analysis of the socket bone wall dimensions in the upper maxilla in relation to immediate implant placement. Clin Oral Implants Res 2010;21:37–42.

40. Fuchigami K, Munakata M, Kitazume T, Tachikawa N, Kasugai S, Kuroda S. A diversity of peri-implant mucosal thickness by site. Clin Oral Implants Res 2017;28:171–176.

41. Grunder U. Crestal ridge width changes when placing implants at the time of tooth extraction with and without soft tissue augmentation after a healing period of 6 months: Report of 24 consecutive cases. Int J Periodontics Restorative Dent 2011;31:9–17.

42. Wöhrle PS. Single-tooth replacement in the aesthetic zone with immediate provisionalization: Fourteen consecutive case reports. Pract Periodontics Aesthet Dent 1998;10:1107–1114.

43. Rompen E, Raepsaet N, Domken O, Touati B, Van Dooren E. Soft tissue stability at the facial aspect of gingivally converging abutments in the esthetic zone: A pilot clinical study. J Prosthet Dent 2007;97(6 suppl):S119–S125.

44. Patil R, van Brakel R, Iyer K, Huddleston Slater J, de Putter C, Cune M. A comparative study to evaluate the effect of two different abutment designs on soft tissue healing and stability of mucosal margins. Clin Oral Implants Res 2013;24:336–341.

45. Galindo-Moreno P, León-Cano A, Ortega-Oller I, et al. Prosthetic abutment height is a key factor in peri-implant marginal bone loss. J Dent Res 2014;93(7 suppl):80S–85S.

46. Fugazzotto PA. Shorter implants in clinical practice: Rationale and treatment results. Int J Oral Maxillofac Implants 2008;23:487–496.

47. Camps-Font O, Burgueño-Barris G, Figueiredo R, Jung RE, Gay-Escoda C, Valmaseda-Castellón E. Interventions for dental implant placement in atrophic edentulous mandibles: Vertical bone augmentation and alternative treatments. A meta-analysis of randomized clinical trials. J Periodontol 2016;87:1444–1457.

48. Moon SH, Um HS, Lee JK, Chang BS, Lee MK. The effect of implant shape and bone preparation on primary stability. J Periodontal Implant Sci 2010;40:239–243.

49. Araújo MG, Sukekava F, Wennström JL, Lindhe J. Ridge alterations following implant placement in fresh extraction sockets: An experimental study in the dog. J Clin Periodontol 2005;32:645–652.

50. Wilson TG Jr, Schenk R, Buser D, Cochran D. Implants placed in immediate extraction sites: A report of histologic and histometric analyses of human biopsies. Int J Oral Maxillofac Implants 1998;13:333–341.

51. Kahnberg KE. Immediate implant placement in fresh extraction sockets: A clinical report. Int J Oral Maxillofac Implants 2009;24:282–288.

52. Artzi Z, Nemcovsky CE, Tal H, Kozlovsky A. Timing of implant placement and augmentation with bone replacement material: Clinical assessment at 8 and 16 months. Clin Implant Dent Relat Res 2013;15:121–129.

53. Becker BE, Becker W, Ricci A, Geurs N. A prospective clinical trial of endosseous screw-shaped implants placed at the time of tooth extraction without augmentation. J Periodontol 1998;69:920–926.

54. Al-Shabeeb MS, Al-Askar M, Al-Rasheed A, et al. Alveolar bone remodeling around immediate implants placed in accordance with the extraction socket classification: A three-dimensional microcomputed tomography analysis. J Periodontol 2012;83:981–987.

55. Covani U, Chiappe G, Bosco M, Orlando B, Quaranta A, Barone A. A 10-year evaluation of implants placed in fresh extraction sockets: A prospective cohort study. J Periodontol 2012;83:1226–1234.

56. Cosyn J, De Bruyn H, Cleymaet R. Soft tissue preservation and pink aesthetics around single immediate implant restorations: A 1-year prospective study. Clin Implant Dent Relat Res 2013;15:847–857.

57. Chen ST, Darby IB, Reynolds EC, Clement JG. Immediate implant placement postextraction without flap elevation. J Periodontol 2009;80:163–172.

58. Cappiello M, Luongo R, Di Iorio D, Bugea C, Cocchetto R, Celletti R. Evaluation of peri-implant bone loss around platform-switched implants. Int J Periodontics Restorative Dent 2008;28:347–355.

59. Canullo L, Goglia G, Iurlaro G, Iannello G. Short-term bone level observations associated with platform switching in immediately placed and restored single maxillary implants: A preliminary report. Int J Prosthodont 2009;22:277–282.

60. Strietzel FP, Reichart PA, Kale A, Kulkarni M, Wegner B, Küchler I. Smoking interferes with the prognosis of dental implant treatment: A systematic review and meta-analysis. J Clin Periodontol 2007;34:523–544.

61. Moy PK, Medina D, Shetty V, Aghaloo TL. Dental implant failure rates and associated risk factors. Int J Oral Maxillofac Implants 2005;20:569–577.

62. Aguirre-Zorzano LA, Estefania-Fresco R, Telletxea O, Bravo M. Prevalence of peri-implant inflammatory disease in patients with a history of periodontal disease who receive supportive periodontal therapy. Clin Oral Implants Res 2015;26:1338–1344.

63. Liddelow G, Klineberg I. Patient-related risk factors for implant therapy. A critique of pertinent literature. Aust Dent J 2011;56:417–426.

64. Heitz-Mayfield LJA, Salvi GE. Peri-implant mucositis. J Periodontol 2018;89(suppl 1):S257–S266.

65. Misch CE, Perel ML, Wang HL, et al. Implant success, survival, and failure: The International Congress of Oral Implantologists (ICOI) Pisa Consensus Conference. Implant Dent 2008;17:5–15.

66. Renvert S, Persson GR, Pirih FQ, Camargo PM. Peri-implant health, peri-implant mucositis, and peri-implantitis: Case definitions and diagnostic considerations. J Periodontol 2018;89(suppl 1):S304–S312.

67. Listgarten MA, Lang NP, Schroeder HE, Schroeder A. Periodontal tissues and their counterparts around endosseous implants [corrected and republished with original paging, article orginally printed in Clin Oral Implants Res 1991 Jan-Mar;2(1):1–19]. Clin Oral Implants Res 1991;2:1–19.

68. Aoki M, Takanashi K, Matsukubo T, Yajima Y, Okuda K, Sato T, Ishihara K. Transmission of periodontopathic bacteria from natural teeth to implants. Clin Implant Dent Relat Res 2012:406–411.

69. Meyer S, Giannopoulou C, Courvoisier D, Schimmel M, Müller F, Mombelli A. Experimental mucositis and experimental gingivitis in persons aged 70 or over. Clinical and biological responses. Clin Oral Implants Res 2017;28:1005–1012.

70. Salvi GE, Aglietta M, Eick S, Sculean A, Lang NP, Ramseier CA. Reversibility of experimental peri-implant mucositis compared with experimental gingivitis in humans. Clin Oral Implants Res 2012;23:182–190.

71. Wong RL, Hiyari S, Yaghsezian A, et al. Early intervention of peri-implantitis and periodontitis using a mouse model. J Periodontol 2018;89:669–679.

72. Linkevicius T, Puisys A, Vindasiute E, Linkeviciene L, Apse P. Does residual cement around implant-supported restorations cause peri-implant disease? A retrospective case analysis. Clin Oral Implants Res 2013;24:1179–1184.

73. Jepsen S, Berglundh T, Genco R, et al. Primary prevention of peri-implantitis: Managing peri-implant mucositis. J Clin Periodontol 2015;42(suppl 16):S152–S157.

74. Wilson TG Jr, Valderrama P, Burbano M, et al. Foreign bodies associated with peri-implantitis human biopsies. J Periodontol 2015;86:9–15.

75. Canullo L, Tallarico M, Radovanovic S, Delibasic B, Covani U, Rakic M. Distinguishing predictive profiles for patient-based risk assessment and diagnostics of plaque induced, surgically and prosthetically triggered peri-implantitis. Clin Oral Implants Res 2016;27:1243–1250.

76. Heitz-Mayfield LJ, Salvi GE, Botticelli D, Mombelli A, Faddy M, Lang NP; Implant Complication Research Group. Anti-infective treatment of peri-implant mucositis: A randomized controlled clinical trial. Clin Oral Implants Res 2011;22:237–241.

77. Laine ML, Leonhardt A, Roos-Jansåker AM, et al. IL-1RN gene polymorphism is associated with peri-implantitis. Clin Oral Implants Res 2006;17:380–385.

78. Quirynen M, Vogels R, Alsaadi G, Naert I, Jacobs R, van Steenberghe D. Predisposing conditions for retrograde peri-implantitis, and treatment suggestions. Clin Oral Implants Res 2005;16:599–608.

79. Heitz-Mayfield LJ. Peri-implant diseases: Diagnosis and risk indicators. J Clin Periodontol 2008;35(8 suppl):292–304.

80. Fretwurst T, Nelson K, Tarnow DP, Wang HL, Giannobile WV. Is metal particle release associated with peri-implant bone destruction? An emerging concept. J Dent Res 2018;97:259–265.

81. Monje A, Wang HL, Nart J. Association of preventive maintenance therapy compliance and peri-implant diseases: A cross-sectional study. J Periodontol 2017;88:1030–1041.

82. Koldsland OC, Scheie AA, Aass AM. The association between selected risk indicators and severity of peri-implantitis using mixed model analyses. J Clin Periodontol 2011;38:285–292.

83. Berglundh T, Gotfredsen K, Zitzmann NU, Lang NP, Lindhe J. Spontaneous progression of ligature induced peri-implantitis at implants with different surface roughness: An experimental study in dogs. Clin Oral Implants Res 2007;18:655–661.

84. Stern JK, Rosenberg ES, Evian CI, Waasdorp J. Implant failure: Prevalence, risk factors, management, and prevention. In: Froum SJ (ed). Dental Implant Complications: Etiology, Prevention, and Treatment. Oxford: Wiley-Blackwell, 2010:110–118.

85. Esposito M, Hirsch JM, Lekholm U, Thomsen P. Biological factors contributing to failures of osseointegrated oral implants. (I). Success criteria and epidemiology. Eur J Oral Sci 1998;106:527–551.

86. Berglundh T, Persson L, Klinge B. A systematic review of the incidence of biological and technical complications in implant dentistry reported in prospective longitudinal studies of at least 5 years. J Clin Periodontol 2002;29:197–212.

87. Eckert SE, Choi YG, Sánchez AR, Koka S. Comparison of dental implant systems: Quality of clinical evidence and prediction of 5-year survival. Int J Oral Maxillofac Implants 2005;20:406–415.

88. Ferreira CF, Buttendorf AR, de Souza JG, Dalago H, Guenther SF, Bianchini MA. Prevalence of peri-implant diseases: Analyses of associated factors. Eur J Prosthodont Restor Dent 2015;23:199–206.

89. Ferreira SD, Silva GL, Cortelli JR, Costa JE, Costa FO. Prevalence and risk variables for peri-implant disease in Brazilian subjects. J Clin Periodontol 2006;33:929–935.

90. Costa FO, Takenaka-Martinez S, Cota LO, Ferreira SD, Silva GL, Costa JE. Peri-implant disease in subjects with and without preventive maintenance: A 5-year follow-up. J Clin Periodontol 2012;39:173–181.

91. Shi Q, Xu J, Huo N, Cai C, Liu H. Does a higher glycemic level lead to a higher rate of dental implant failure?: A meta-analysis. J Am Dent Assoc 2016;147:875–881.

92. Lecture by Dr. Greenwell at the American Academy of Periodontology 10/29/18.

93. Lindhe J, Meyle J; Group D of European Workshop on Periodontology. Peri-implant diseases: Consensus Report of the Sixth European Workshop on Periodontology. J Clin Periodontol 2008;35(8 suppl):282–285.

94. Fransson C, Tomasi C, Pikner SS, et al. Severity and pattern of peri-implantitis-associated bone loss. J Clin Periodontol 2010;37:442–448.

95. Menezes KM, Fernandes-Costa AN, Silva-Neto RD, Calderon PS, Gurgel BC. Efficacy of 0.12% chlorhexidine gluconate for non-surgical treatment of peri-implant mucositis. J Periodontol 2016;87:1305–1313.

96. Schwarz F, Becker K, Sager M. Efficacy of professionally administered plaque removal with or without adjunctive measures for the treatment of peri-implant mucositis. A systematic review and meta-analysis. J Clin Periodontol 2015;42(suppl 16):S202–S213.

97. Byrne G. Effectiveness of different treatment regimens for peri-implantitis. J Am Dent Assoc 2012;143:391–392.

98. Lang NP, Berglundh T, Heitz-Mayfield LJ, Pjetursson BE, Salvi GE, Sanz M. Consensus state-ments and recommended clinical procedures regarding implant survival and complications. Int J Oral Maxillofac Implants 2004;19(suppl):150–154.

99. Fletcher P, Tarnow DP. Circumferential Occlusal Access Procedure (COAP): Novel minimally invasive surgical approach for treatment of peri-implantitis—A case series. Compend Contin Educ Dent 2018;39:626–635.

100. Persson LG, Mouhyi J, Berglundh T, Sennerby L, Lindhe J. Carbon dioxide laser and hydrogen peroxide conditioning in the treatment of periimplantitis: An experimental study in the dog. Clin Implant Dent Relat Res 2004;6:230–238.

101. Schwarz F, Hegewald A, John G, Sahm N, Becker J. Four-year follow-up of combined surgical therapy of advanced peri-implantitis evaluating two methods of surface decontamination. J Clin Periodontol 2013;40:962–967.

102. Mengel R, Buns CE, Mengel C, Flores-de-Jacoby L. An in vitro study of the treatment of implant surfaces with different instruments. Int J Oral Maxillofac Implants 1998;13:91–96.

103. Fox SC, Moriarty JD, Kusy RP. The effects of scaling a titanium implant surface with metal and plastic instruments: An in vitro study. J Periodontol 1990;61:485–490.

104. Gay IC, Tran DT, Weltman R, et al. Role of supportive maintenance therapy on implant survival: A university-based 17 years retrospective analysis. Int J Dent Hyg 2016;14:267–271.

105. Ulm CW, Solar P, Krennmair G, Matejka M, Watzek G. Incidence and suggested surgical man-agement of septa in sinus-lift procedures. Int J Oral Maxillofac Implants 1995;10:462–465.

106. Komorniczak M. Paranasal sinuses. Wikimedia Commons. https://upload.wikimedia.org/wikipedia/commons/e/e8/Paranasal_sinuses_numbers.svg. CC BY-SA 3.0 (https://creativecommons.org/licenses/by-sa/3.0/deed.en). Published 21 October 2009. Accessed 6 January 2020.

107. Boyne PJ, James RA. Grafting of the maxillary sinus floor with autogenous marrow and bone. J Oral Surg 1980;38:613–616.

108. Tatum H Jr. Maxillary and sinus implant reconstructions. Dent Clin North Am 1986;30:207–229.

109. Tan WC, Lang NP, Zwahlen M, Pjetursson BE. A systematic review of the success of sinus floor elevation and survival of implants inserted in combination with sinus floor elevation. Part II: Transalveolar technique. J Clin Periodontol 2008;35(8 suppl):241–254.

110. Malet J, Mora F, Bouchard P. Implant Dentistry at-a-Glance. Chichester, West Sussex, UK: Wiley-Blackwell, 2012:89.

111. Wallace SS, Mazor Z, Froum SJ, Cho SC, Tarnow DP. Schneiderian membrane perforation rate during sinus elevation using piezosurgery: Clinical results of 100 consecutive cases. Int J Periodontics Restorative Dent 2007;27:413–419.

112. Toscano NJ, Holtzclaw D, Rosen PS. The effect of piezoelectric use on open sinus lift perfo-ration: A retrospective evaluation of 56 consecutively treated cases from private practices. J Periodontol 2010;81:167–171.

113. Rosen PS. Complications with the bone-added osteotome sinus floor elevation: Etiology, pre-vention, and treatment. In: Froum S (ed). Dental Implant Complications: Etiology, Prevention, and Treatment. Oxford, UK: Blackwell Publishing, 2010:310–324.

114. Wallace SS, Froum SJ. Effect of maxillary sinus augmentation on the survival of endosseous dental implants. A systematic review. Ann Periodontol 2003;8:328–343.

115. Froum SJ, Tarnow DP, Wallace SS, Rohrer MD, Cho SC. Sinus floor elevation using anorganic bovine bone matrix (OsteoGraf/N) with and without autogenous bone: A clinical, histologic, radiographic, and histomorphometric analysis—Part 2 of an ongoing prospective study. Int J Periodontics Restorative Dent 1998;18:528–543.

116. Piero B, Mario V, Niccolò N, Marco F. Implant placement in combination with sinus membrane elevation without biomaterials: A 1-year study on 15 patients. Clin Implant Dent Relat Res 2012;14:682–689.

117. Al-Nawas B, Schiegnitz E. Augmentation procedures using bone substitute materials or au-togenous bone—A systematic review and meta-analysis. Eur J Oral Implantol 2014;7(suppl 2):S219–S234.

118. Bornstein MM, Chappuis V, Von Arx T, Buser D. Performance of dental implants after staged sinus floor elevation procedures: 5-year results of a prospective study in partially edentulous patients. Clin Oral Implants Res 2008;19:1034–1043.

119. Tarnow DP, Wallace SS, Froum SJ, Rohrer MD, Cho SC. Histologic and clinical comparison of bilateral sinus floor elevations with and without barrier membrane placement in 12 patients: Part 3 of an ongoing prospective study. Int J Periodontics Restorative Dent 2000;20:117–125.

120. Tawil G, Mawla M. Sinus floor elevation using a bovine bone mineral (Bio-Oss) with or without the concomitant use of a bilayered collagen barrier (Bio-Gide): A clinical report of immediate and delayed implant placement. Int J Oral Maxillofac Implants 2001;16:713–721.

121. McAllister BS, Haghighat K. Bone augmentation techniques. J Periodontol 2007;78:377–396.

122. Misch CE. Maxillary sinus augmentation for endosteal implants: Organized alternative treatment plans. Int J Oral Implantol 1987;4:49–58.

123. Summers RB. A new concept in maxillary implant surgery: The osteotome technique. Compendium 1994;15:152,154–156,158.

124. Rosen PS, Summers R, Mellado JR, et al. The bone-added osteotome sinus floor elevation technique: Multicenter retrospective report of consecutively treated patients. Int J Oral Maxillofac Implants 1999;14:853–858.

125. Toffler M. Osteotome-mediated sinus floor elevation: A clinical report. Int J Oral Maxillofac Implants 2004;19:266–273.

126. Viña-Almunia J, Maestre-Ferrín L, Alegre-Domingo T, Peñarrocha-Diago M. Survival of implants placed with the osteotome technique: An update. Med Oral Patol Oral Cir Bucal 2012;17:e765–e768.

127. Shi JY, Gu YX, Zhuang LF, Lai HC. Survival of implants using the osteotome technique with or without grafting in the posterior maxilla: A systematic review. Int J Oral Maxillofac Implants 2016;31:1077–1088.

128. Lecture by Neema Bakhshatian 1/20/19.

129. Pal US, Kishor Sharma N , Singh RK, et al. Direct vs. indirect sinus lift procedure: A comparison. Natl J Maxillofac Surg 2012;3:31–37.

130. Torabinejad M, Anderson P, Bader J, et al. Outcomes of root canal treatment and restoration, implant-supported single crowns, fixed partial dentures, and extraction without replacement: A systematic review. J Prosthet Dent 2007;98:285–311.

131. Salinas TJ, Eckert SE. In patients requiring single-tooth replacement, what are the outcomes of implant- as compared to tooth-supported restorations? Int J Oral Maxillofac Implants 2007;22(suppl):71–95.

132. Iqbal MK, Kim S. For teeth requiring endodontic treatment, what are the differences in outcomes of restored endodontically treated teeth compared to implant-supported restorations? Int J Oral Maxillofac Implants 2007;22(suppl):96–116.

133. Scharf DR, Tarnow DP. Success rates of osseointegration for implants placed under sterile versus clean conditions. J Periodontol 1993;64:954–956.

134. Buddula A, Assad DA, Salinas TJ, Garces YI, Volz JE, Weaver AL. Survival of dental implants in irradiated head and neck cancer patients: A retrospective analysis. Clin Implant Dent Relat Res 2012;14:716–722.

Inflammation

14

Background

Q: What are the signs of inflammation?

Rubor (redness), tumor (swelling), calor (heat), dolor (pain), and loss of function are the signs of inflammation.

Q: What is the difference between the innate and the adaptive immune response?

Figure 14-1 presents the characteristics of the innate and adaptive immune responses.

Innate immune response

- Immediate protection through immune cells (macrophages, polymorphonuclear leukocytes [PMNs])
- Not antigen specific

Adaptive immune response

- Recognition of the pathogens (immunologic memory) and a stronger but longer response time through immune cells (B cells and T cells)
- Antigen specific

Fig 14-1 Characteristics of the innate and adaptive immune responses.

Q: Describe the following terms: epigenetics, resolvins, and protectins.

▪ *Epigenetics:* The relationships between environmental settings (such as diet, microbial infections, cigarette smoke, and diabetes) and the genetic background to produce a given phenotypical outcome.[1] Includes all meiotically and mitotically inherited changes in gene expression that are not encoded in the DNA sequence itself (DNA methylation or posttranslational modification of histone proteins).

▪ According to Martinez et al,[1] dietary and environmental factors in the mother may enhance or reduce epigenetic mechanisms, which may be transmitted intergenerationally or transiently and could be involved in the offspring's susceptibility to obesity and inflammation.

▪ In periodontitis, epigenetic modifications during inflammation occur locally at the biofilm/gingival interface around the teeth. It has been reported that the epigenome differs between inflamed periodontal sites and noninflamed sites in the same individual.[2]

▪ Specific cells within the oral mucosa may respond differently to bacterial infection or to the periodontal inflammatory processes. This results in differences in the methylation pattern of a certain gene among cell types.[2]

▪ *Resolvins and protectins:* Control the duration and magnitude of inflammation. They are synthesized by omega-3 fatty acids and can stop neutrophil infiltration and chemotaxis. Resolvins (a term derived from *resolution phase interaction products*) have potent anti-inflammatory and immunoregulatory actions, including neutrophil trafficking reduction, cytokine and reactive oxygen species regulation, and inflammatory response decrease. Protectin and neuroprotectin are 10R,17S-dihydroxy docosatrienes, so named given their general anti-inflammatory and protective effects in neural systems, stroke, animal models of Alzheimer disease, and peritonitis.[3]

Q: Describe the five major classes of immunoglobulin (Ig).

IgA

▪ Important in mucosal immunity
▪ Found in tears and saliva
▪ Activates the alternative pathway

IgD

▪ Found on B lymphocytes
▪ Usually found with IgM →

IgE

- Elicits an immune response by binding to Fc receptors found on the surface of mast cells and basophils and is also found on eosinophils, monocytes, macrophages, and platelets in humans
- Involved in allergies

IgG

- Antibodies are involved in the secondary immune response
- Presence corresponds to maturation of the antibody response
- Can pass through the human placenta, thereby providing protection to the fetus in utero
- Involved in the classic pathway

IgM

- Largest antibody; produced by B cells
- Appears early in infection
- Involved in the classic pathway

Pro-inflammatory Molecules

Q: Which molecules have been associated with bone loss in periodontal disease?

Interleukin-1 (IL-1) and tumor necrosis factor α (TNF-α) are the molecules associated with periodontal disease primarily.[4] Antigen-stimulated lymphocytes (B cells and T cells) also seem to be important. The cascade of events is illustrated in Fig 14-2.

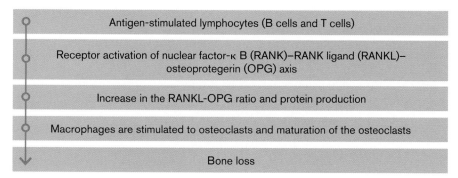

Fig 14-2 Cascade of events leading to bone loss.

Q: Describe the pro-inflammatory molecules.

- IL-1: Both IL-1α and IL-1β are produced by macrophages, monocytes, fibroblasts, and dendritic cells. They form an important part of the inflammatory response of the body against infection. They can promote bone resorption.
- IL-2: Produced by CD4 cells and part of the body's natural response to microbial infection.
- IL-4: Involved in differentiation of CD4$^+$ T cells into T-helper type 2 (Th2) cells.
- IL-6: Secreted by T cells and macrophages to stimulate the immune response. It can stimulate osteoclasts and plasma cells.
- IL-8: Primary function is the induction of chemotaxis in its target cells. It serves as a chemical signal that attracts neutrophils at the site of inflammation.
- IL-10: Anti-inflammatory cytokine.
- C-reactive protein (CRP): Rapid, marked increases in CRP occur with inflammation, infection, trauma and tissue necrosis, malignancies, and autoimmune disorders. An elevated CRP level can provide support for the presence of an inflammatory disease. CRP levels are elevated in patients with periodontitis and may decrease after periodontal therapy.[5]
- Prostaglandin E$_2$ (PGE$_2$): Stimulates osteoblasts to release factors that stimulate bone resorption by osteoclasts and matrix metalloproteinase (MMP) secretion. Elevated levels of prostaglandins such as PGE$_2$ in inflamed gingiva play a significant role in the tissue destruction caused by periodontitis, in part by targeting local fibroblasts.[6]
- Bradykinin: Increases vascular permeability.
- Interferon-γ (IFN-γ): IFN-γ released by Th1 cells recruits leukocytes to a site of infection, resulting in increased inflammation.
- TNF family: A group of cytokines that can cause cell death (apoptosis).
- Transforming growth factor β (TGF-β): TGF-β1 is the most potent chemoattractant described for human peripheral blood neutrophils (PMNs), suggesting that TGF-β may play a role in the recruitment of PMNs during the initial phase of the inflammatory response.[7]
- MMPs: The collagenases are capable of degrading collagens into distinctive $\frac{3}{4}$- and $\frac{1}{4}$-length fragments. These collagens are the major components of bone, cartilage, and dentin.

Q: Which pro-inflammatory molecules have shown an association with diabetes?

Pradhan et al[8] found that elevated levels of CRP and IL-6 can predict the development of type 2 diabetes.

Choi et al[9] found the relationship between periodontitis and diabetes was stronger in people having higher serum CRP and *Porphyromonas gingivalis* titers. This may indicate that chronic inflammatory conditions could increase the effect of periodontitis on hyperglycemic status.

Costa et al[10] reported MMP-8, a neutrophil collagenase involved in the degradation of the extracellular matrix, having the highest concentrations in patients with diabetes.

Q: Describe the interaction of CD4 cells with other molecules.

Table 14-1 presents the interaction of CD4 cells (T-helper cells) with other molecules.

Table 14-1	Interaction of CD4 cells with other molecules	
	Th1 cell	**Th2 cell**
Partner	Macrophage	B cell
Cytokine	IL-1β, PGE$_2$, IL-8, and IFN-γ	IL-10, IFN-4, IFN-5, and IFN-6

Q: Can inhibition of IL-1 and TNF reduce the progression of periodontal disease?

Yes, it can. Clinical, radiographic, and biochemical findings by Deo and Bhongade[11] showed in animal models that antagonists to IL-1 and TNF-α block inflammatory cell infiltrate advancement toward the alveolar crest as well as the recruitment of osteoclasts.

Q: Can inhibition of the host response contribute to periodontal tissue destruction?

Yes, neutrophil depletion contributes to periodontal destruction.

Periodontal Disease and Inflammation

Q: Describe the stages from an initial to an advanced lesion.

Figure 14-3 presents the stages from an initial to an advanced lesion.[12]

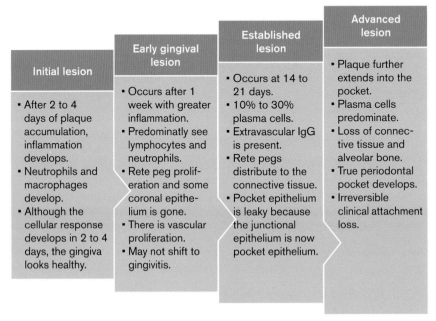

Initial lesion	Early gingival lesion	Established lesion	Advanced lesion
• After 2 to 4 days of plaque accumulation, inflammation develops. • Neutrophils and macrophages develop. • Although the cellular response develops in 2 to 4 days, the gingiva looks healthy.	• Occurs after 1 week with greater inflammation. • Predominatly see lymphocytes and neutrophils. • Rete peg proliferation and some coronal epithelium is gone. • There is vascular proliferation. • May not shift to gingivitis.	• Occurs at 14 to 21 days. • 10% to 30% plasma cells. • Extravascular IgG is present. • Rete pegs distribute to the connective tissue. • Pocket epithelium is leaky because the junctional epithelium is now pocket epithelium.	• Plaque further extends into the pocket. • Plasma cells predominate. • Loss of connective tissue and alveolar bone. • True periodontal pocket develops. • Irreversible clinical attachment loss.

Fig 14-3 Stages from an initial to an advanced lesion.

Q: What are the theories for periodontal disease progression?

- *The continuous model:* Most common forms of destructive periodontal disease have been thought to slowly and continuously progress until treatment is provided or tooth loss occurs.
- *Random burst or recurrent acute episodes:* Rates of attachment loss in individual sites are faster than those consistent with the continuous disease hypothesis or slower than those expected from estimates of prior loss rates. Bursts of activity occur for short periods of time in individual sites.[13]

Q: Describe the inflammatory process of periodontitis.

The inflammatory process of periodontitis is presented in Fig 14-4.

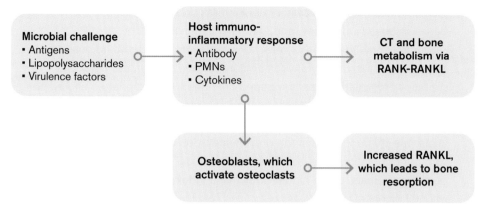

Fig 14-4 Inflammatory process of periodontitis.

Q: How does caloric restriction affect periodontitis?

Reynolds et al[14] found significantly fewer periodontal pockets, a reduced IgG antibody response, and lower IL-8 and β-glucuronidase levels in male patients who had caloric restriction.

Branch-Mays et al[15] found that caloric restriction has anti-inflammatory effects. The study also suggested that caloric restriction decreases the inflammatory response and reduces active periodontal breakdown associated with an acute microbial challenge.

Abnormalities Associated with Chronic Inflammation

Q: Describe metabolic disorders and their relationship with inflammation.

Metabolic disorders are abnormalities that include obesity, high blood pressure, high blood glucose, dyslipidemia, and cardiovascular disease. At the heart of these abnormalities is a pro-inflammatory state.

Obesity, insulin resistance, and type 2 diabetes are closely associated with chronic inflammation characterized by abnormal cytokine production, increased acute-phase reactants and other mediators, and activation of a network of inflammatory signaling pathways.[16] The finding that TNF is →

overexpressed in the fat cells of obese mice provided the first clear link between obesity, diabetes, and chronic inflammation.[17]

Studies show that cross interactions between T cells and adipose tissue shapes the inflammatory environment in obesity-associated metabolic diseases.[18] Similarly, obesity-induced changes to macrophages and adipocytes may cause insulin resistance and chronic inflammation.[19]

A meta-analysis from 57 independent study populations found an approximate one-third increase in the prevalence odds of obesity among subjects with periodontal disease, a greater mean clinical attachment loss among obese individuals, and a higher body mass index among subjects with periodontal disease.[20]

Q: Describe the relationship between diabetes and inflammation.

Figures 14-5 and 14-6 present two depictions of the relationship between inflammation and diabetes.

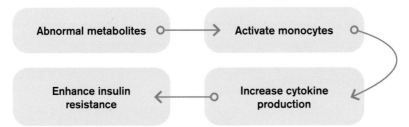

Fig 14-5 Inflammation leading to insulin resistance.

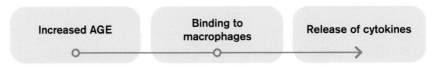

Fig 14-6 Advanced glycation end product (AGE) leading to the release of cytokines and inflammation.

- Advanced glycation end products (AGEs) and their key receptor, receptor for advanced glycation end products (RAGE), is thought to play a major role in the development of complications associated with hyperglycemia.[21]
- AGEs and RAGE are elevated in patients with diabetes and have periodontitis.[22] →

- AGEs can also prevent development of macrophages involved in repair and thereby delay wound healing.
- When a patient has hyperglycemia, there is a hyperinflammatory response to a bacterial challenge, which can change the host response (neutrophil defects, responsive monocytes, increased cytokines, impaired healing, and oxidative stress).
- The association between diabetes and periodontitis is bidirectional, as "periodontitis has been reported to adversely affect glycemic control in patients with diabetes mellitus and to contribute to the development of diabetic complications. In addition, meta-analyses conclude that periodontal therapy in individuals with diabetes mellitus can result in a modest improvement of glycemic control."[22]

It has also been shown that obesity can increase inflammatory mediators and increase insulin resistance.[23]

Q: What is the relationship between Alzheimer disease (AD) and inflammation?

Dominy et al[24] analyzed brain tissue, spinal fluid, and saliva from patients (both living and deceased) with AD and discovered evidence of *P gingivalis*. Gingipains, the toxic enzyme secreted by *P gingivalis*, were obtained in 96 percent of the 53 brain tissue samples inspected, with higher levels noticed in those with the pathology and symptoms of AD.

The presence of *P gingivalis* increased the production of amyloid beta, a component of the amyloid plaques whose buildup contributes to AD. The study confirmed via animal testing that *P gingivalis* can go from the mouth to the brain and that the associated gingipains can destroy brain neurons. These findings are remarkable in that they imply a biologic mechanism for how periodontal disease bacteria may play a role in the progress and progression of AD.

Cojocaru et al[25] found that patients with AD had increased production of the IL-6 cytokine, which indicates that an abnormal cellular immunity may be present. IL-6, which is involved in the pathogenesis of AD, may account for the serum acute-phase proteins found in patients with AD.

Q: Describe the relationship between arthritis and inflammation.

Osteoarthritis (OA) is a multifactorial disorder in which obesity is one of the most influential but modifiable risk factors. Although it has been postulated →

that obesity is a risk factor simply because it increases mechanical stress on the joints, OA is also prevalent in non-weightbearing areas, such as finger joints, in obese individuals, suggesting another link between obesity and OA—inflammation. Adipose tissues and the infrapatellar fat pad contain cytokines, chemokines, and adipokines (or adipocytokines), which have been shown to have catabolic and pro-inflammatory properties and to coordinate the pathophysiologic processes involved in OA.[26]

Mangge et al[27] found an association between juvenile rheumatoid arthritis and consistent significant fluctuations in serum levels of inflammatory cytokines and soluble receptors.

Q: Is periodontitis more common in patients with rheumatoid arthritis (RA) or osteoarthritis?

In a cohort of US veterans, periodontitis was more common and severe in patients with RA (51%) compared to patients with OA (26%).[28]

Q: Is there a relationship between osteoporosis and periodontitis?

A systematic review and meta-analysis found postmenopausal women with osteoporosis or osteopenia exhibit greater clinical attachment loss compared with women with normal bone mineral density.[29]

Miscellaneous

Q: Describe the major histocompatibility complex (MHC) proteins.

- *Class I MHC proteins:* Found on virtually all cell types and are responsible for presenting fragments of proteins that are synthesized inside the cell. The peptide antigens presented in this manner are checked by killer T cells, which have receptors for the class I MHC proteins. The purpose of this surveillance system is to identify abnormal body cells, such as those infected with viruses or those that have turned malignant.
- *Class II MHC proteins:* Found only on immune cells such as phagocytes that engulf foreign particles such as bacteria. These cells are specially designed to present peptide antigens derived from such digested particles.

$\rightarrow$

The antigens are presented to helper T cells, which have receptors for class II MHC proteins. The purpose of this surveillance system is to stop the immune system from running out of control and attacking the body's own cells.

References

1. Martínez JA, Cordero P, Campión J, Milagro FI. Interplay of early-life nutritional programming on obesity, inflammation and epigenetic outcomes. Proc Nutr Soc 2012;71:276–283.
2. Larsson L, Castilho RM, Giannobile WV. Epigenetics and its role in periodontal diseases: A state-of-the-art review. J Periodontol 2015;86:556–568.
3. Ariel A, Serhan CN. Resolvins and protectins in the termination program of acute inflammation. Trends Immunol 2007;28:176–183.
4. Cochran DL. Inflammation and bone loss in periodontal disease. J Periodontol 2008;79(8 suppl):1569–1576.
5. Dasanayake AP. C-reactive protein levels are elevated in patients with periodontitis and their CRP levels may go down after periodontal therapy. J Evid Based Dent Pract 2009;9:21–22.
6. Weinberg E, Zeldich E, Weinreb MM, Moses O, Nemcovsky C, Weinreb M. Prostaglandin E2 inhibits the proliferation of human gingival fibroblasts via the EP2 receptor and Epac. J Cell Biochem 2009;108:207–215.
7. Parekh T, Saxena B, Reibman J, Cronstein BN, Gold LI. Neutrophil chemotaxis in response to TGF-beta isoforms (TGF-beta 1, TGF-beta 2, TGF-beta 3) is mediated by fibronectin. J Immunol 1994;152:2456–2466.
8. Pradhan AD, Manson JE, Rifai N, Buring JE, Ridker PM. C-reactive protein, interleukin 6, and risk of developing type 2 diabetes mellitus. JAMA 2001;286:327–334.
9. Choi YH, McKeown RE, Mayer-Davis EJ, Liese AD, Song KB, Merchant AT. Serum C-reactive protein and immunoglobulin G antibodies to periodontal pathogens may be effect modifiers of periodontitis and hyperglycemia. J Periodontol 2014;85:1172–1181.
10. Costa PP, Trevisan GL, Macedo GO, et al. Salivary interleukin-6, matrix metalloproteinase-8, and osteoprotegerin in patients with periodontitis and diabetes. J Periodontol 2010;81:384–391.
11. Deo V, Bhongade ML. Pathogenesis of periodontitis: Role of cytokines in host response. Dent Today 2010;29(9):60–62,64–66.
12. Page RC, Schroeder HE. Pathogenesis of inflammatory periodontal disease. A summary of current work. Lab Invest 1976;34:235–249.
13. Socransky SS, Haffajee AD, Goodson JM, Lindhe J. New concepts of destructive periodontal disease. J Clin Periodontol 1984;11:21–32.
14. Reynolds MA, Dawson DR, Novak KF, et al. Effects of caloric restriction on inflammatory periodontal disease. Nutrition 2009;25:88–97.
15. Branch-Mays GL, Dawson DR, Gunsolley JC, et al. The effects of a calorie-reduced diet on periodontal inflammation and disease in a non-human primate model. J Periodontol 2008;79:1184–1191.
16. Wellen KE, Hotamisligil GS. Inflammation, stress, and diabetes. J Clin Invest 2005;115:1111–1119.
17. Hotamisligil GS, Shargill NS, Spiegelman BM. Adipose expression of tumor necrosis factor-alpha: Direct role in obesity-linked insulin resistance. Science 1993;259(5091):87–91.
18. Becker M, Levings MK, Daniel C. Adipose-tissue regulatory T cells: Critical players in adipose-immune crosstalk. Eur J Immunol 2017;47:1867–1874.
19. Thomas D, Apovian C. Macrophage functions in lean and obese adipose tissue. Metabolism 2017;72:120–143.

20. Chaffee BW, Weston SJ. Association between chronic periodontal disease and obesity: A systematic review and meta-analysis. J Periodontol 2010;81:1708–1724.

21. Del Turco S, Basta G. An update on advanced glycation endproducts and atherosclerosis. Biofactors 2012;38:266–274.

22. Lalla E, Papapanou PN. Diabetes mellitus and periodontitis: A tale of two common interrelated diseases. Nat Rev Endocrinol 2011;7:738–748.

23. Cohen DH, Leroith D. Obesity, type 2 diabetes, and cancer: The insulin and IGF connection. Endocr Relat Cancer 2012;19(5):F27–F45.

24. Dominy SS, Lynch C, Ermini F, et al. *Porphyromonas gingivalis* in Alzheimer's disease brains: Evidence for disease causation and treatment with small-molecule inhibitors. Sci Adv 2019;5:eaau3333.

25. Cojocaru IM, Cojocaru M, Miu G, Sapira V. Study of interleukin-6 production in Alzheimer's disease. Rom J Intern Med 2011;49:55–58.

26. Rai MF, Sandell LJ. Inflammatory mediators: Tracing links between obesity and osteoarthritis. Crit Rev Eukaryot Gene Expr 2011;21:131–142.

27. Mangge H, Kenzian H, Gallistl S, et al. Serum cytokines in juvenile rheumatoid arthritis. Correlation with conventional inflammation parameters and clinical subtypes. Arthritis Rheum 1995;38:211–220.

28. Dissick A, Redman RS, Jones M, et al. Association of periodontitis with rheumatoid arthritis: A pilot study. J Periodontol 2010;81:223–230.

29. Penoni DC, Fidalgo TK, Torres SR, et al. Bone density and clinical periodontal attachment in postmenopausal women: A systematic review and meta-analysis. J Dent Res 2017;96:261–269.

Oral Medicine

Laboratory Work

Q: What are some important laboratory values?

- Platelet count: 150,000 to 400,000 is normal
- Bleeding time: 2.5 to 8 minutes is normal
- High-density lipoprotein (HDL): > 50 mg/dL is normal
- Low-density lipoprotein (LDL): < 100 mg/dL is normal
- International normalized ratio (INR): 1 to 1.5 is normal
  - Can treat an INR < 3.5
- Fasting blood sugar:
  - 75 to 100 mg/dL is normal
  - 126 mg/dL indicates diabetes
  - < 72 mg/dL indicates hypoglycemia
- Hemoglobin A1c: 4% to 6% is normal
  - Can treat patients < 7%
- Body mass index:
  - 25 kg/m³ indicates overweight
  - 30 kg/m³ indicates obese
- White blood cell count: 4×10^9 to 1.1×10^{10} per liter of blood is normal
- Red blood cell count: 4×10^6 to 6×10^6 is normal
- CD4 counts: 500×10^6 to $1,200 \times 10^6$ is normal
- Neutropenia in adults: count of 1,700 or fewer neutrophils per microliter of blood $\rightarrow$

- Hemoglobin levels:
    - Adult men: 14 to 18 g/dL is normal
    - Adult women: 12 to 16 g/dL is normal

Q: What is the normal heart rate?

- Normal heart rate: 60 to 110 beats per minute (bpm)[1]
- Bradycardia: < 60 bpm
- Tachycardia: > 110 bpm

Blood Pressure

Q: What is the difference between primary and secondary hypertension?

- Primary hypertension: Most patients (90% to 95%) have primary hypertension. It is idiopathic.
- Secondary hypertension: It may be caused by kidney disease, primary hyperaldosteronism, and pheochromocytoma.

Q: What are the values for normal blood pressure, prehypertension, and stage 1 and 2 hypertension?

- Normal blood pressure: 120/80
- Prehypertension: 120 to 139/80 to 89
- Stage 1 hypertension: 140 to 159/90 to 99
- Stage 2 hypertension: 160/100

Q: What is the classification of blood pressure according to the American Society of Anesthesiologists (ASA)?

- ASA 1: < 140/< 90
- ASA 2: 140 to 159/90 to 94
- ASA 3: 160 to 199/95 to 114
- ASA 4: > 200/> 115

Q: **Does it make a difference on which arm blood pressure is taken?**

The arm on which blood pressure is measured only makes a difference if the patient has aortic stenosis or a mastectomy.

Q: **Are electronic devices as accurate as manual ones in determining the blood pressure of a patient?**

Electronic devices are usually accurate to within 3% of a manual sphygmomanometer.[2]

Q: **What can cause errors in blood pressure measurements?**

The following factors may cause errors in blood pressure measurements:

- Stress
- Blood pressure may decrease following a big meal
- Caffeine may increase blood pressure

Q: **What are the concerns regarding hypertension?**

Hypertension can lead to heart disease, stroke, kidney failure, and heart attack.

Q: **Describe how hypertension can lead to thrombosis.**

Figure 15-1 presents the process by which hypertension can lead to thrombosis.

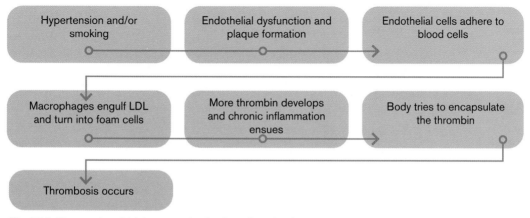

Fig 15-1 Process by which hypertension leads to thrombosis.

Stroke

Q: Describe the two types of stroke.

A stroke is a medical condition in which poor blood flow to the brain results in cell death. There are two main types of stroke: ischemic, due to lack of blood flow (blockage of a blood vessel), and hemorrhagic, due to bleeding (bleeding directly into the brain or into the space between the brain's membranes.)

The main risk factor is high blood pressure.

Q: What are the symptoms of stroke?

- Numbness or weakness in your face, arm, or leg, especially on one side (drooping eyelid)
- Confusion or trouble understanding other people
- Difficulty speaking
- Trouble seeing with one or both eyes
- Problems walking or staying balanced or coordinated
- Dizziness
- Severe headache that comes on for no reason[3]

Cardiovascular Disease

Q: What are risk factors for cardiovascular disease?

- Patient older than 65 years old
- Smoking
- Systemic blood pressure greater than 140 and diastolic blood pressure greater than 90
- LDL greater than 160
- HDL less than 40
- Fasting blood glucose greater than 120
- Periodontal disease
- Genetics
- Obesity

Q: What does the evidence show about the relationship between cardiovascular disease and periodontal disease?

- A review by Humphrey et al[4] reported on several studies that revealed an independent association of periodontal disease with increased risk for coronary heart disease (CHD). Summary relative risk estimates ranged from 1.24 to 1.34 for different types of periodontal disease (including periodontitis, tooth loss, gingivitis, and bone loss).
- In a meta-analysis of five prospective cohort studies (including 86,092 patients), Bahekar et al[5] found a 1.14-fold increase in risk of developing CHD in individuals with periodontitis compared with controls.
- Beck et al[6] concluded that periodontitis could be considered a risk factor for atherosclerosis/CHD based on the study's finding of an incidence odds ratio of approximately 2.0. Beck et al[7] also found that severe periodontitis was associated with carotid artery intima-media wall thickness $\geq$ 1 mm.
- In a study on 9,760 individuals, DeStefano et al[8] found that those with periodontitis had a 25% increased risk of CHD compared with those who had minimal periodontal disease.

Q: What are the four main theories about the relationship between cardiovascular disease and periodontitis?

1. Direct invasion: Several groups have identified specific oral pathogens in atheromatous tissue.
2. Immunologic sounding: Cytokines and chemokines play a role in activation of endothelium and monocytes associated with developing atheroma[9] (Fig 15-2).
3. Pathogen trafficking: Trafficking of pathogens from the local site of infection to the developing atheroma via inflammatory cells.
4. Autoimmune response: Stimulation of an autoimmune response via molecular mimicry.

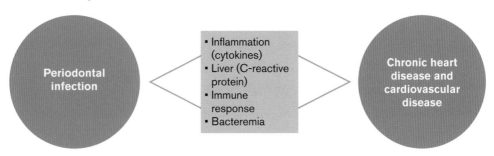

Fig 15-2 Immunologic sounding.

315

Q: **What are the recommendations for patients who have cardiovascular or periodontal disease?**

Following are the recommendations for patients with cardiovascular or periodontal disease[10]:

- Patients with moderate to severe periodontitis: Patients should be informed that there may be an increased risk for atherosclerotic cardiovascular disease associated with periodontitis.
- Patients with moderate to severe periodontitis who have one known major atherosclerotic cardiovascular disease risk factor (including smoking, immediate family history of cardiovascular disease, or history of dyslipidemia): These patients should consider a medical evaluation if they have not had one in the past 12 months.
- Patients with periodontitis who have two known major atherosclerotic cardiovascular disease risk factors: These patients should be referred for medical evaluation if they have not had one in the past 12 months.

Q: **What are the symptoms of congestive heart failure?**

Fatigue, limited activity, edema, and shortness of breath are symptoms of congestive heart failure. It is important to be aware of orthostatic hypotension with these patients.

Q: **What is the difference between congestive heart failure and a heart attack?**

- Congestive heart failure: The pump and cardiac muscles do not work properly.
- Heart attack/myocardial infarction (MI): There is death of the tissue due to lack of oxygen. There is an interruption of blood supply.

Diabetes

Q: **Describe the two types of diabetes.**

Defining characteristics of the two types of diabetes are described in Fig 15-3. →

Type 1 diabetes	Type 2 diabetes
• Formerly called *insulin-dependent diabetes mellitus* • 5% to 10% of diabetic cases; first discovered when patients are young • Immune-mediated destruction of the pancreatic β cells that secrete insulin	• Formerly called *non–insulin-dependent diabetes* • 90% to 95% of diabetic patients; discovered midlife and in obese patients • Insulin resistance

Fig 15-3 Defining characteristics of type 1 and type 2 diabetes.

Q: How prevalent is diabetes?

According to the World Health Organization, "Globally, an estimated 422 million adults were living with diabetes in 2014, compared to 108 million in 1980. The global prevalence (age-standardized) of diabetes has nearly doubled since 1980, rising from 4.7% to 8.5% in the adult population."[11]

Q: What does hemoglobin A1c measure?

Glycosylate hemoglobin measures the amount of glucose bound to hemoglobin in the red blood cell. Hemoglobin A1c values of 4% to 6% are normal. Patients can be treated in the dental office with a value of 7% or less. This laboratory result indicates diabetic control over the last 3 months.

Q: What are the possible oral manifestations of diabetes?

The possible oral manifestations of diabetes are shown in Fig 15-4.

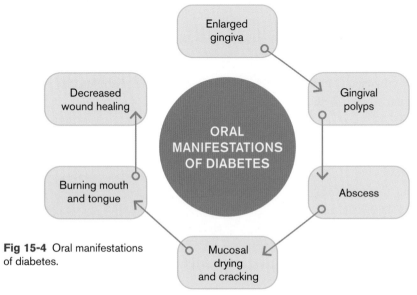

Fig 15-4 Oral manifestations of diabetes.

Q: How should patients with diabetes be managed?

- Ask the patients about their blood sugar values.
- Ask them to bring in their hemoglobin A1c lab values.
- If the values are too high, a medical consult should be obtained (regarding changing the type or dosage of medication).
- Be aware that these patients have poor wound healing and must be monitored for a possible medical emergency (see chapter 18).

Q: How can hyperglycemia lead to a diabetic coma?

Figure 15-5 describes the process by which hyperglycemia can lead to a diabetic coma.

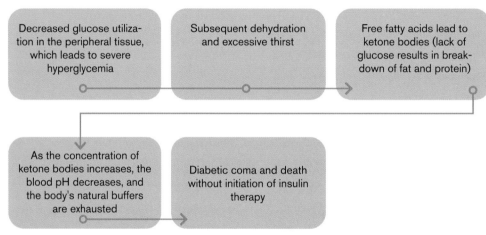

Fig 15-5 Process by which hyperglycemia leads to a diabetic coma.

Q: What are the possible macrovascular and microvascular complications of diabetes?

The macrovascular and microvascular complications of diabetes are presented in Fig 15-6.

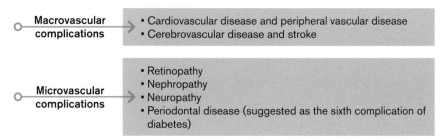

Fig 15-6 Macrovascular and microvascular complications of diabetes.

Organs and Their Functions

Q: Describe the functions of selected body organs.

Pancreas:

- Alpha cells produce glucagon (converts glycogen to glucose)
- Beta cells produce insulin and amylin
- Delta cells produce somatostatin (growth hormone)
- Acini produce digestive enzymes (eg, trypsin)

Adrenal gland:

- Adrenal cortex secretes corticosteroids (eg, testosterone and aldosterone)
- Adrenal medulla releases catecholamines (eg, tyrosine)

Thyroid:

- Involved in metabolism
- Produces calcitonin, which plays a role in calcium homeostasis

Spleen:

- White pulp: Active in immune response
- Red pulp: Filters red blood cells

Kidneys:

- Creatinine clearance
- Activate vitamin D
- Essential in the urinary system and also serve homeostatic functions such as the regulation of electrolytes, maintenance of acid-base balance, and regulation of blood pressure
- Serve as a natural filter of the blood and remove wastes, which are diverted to the urinary bladder
- Produce hormones including calcitriol and erythropoietin and the enzyme renin

Liver:

- The liver, an accessory digestive gland, has a broad range of functions in maintaining homeostasis and health, detoxifies various metabolites, synthesizes proteins, and produces biochemicals necessary for digestion.
- It synthesizes most essential serum proteins (albumin; transporter proteins; blood coagulation factors V, VII, IX, and X; prothrombin; and fibrinogen, as well as many hormone and growth factors).
- The liver produces bile, an alkaline compound which helps the breakdown of fat. $\rightarrow$

Stomach:

- Gastrin, a peptide hormone, stimulates secretion of gastric acid (HCl) by the parietal cells of the stomach and aids in gastric motility.
- Gastric inhibitory peptide decreases both gastric acid release and motility.
- Pepsin, an enzyme whose zymogen (pepsinogen) is released by the chief cells in the stomach, degrades food into peptides.

Anterior pituitary gland:

- Luteinizing hormone (LH) is produced by the anterior pituitary gland. In women, an acute rise of LH triggers ovulation and development of the corpus luteum. In men, it stimulates Leydig cell production of testosterone.
- Follicle-stimulating hormone (FSH) is a hormone found in humans and other animals. FSH regulates the development, growth, pubertal maturation, and reproductive processes of the body. FSH and LH act synergistically in reproduction.

Blood

Q: What is the mechanism of action of warfarin? Heparin?

- Warfarin: Also known as *coumadin*, warfarin inhibits the vitamin K–dependent synthesis of biologically active forms of the calcium-dependent clotting factors II, VII, IX, and X.
- Heparin: Heparin binds to the enzyme inhibitor antithrombin III, causing a conformational change that results in its activation through an increase in the flexibility of its reactive site loop. The activated antithrombin then inactivates thrombin and other proteases involved in blood clotting, most notably factor Xa.

Q: What patients are most often treated with anticoagulants?

The patients most often given anticoagulants are those with:

- Atrial fibrillation
- Valvular heart disease
- Mechanical heart valves
- MI
- Recurrent systemic embolism

Q: What is the difference between prothrombin time (PT) and partial prothrombin time (PTT)?

Figure 15-7 presents the differences between PT and PTT.

PT	PTT
• Measures the extrinsic pathway of coagulation. • Measures factors I, II, V, VII, and X. • The reference range is usually around 10 to 13 seconds.	• Measures the intrinsic pathway of coagulation. • Typically between 25 and 39 seconds. • Normal PTT times require the presence of the following coagulation factors: I, II, V, VIII, IX, X, XI, and XII. Notably, deficiencies in factors VII or XIII will not be detected with the PTT test.

Fig 15-7 Differences between PT and PTT.

See chapter 5 for more information about anticoagulation and antiplatelet medications.

Liver Disease

Q: What are the signs and symptoms of liver disease?

- Jaundice and yellow conjunctiva
- Tender and shrunken liver (accumulation of fluids)
- Peripheral edema
- Prolonged PT
- In situations of advanced liver disease, the vitamin K levels can be significantly lowered, thus giving rise to a reduction in the production of blood coagulation factors
- Patients with alcoholic hepatitis can present glossitis, angle cheilitis, and gingivitis, particularly in combination with nutritional deficiencies.[12]

Liver diseases are very common, and the main underlying causes are viral infections, alcohol abuse, and lipid and carbohydrate metabolic disorders. The patient drug metabolizing capacity can be evaluated based on the analysis of enzymes such as alanine aminotransferase (ALT) or aspartate aminotransferase (AST) and other liver function tests.[12]

Q: What are some drugs that are metabolized in the liver?

Local anesthetics:

- Lidocaine
- Prilocaine
- Mepivacaine
- Bupivacaine

Analgesics:

- Aspirin
- Acetaminophen (paracetamol)
- Ibuprofen
- Codeine
- Meperidine

Sedatives:

- Diazepam
- Barbiturates

Antibiotics:

- Erythromycin
- Clindamycin
- Tetracycline

Antifungals:

- Ketoconazole
- Fluconazol

The drugs above must be used with caution or avoided in patients with advanced stage liver disease.[12]

Immune System

Q: What are the five major classes of immunoglobulin (Ig)?

1. IgA
2. IgD
3. IgE
4. IgG
5. IgM

See chapter 14 (pages 300–301) for descriptions of the five major classes of Ig.

Q: Describe the host defense against plaque.

The host defense against plaque[9] is presented in Fig 15-8.

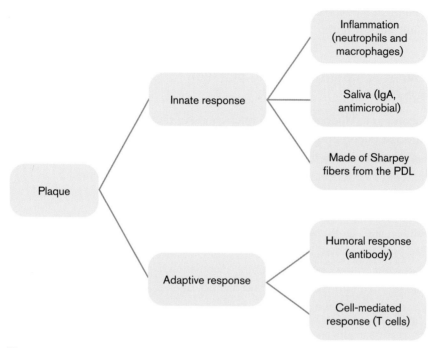

Fig 15-8 Host defense against plaque. PDL, periodontal ligament.

Miscellaneous

Q: What are some of the causes and treatment of oral malodor?

Causes:

- Bacteria (most common cause)
- Volatile sulfide compounds
- Gastrointestinal tract problems
- Deep caries, purulent discharge
- Denture left in the mouth overnight →

Treatment:

- Chlorhexidine 0.12%
- Good oral hygiene regimen
- Referral to medical doctor
- Metal salt solution

Q: What precautions should be taken for a patient who is pregnant?

- According to Huebner et al,[13] comprehensive dental care should be provided during pregnancy not only to prevent pregnancy-specific oral health problems for the mother but also to prevent early childhood caries.
- The best time to treat a pregnant patient is in the second trimester.[14]
- It is a good idea to contact the medical doctor by fax with the treatment plan, including the drugs to be used, quantity, and dosage.
- Tetracycline, vancomycin, and streptomycin should not be used.
- Radiographs should be limited.
- According to the California Dental Association,[15] periodontal treatment is safe for the mother and fetus and has not been shown to cause preterm labor or low birth weight.

References

1. Malamed S. Medical Emergencies in the Dental Office, ed 5. St Louis: Mosby, 2000:34.
2. Burket LW, Greenberg MS, Glick M. Burket's Oral Medicine: Diagnosis and Treatment, ed 10. Hamilton, Ontario: Decker, 2003:14.
3. WebMD. The warning signs of a stroke. https://www.webmd.com/stroke/guide/signs-of-stroke. Accessed 21 Oct 2019.
4. Humphrey LL, Fu R, Buckley DI, Freeman M, Helfand M. Periodontal disease and coronary heart disease incidence: A systematic review and meta-analysis. J Gen Intern Med 2008;23:2079–2086.
5. Bahekar AA, Singh S, Saha S, Molnar J, Arora R. The prevalence and incidence of coronary heart disease is significantly increased in periodontitis: A meta-analysis. Am Heart J 2007;154:830–837.
6. Beck JD, Offenbacher S, Williams R, Gibbs P, Garcia R. Periodontitis: A risk factor for coronary heart disease? Ann Periodontol 1998;3:127–141.
7. Beck JD, Elter JR, Heiss G, Couper D, Mauriello SM, Offenbacher S. Relationship of periodontal disease to carotid artery intima-media wall thickness: The atherosclerosis risk in communities (ARIC) study. Arterioscler Thromb Vasc Biol 2001;21:1816–1822.
8. DeStefano F, Anda RF, Kahn HS, Williamson DF, Russell CM. Dental disease and risk of coronary heart disease and mortality. BMJ 1993;306:688–691.
9. Clerehugh V, Tugnait A, Genco RJ. Periodontology at a Glance. Oxford: Wiley-Blackwell, 2009.
10. Friedewald VE, Kornman KS, Beck JD, et al. The American Journal of Cardiology and Journal of Periodontology editors' consensus: Periodontitis and atherosclerotic cardiovascular disease. J Periodontol 2009;80:1021–1032.

11. World Health Organization. Global report on diabetes. https://apps.who.int/iris/bitstream/handle/10665/204871/9789241565257_eng.pdf;jsessionid=32C527AE4B0576E3E7A9F-C01FF22DD7E?sequence=1. Accessed 21 Oct 2019.

12. Cruz-Pamplona M, Margaix-Muñoz M, Gracia Sarrión-Pérez MG. Dental considerations in patients with liver disease. J Clin Exp Dent 2011;3:e127–e134.

13. Huebner CE, Milgrom P, Conrad D, Lee RS. Providing dental care to pregnant patients: A survey of Oregon general dentists. J Am Dent Assoc 2009;140:211–222.

14. Task Force on Periodontal Treatment of Pregnant Women of the American Academy of Periodontology. American Academy of Periodontology statement regarding periodontal management of the pregnant patient. J Periodontol 2004;75:495.

15. CDA Foundation publishes guidelines for dental care during pregnancy. J Calif Dent Assoc 2010;38:85,87.

Oral Pathology

16

Staging System for Tumors

Q: Describe the TNM staging system for tumors.

T (size or direct extent of the primary tumor):

- T0: No signs of tumor
- Tis: Carcinoma in situ
- T1: Tumor is less than 2 cm
- T2: Tumor is 2 to 4 cm
- T3: Tumor is greater than 4 cm
- T4: Tumor invades adjacent structures

N (degree of spread to regional lymph nodes):

- N0: Tumor cells absent from regional lymph nodes/not palpable
- N1: Regional lymph node metastasis present (at some sites: tumor spread to closest or small number of regional lymph nodes)
- N2: Tumor spread to an extent between N1 and N3
- N3: Tumor spread to more distant or numerous regional lymph nodes and palpable

M (presence of metastasis):

- M0: No distant metastasis
- M1: Metastasis to distant organs (beyond regional lymph nodes)

Biopsies

Q: What are important rules to know when performing biopsies?

- Biopsy of lesion smaller than 1 cm: Excisional biopsy (removal of the whole lesion)
- Biopsy of lesion greater than 1 cm: Incisional biopsy (surgical removal of part of the lesion; can be done with a biopsy punch)
- Biopsy a part of the normal tissue around the lesion
- Never perform an incisional biopsy of a suspected pigmented lesion
- Try to put the specimen in a formalin solution

Ulcers and Cysts

Q: What are aphthous ulcers (also known as canker sores)?

Aphthous ulcers are painful superficial ulcers of the oral gland-bearing mucosa, usually sparing the hard palate, attached gingiva, and dorsum of the tongue.[1] They may occur from a deficiency of vitamin B_{12}, folic acid, trauma, allergens, anemia, chemicals like sodium lauryl sulphate (which is used in toothpaste), or inflammatory bowel syndrome.[2]

Q: What is the treatment for aphthous ulcers?

Chlorhexidine rinses have shown short-term relief in some patients. Vitamin supplements have also been shown to be helpful. Oral lesions may need topical steroid application such as Kenalog (Bristol-Myers Squibb) or Lidex (Medicis Pharmaceutical).

Q: What is the difference between aphthous ulcers and herpetic lesions?

Table 16-1 presents the differences between aphthous ulcers and herpetic lesions. A cytologic smear can be performed to rule out a viral etiology.[3]

Figure 16-1 is a case of primary herpes. Figure 16-2 shows a case of herpetic whitlow on a finger. It can occur on a finger or thumb, and it is caused by the herpes simplex virus. It is a painful infection. $\rightarrow$

Table 16-1	Aphthous ulcers and herpetic lesions	
	Aphthous ulcers	**Herpetic lesions**
Movement	Movable	Bound
Area found	Mucosa	Keratinized and gland-bearing tissue
Coalescence	Do not coalesce	Coalesce
Forms	Major (> 1 cm), minor (< 1 cm) and herpetiform (may be on keratinized mucosa)	Primary/recurrent

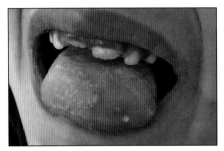

Fig 16-1 A 6-year-old boy with primary herpetic lesions.

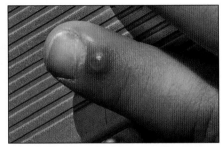

Fig 16-2 Herpetic whitlow of a 6-year-old boy.

Q: What is the treatment for herpetic lesions?

5% acyclovir cream can shorten the duration of the episode. 1% penciclovir was shown to be more effective than 5% acyclovir in reducing the healing time and duration of the painful phase.[4]

The lesions are self-limiting and run a course of 7 to 14 days.[3]

Q: Describe the lateral periodontal cyst and the odontogenic keratocyst.

Characteristics of the lateral periodontal cyst and the odontogenic keratocyst are presented in Fig 16-3. →

Lateral periodontal cyst	Odontogenic keratocyst
• An odontogenic cyst derived from rests of the dental lamina. • It is most often found in the mandibular premolar region. • The treatment is enucleation.	• Also derived from rests of dental lamina. • It is a cyst that occurs most often in the posterior body and ramus area. • It is one of the features of nevoid basal cell carcinoma. • It is treated by surgical enucleation.

Fig 16-3 Characteristics of the lateral periodontal cyst and the odontogenic keratocyst.

Epithelial Disorders

Q: Describe pseudoepitheliomatous hyperplasia.

Pseudoepitheliomatous hyperplasia is increased cell production of the squamous epithelium that is similar to squamous cell carcinoma. It is seen in chronic candidiasis and papillary hyperplasia.

Q: What is leukoplakia?

Leukoplakia is a clinical term used to denote mucosal conditions that produce coloration of the mucous membranes that is whiter than normal and cannot be characterized as any other definable lesion. Malignant transformation rate of oral leukoplakia varies from 0.13% to 34%,[5] and 5.4% to turn into squamous cell carcinoma. It is usually found in the buccal mucosa, the floor of the mouth, the labial commissures, the lateral borders of the tongue, and the mandibular and maxillary alveolar ridges.[1]

Q: What is proliferative (verrucous) leukoplakia?

Proliferative (verrucous) leukoplakia is an uncommon leukoplakia that creates white papillary areas covered with a thick keratinized surface that have the potential to develop into verrucous or squamous cell carcinoma. The treatment of choice is local excision.

Q: What is erythroplakia?

Erythroplakia is a painless, red, velvety, and plaque-like lesion of the mucous membranes that does not rub off. It is caused by epithelial dysplasia, carcinoma in situ, or squamous cell carcinoma. Histologic analysis shows that 60% to 90% of erythroplakias are epithelial dysplasia, carcinoma in situ, or squamous cell carcinoma.[1] It usually occurs on the floor of the mouth, ventral tongue, and soft palate. Depending on the stage, these lesions are usually excised.

Q: What is the most common malignant neoplasm of the oral cavity? What are its causes?

Squamous cell carcinoma represents 90% of all oral cancers. It is most often seen on the lower lip, lateral and ventral areas of the tongue, and the floor of the mouth. Mobility of adjacent teeth is common, and the invasion of the alveolar bone is seen in 50% of cases.[6] The causes are illustrated in Fig 16-4.

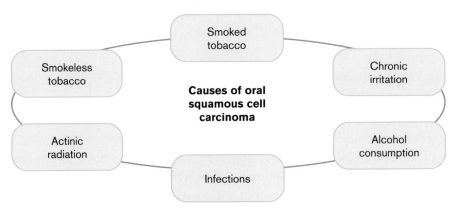

Fig 16-4 Causes of squamous cell carcinoma.

Q: How is squamous cell carcinoma treated?

Depending on the stage, it is usually treated by excision, radiation, or both.

Q: What sites metastasize to the mandible?

The kidney, breast, prostate, and lungs metastasize to the mandible.[7]

Q: Explain the ABCDE staging system for melanoma.

The ABCDE staging system for melanoma is presented in Fig 16-5.

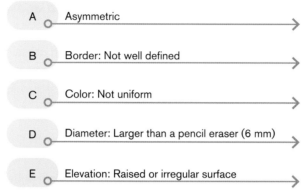

Fig 16-5 ABCDE staging for skin cancer.

Connective Tissue Lesions

Q: Describe a pyogenic granuloma (telangiectatic granuloma, pregnancy granuloma, pregnancy tumor, vascular epulis).

A *pyogenic granuloma* is a small, fast-growing rounded mass of inflamed tissue made of endothelial cells usually found on the gingiva. They are also known as pregnancy tumors because they often occur during the second and third trimesters of pregnancy. The lesion should be excised and curetted.

Q: Describe inflammatory papillary hyperplasia.

Inflammatory papillary hyperplasia is an overgrowth of fibrous connective tissue beneath a loose or ill-fitting denture. Usually the chronic inflammation is confined to the palatal vault. The hyperplastic tissue needs to be removed before a new denture is made.

Odontogenic Tumors

Q: What is the difference between a compound and a complex odontoma?

An odontoma is found predominantly in young adults and contains enamel, dentin, pulp, and cementum. A *compound odontoma* is tooth shaped and found in the anterior of the mouth. A *complex odontoma* is a solid mass and found in the posterior of the mouth. Treatment is enucleation.

Q: Describe the characteristics of an ameloblastoma.

An *ameloblastoma* is a slow-growing and aggressive tumor with a broad spectrum of histologic features. It is multicystic, has a soap bubble appearance on radiographs (Fig 16-6), and occurs most frequently in the mandible. It is rare for an ameloblastoma to metastasize. Treatment is marginal or block resection due to their high recurrence rate.

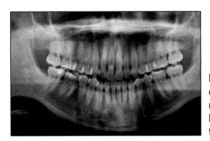

Fig 16-6 Panoramic radiograph showing a radiolucency at the mesial aspect of the root of the mandibular right second premolar to the mesial buccal of the mandibular right first molar. Differential diagnosis includes ameloblastoma.

Immune-Mediated Disorders

Q: What is desquamative gingivitis?

Desquamative gingivitis is characterized by scooped-out gingiva, diffuse gingival erythema, and mucosal sloughing and erosion. Approximately 50% of desquamative gingivitis cases are localized to the gingiva, and 75% of desquamative gingivitis cases have a dermatologic genesis.[8] It may be found in lichen planus, pemphigus vulgaris, mucous membrane pemphigoid, and lupus.

Q: Describe the differences between pemphigus vulgaris and mucous membrane pemphigoid.

The differences between pemphigus vulgaris and mucous membrane pemphigoid are shown in Fig 16-7.

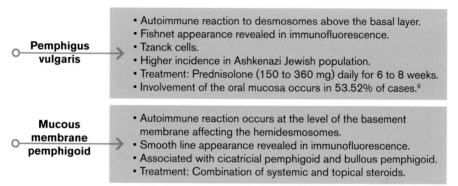

Pemphigus vulgaris →
- Autoimmune reaction to desmosomes above the basal layer.
- Fishnet appearance revealed in immunofluorescence.
- Tzanck cells.
- Higher incidence in Ashkenazi Jewish population.
- Treatment: Prednisolone (150 to 360 mg) daily for 6 to 8 weeks.
- Involvement of the oral mucosa occurs in 53.52% of cases.[9]

Mucous membrane pemphigoid →
- Autoimmune reaction occurs at the level of the basement membrane affecting the hemidesmosomes.
- Smooth line appearance revealed in immunofluorescence.
- Associated with cicatricial pemphigoid and bullous pemphigoid.
- Treatment: Combination of systemic and topical steroids.

Fig 16-7 Characteristics of pemphigus vulgaris and mucous membrane pemphigoid.

Q: What is the Nikolsky test?

The *Nikolsky test* consists of rubbing the tissue with a blunt instrument and observing whether a blister forms in minutes. Blister formation indicates that the clinical test is positive. The test is positive in patients with disorders in cell cohesion at the basement membrane (eg, mucous membrane pemphigoid).

Q: What is erythema multiforme?

Erythema multiforme is a hypersensitivity reaction that is centered on superficial vessels of the skin and is of immune origin. It clinically presents as ulcerations on any mucosal site, and it is most common in young adult men. The immunofluorescent pattern is perivascular. It can be incited by the following[10]:

- Drugs (penicillin and sulfa)
- Gastrointestinal conditions (Crohn disease and ulcerative colitis)
- Infections (herpes)
- Recent vaccinations

Treatment is to find the inciting factor and neutralize it. The condition is usually self-limiting.

Q: Describe lichen planus.

Oral lichen planus (OLP) is the most common mucosal localization of lichen planus, affecting about 1% to 2% of the population. It is associated with skin lesions in 60% to 70% of cases, while arising as the only manifestation in 15% to 25% of patients,[11] with a noticeable T lymphocyte reaction in the connective tissue. The chance for malignant transformation is 0.4% to 2%. The immunofluorescent pattern demonstrates a deposit of fibrinogen in a shaggy pattern at the basement membrane. Six types of clinical manifestation have been described[12,13] (Table 16-2; see next page). Mucosal lesions, which are numerous, generally have a symmetric distribution, particularly on the mucosa of the cheeks, adjacent to molars, and on the mucosa of the tongue. It is seen less frequently on the mucosa of the lips (lichenous cheilitis) and on the gums (the atrophic and erosive forms localized on the gums manifest as a desquamative gingivitis), seldom on the floor of the mouth and palate.[14]

A recent randomized controlled study found that a plaque control program (patients received oral hygiene instruction using a powered toothbrush and provided with interdental cleaning aids) was more effective than the control (continued with their normal plaque control regimen and did not receive any advice) in managing patients with gingival manifestations of OLP. At 20 weeks, patients in the plaque control group showed significantly better clinical measures when compared with those in the control.[15]

Q: Describe the characteristics of lupus erythematosus (LE).

Lupus erythematosus is a group of autoimmune disorders with chronic inflammation of the skin, connective tissues, and internal organs. It is commonly found in middle-aged women. It is thought that antibodies target DNA. There are two major forms: discoid LE (DLE) and systemic LE (SLE). DLE is a mild chronic form; it is characterized in the mouth with buccomucosal lesions and occasionally the gingiva. The usual lesion presents as a central atrophic area with small white dots surrounded by fine white striae. The systemic type includes lesions on the face (characteristic red butterfly lesions on bridge of the nose and cheeks) and tend to spread all over the body.[6] It is usually treated with topical steroids, antimalarial agents, and sulfones.

Table 16-2	Forms of lichen planus[12,13]					
	Papular	**Reticular (most common)**	**Ulcerative (erosive)**	**Plaque**	**Bullous (vesicles)**	**Erythematous (atrophic)**
Description	Mainly in the initial phase and has a transitory course.	Wickham striae: raised, thin, white lines that have a reticular pattern.	Painful erythematous or white pseudomembranous areas. More persistent and shows a short-term course.	White raised or flattened area. More constant form, but also demonstrated many newly established infections.	Usually develop in the context of preexisting lichen planus lesions.	Fluctuating with many remissions and newly established infections.

Q: What are some preventive treatments to consider for patients with Sjögren syndrome?

Sjögren syndrome is a chronic autoimmune disease that attacks the exocrine glands that produce tears and saliva. Maintenance is as follows:

- Four-month recall: 1.23% acidulated phosphate sodium fluoride gel in a fluoride tray for 4 minutes or 2.25% fluoride varnish.
- Patient should brush with a fluoride dentifrice (PreviDent 5000 Plus, Colgate-Palmolive).
- Chlorhexidine 0.12% rinse for 30 seconds at night.

Q: Compare and contrast erosive lichen planus, mucous membrane pemphigoid, pemphigus vulgaris, and erythema multiforme.

Table 16-3 describes the differences between the erosive lesions of the mouth (see next page).[10]

Salivary Gland Disorders

Q: What is the difference between a mucocele and a mucus retention cyst?

Table 16-4 presents the defining characteristics of mucoceles and mucus retention cysts (see next page).

Oral Infections

Q: How does herpes zoster manifest itself in the oral cavity?

Herpes zoster can appear as a vesicular eruption on the mucosa as well as on the skin. The lesions can arise along the ophthalmic, maxillary, and mandibular distribution of the nerve. Herpes zoster can be very painful.

Table 16-3	Differences between the erosive lesions of the mouth			
	Location	**Antigen**	**Direct immunofluo-rescence**	**Treatment**
Erosive lichen planus	Basal cell/base-ment membrane	Unknown	Shaggy, fibrinogen	If symptomatic, persistent or widespread, topical or systemic steroids.
Mucous membrane pemphigoid	Hemidesmosome	BP-1, -2, laminin-5	IgG, C3, smooth linear	Systemic and topical steroids.
Pemphigus vulgaris	Desmosomes	Desmoglein 3	IgG; fishnet appearance	Prednisone (150 to 360 mg) daily for 6 to 8 weeks.
Erythema multiforme	Blood vessel wall/basement membrane	Immune complexes	IgM, C3, perivascular	Acyclovir if the episode follows a herpes attack. Patients should be transferred to ICU or burn center to reduce risk of infection and mortality.

Ig, immunoglobulin; ICU, intensive care unit.

Table 16-4	Characteristics of mucoceles and mucus retention cysts	
	Mucocele	**Mucus retention cyst**
Definition	Swelling in the mouth when a salivary duct is severed	Cyst caused by an obstruction of a duct
Lining	Granulation tissue	Lined by epithelium
Common location	Lower lip	Lower lip and buccal mucosa
Differential	Mucus retention cyst, fibroma, neuroma, and mucoepidermoid carcinoma	Mucocele and mucoepidermoid carcinoma

Q: Describe the features of necrotizing periodontal diseases (an extension of necrotizing gingivitis).

Necrotizing periodontitis is a necrotizing disease that extends to the gingiva and bone. The features of necrotizing periodontal diseases[16] are presented in Fig 16-8.

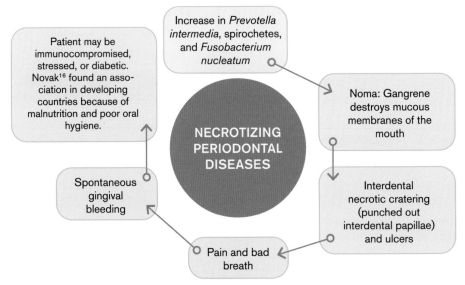

Fig 16-8 Features of necrotizing periodontal diseases.

Q: What is the treatment for necrotizing periodontal diseases?

Treatment consists of chlorhexidine, metronidazole (250 mg taken four times per day), and local debridement. Novak[16] noted that adjunctive systemic metronidazole therapy has been shown to effectively manage HIV-associated periodontitis and control spirochetal infection but warned of the risk of super-infection with oral *Candida* associated with the use of systemic antibiotics, particularly in the treatment of patients with HIV.

Q: Describe the symptoms of atrophic candidiasis.

- Most commonly found on the palate under a denture
- A continuous painful burning feeling
- Increased sensitivity

Papillon-Lefèvre Syndrome

Q: Describe Papillon-Lefèvre syndrome.

Papillon-Lefèvre syndrome is an autosomal recessive disorder caused by deficiency of cathepsin C. Severe periodontal disease affects the primary teeth (by 4 years of age, most of the primary teeth are lost) and permanent teeth (by 14 years of age, most of the permanent teeth are lost).[1] There is also hyperkeratosis of the palms of the hands and soles of the feet.

Differential Diagnosis

Q: What is the differential diagnosis for a bump?

The differential diagnosis for a bump includes[10]:

- Fibroma
- Traumatic neuroma (painful nodular proliferation of nerve and fibrous tissue of the nerve sheath resulting from the unsuccessful attempt of nerve fibers to reunite with their severed distal portion)
- Neurofibroma (demarcated or diffuse benign proliferation of fibroblasts that are oriented in a random or nodular pattern with a myxoid background)
- Giant cell fibroma (a variant of focal fibrous hyperplasia)
- Peripheral fibroma
- Peripheral ossifying fibroma (a gingival nodule consisting of a reactive hyperplasia of connective tissue containing focal areas of bone)
- Pyogenic granuloma (a fast-growing reactive proliferation of endothelial cells usually on the gingiva and commonly in response to constant irritation; also known as *pregnancy tumor*)
- Periodontal abscess (parulis)
- Ranula (mucocele of the floor of the mouth)
- Lymphangioma (a benign production of lymphatic vessels that occurs as a focal superficial lesion in the oral cavity and as a big diffuse lesion in the neck, eg, cystic hygroma)
- Salivary gland enlargement
- Lipoma (a benign neoplasm of normal fat cells that appear as a soft, movable swelling; usually yellowish) →

- Leiomyoma (a benign neoplasm of smooth muscle within the oral cavity that looks firm, movable, and commonly of the blood vessels)
- Rhabdomyoma (a tumor of striated muscle, usually in the heart and tongue)
- Hemangioma (a production of large or small vascular channels usually found in children; individual lesions with variable clinical courses)
- Granular cell tumor (a mass of large cells of either muscle or nerve origin with a cytoplasm of densely packed eosinophilic granules; usually found on the dorsal surface of the tongue)
- Schwannoma

Q: What is the differential diagnosis for a circumscribed flat lesion? Circumscribed elevated lesion?

Flat:

- Ephelis
- Junctional nevus
- Café au lait spots or macules
- Lentigo
- Melanotic macule

Elevated:

- Nevi
- Seborrheic keratosis
- Melanoma

Q: What is the differential diagnosis for a nonspecific ulcer?

- Aphthae
- Squamous cell carcinoma
- Herpetic ulcer
- Traumatic ulcer
- Traumatic granuloma
- Primary/secondary syphilis
- Necrotizing ulcerative gingivitis
- Herpangina

Q: What is the differential diagnosis for a pericoronal radiolucency?

- Dentigerous cyst
- Odontogenic keratocyst
- Ameloblastoma

Q: What are the differential diagnoses for pigmented, white, and red lesions?

Figure 16-9 presents the differential diagnoses for pigmented, white, and red lesions.

Pigmented lesions	White lesions	Red lesions
• Amalgam tattoo • Mucosal nevi • Vascular malformation • Melanotic macule • Melanoma • Blue nevus • Kaposi sarcoma • Black hairy tongue	• Epithelial hyperplasia • Frictional keratosis • Plaque-type lichen planus • Chronic hyperplastic *Candida* • Tobacco-related leukoplakia • Hairy leukoplakia • Snuff dipper's pouch • Hyperkeratosis • Squamous cell carcinoma • Proliferative verrucous leukoplakia • Leukoedema • Fordyce granules	• Squamous cell carcinoma • Erythematous *Candida* • Contact stomatitis • Drug reaction • Geographic tongue • Osteosarcoma • Ecchymosis • Kaposi sarcoma • Angular cheilitis • Erythroplakia • Atrophic glossitis

Fig 16-9 Differential diagnoses for pigmented, white, and red lesions.

Q: What is the differential diagnosis for a papillary lesion?

The differential diagnosis for a papillary lesion[3] includes:

- Oral papilloma
- Verruca vulgaris
- Verrucas carcinoma
- Squamous papilloma
- Inflammatory papillary hyperplasia
- Condyloma acuminatum
- Focal epithelial hyperplasia

Q: What is the differential diagnosis for a lump in the midline of the neck? Lateral neck?

The differential diagnoses for a lump in the midline of the neck and in the lateral neck are presented in Fig 16-10.

Midline of the neck
- Thyroglossal duct cyst
- Thyroiditis
- Goiter
- Thyroid tumors
- Hashimoto disease

Lateral neck
- Branchial cleft cyst
- Lymphadenitis
- Hodgkin and non-Hodgkin lymphoma

Fig 16-10 Differential diagnoses for a lump in the midline and lateral region of the neck.

Q: What is the differential diagnosis for apical radiolucencies?

According to Blicher et al[17]:

- Periapical granuloma
- Periapical cyst
- Periapical scar
- Ameloblastoma
- Ameloblastoma fibroma
- Keratocystic odontogenic tumor
- Odontogenic myxoma
- Dentigerous cyst
- Residual cyst
- Nasopalatine duct cyst
- Globulomaxillary cyst
- Lateral periodontal cyst
- Traumatic bone cyst
- Stafne bone defect
- Central giant cell lesion
- Langerhans cell histiocytosis
- Brown tumor
- Cemento-osseous dysplasia (early)
- Vitamin D-resistant rickets
- Neurofibromatosis
- Malignancy →

Sirotheau Corrêa Pontes et al[18] did a study of cases referred from a reference service in oral pathology that were initially misdiagnosed as periapical lesions of endodontic origin. They found 66% of non-endodontic lesions were benign (most common were ameloblastomas and nasopalatine duct cysts), 29% were malignant (most common were metastatic lesions and carcinomas), and 5% were stafne bone cavities.

Miscellaneous

Q: What is the difference between osteogenesis imperfecta and dentinogenesis imperfecta?

Table 16-5 presents the characteristics of osteogenesis imperfecta and dentogenesis imperfecta.

Table 16-5	Osteogenesis imperfecta and dentinogenesis imperfecta	
	Osteogenesis imperfecta (OI)	**Dentinogenesis imperfecta (DI)**
Definition	• Alteration in formation of bone • Inability of the matrix to mineralize	Undermineralized dentin obliterates pulp chambers and canals
Characteristics	Blue sclera	• Opalescent teeth • Dentin is soft
Treatment	Orthopedic treatment is usually nonsurgical	Appropriate restorations are made to prevent further loss of enamel
Relation to one another	25% have DI	• Type 1: Patients have OI • Type 2: Patients do not have OI • Type 3: Mostly in Maryland, primary teeth have multiple pulp exposures

Q: **What is the difference between actinic cheilitis and angular cheilitis?**

Table 16-6 presents the characteristics and treatment of actinic cheilitis and angular cheilitis.

Table 16-6	Definition and treatment of actinic cheilitis and angular cheilitis	
	Actinic cheilitis	**Angular cheilitis**
Definition	• Red and white patches with telangiectasia • Caused by prolonged exposure to sunlight • Premalignant squamous cell carcinoma occurs in 10% of cases	• Bilateral fissures at the corners of the mouth usually caused by *Candida albicans* • May have secondary infection with bacteria
Treatment	Superficial surgical removal of the damaged tissue unless metastasis has occurred	Antifungal ointment alone or in combination with antibiotics

Q: **What is PFAPA syndrome?**

Periodic fever, aphthous stomatitis, pharyngitis, and adenitis or *periodic fever aphthous pharyngitis and cervical adenopathy* (PFAPA) syndrome is a medical condition, typically starting in young children, in which high fever occurs periodically at intervals of about 3 to 5 weeks, frequently accompanied by aphthous ulcers, pharyngitis, or adenitis. A possible treatment is a dose of prednisone.

Q: **What are the comorbidities found in patients with AIDS?**

- Hairy leukoplakia
- *Candida*/angular cheilitis
- Atrophic *Candida*
- Kaposi sarcoma
- Non-Hodgkin lymphoma
- Linear gingivitis
- Herpes simplex/herpes zoster

Q: What is mucoepidermoid carcinoma?

Mucoepidermoid carcinoma is the most common salivary gland carcinoma and the malignant tumor most frequently found in individuals younger than 20 years. It does not have a capsule and is composed of mucus-secreting and stratified squamous epithelial cells. About two-thirds of mucoepidermoid carcinomas are found within the parotid gland; the remaining one-third are located within the minor salivary glands.[19] The treatment is based on its grade. If it is found in the parotid gland, lobectomy and cervical node dissection are indicated if the nodes are palpable.

Q: Do cemento-osseous lesions need to be treated?

Cemento-osseous lesions, which are common in the black population, do not need to be treated. They consist of calcifications at the apices of the teeth, and patients have no symptoms.

References

1. Sapp JP, Eversole LR, Wysocki GP. Contemporary Oral and Maxillofacial Pathology, ed 2. St Louis: Mosby, 2004:40,174,183,253.
2. Woo SB, Sonis ST. Recurrent aphthous ulcers: A review of diagnosis and treatment. J Am Dent Assoc 1996;127:1202–1213.
3. Newland JR, Meiller TF, Wynn RL, Crossley HL. Oral Soft Tissue Diseases: A Reference Manual for Diagnosis and Management, ed 2. Hudson, Ohio: Lexi-Comp, 2002:29,48,53,87.
4. Snoeck R. Antiviral therapy of herpes simplex. Int J Antimicrob Agents 2000;16:157–159.
5. Anderson A, Ishak N. Marked variation in malignant transformation rates of oral leukoplakia. Evid Based Dent 2015;16:102–103.
6. Holmstrup P, Plemons J, Meyle J. Non-plaque-induced gingival diseases. J Periodontol 2018;89(suppl 1):S28–S45.
7. Kumar G, Manjunatha B. Metastatic tumors to the jaws and oral cavity. J Oral Maxillofac Pathol 2013;17:71–75.
8. Aguirre, A,Vasquez JLT, Nisengard RJ. Desquamative gingivitis. In: Newman MG, Takei HH, Klokkevold PR, Carranza FA. Carranza's Clinical Periodontology, ed 10. St Louis: Saunders, 2006:411–433.
9. Shamim T, Varghese VI, Shameena PM, Sudha S. Pemphigus vulgaris in oral cavity: Clinical analysis of 71 cases. Med Oral Patol Oral Cir Bucal 2008;13:E622–E626.
10. Sapp JP, Eversole LR, Wysocki GP. Contemporary Oral and Maxillofacial Pathology, ed 2. St Louis: Mosby, 2004.
11. Giannetti L, Dello Diago AM, Spinas E. Oral lichen planus. J Biol Regul Homeost Agents 2018;32:391–395.
12. Liakopoulou A, Rallis E. Bullous lichen planus—A review. J Dermatol Case Rep 2017 31;11:1–4.
13. Thorn JJ, Holmstrup P, Rindum J, Pindborg JJ. Course of various clinical forms of oral lichen planus. A prospective follow-up study of 611 patients. J Oral Pathol 1988;17:213–218.

14. Boorghani M, Gholizadeh N, Taghavi Zenouz A, Vatankhah M, Mehdipour M. Oral lichen planus: Clinical features, etiology, treatment and management; a review of literature. J Dent Res Dent Clin Dent Prospects 2010;4:3–9.
15. Stone SJ, McCracken GI, Heasman PA, Staines KS, Pennington M. Cost-effectiveness of personalized plaque control for managing the gingival manifestations of oral lichen planus: A randomized controlled study. J Clin Periodontol 2013;40:859–867.
16. Novak MJ. Necrotizing ulcerative periodontitis. Ann Periodontol 1999;4:74–78.
17. Blicher B, Pryles RL, Lin J. Endodontics Review: A Study Guide. Chicago: Quintessence, 2016:58.
18. Sirotheau Corrêa Pontes F, Paiva Fonseca F, Souza de Jesus A, et al. Nonendodontic lesions misdiagnosed as apical periodontitis lesions: Series of case reports and review of literature. J Endod 2014;40:16–27.
19. Mucoepidermoid Carcinoma. http://www.thedoctorsdoctor.com/diseases/mucoepidermoid_ca.htm. Accessed 2 October 2012.

Lasers

Background

Q: What is laser an acronym for?

Laser stands for **l**ight **a**mplification by **s**timulated **e**mission of **r**adiation.

Q: What are the most common types of lasers used in periodontics?

The most common types of laser used in periodontics[1] are presented in Fig 17-1.

Carbon dioxide (CO$_2$)	Neodymium: yttrium-aluminum-garnet (Nd:YAG)	Erbium: yttrium-aluminum-garnet (Er:YAG)
• 10,600-nm wavelength • Useful for soft tissue surgery such as frenectomy, degranulation, biopsy, and gingivectomy	• 1,064-nm wavelength • Affinity for pigmented colors and can penetrate deep beyond the surface • Useful for soft tissue incision, subgingival ablation, and bacterial elimination	• 2,940-nm wavelength for the free-running laser • Useful for soft tissue incision and ablation, subgingival curettage, scaling of root surfaces, osteoplasty, and ostectomy • Highly absorbed in both water and hydroxyapatite

Fig 17-1 Types of lasers.

Q: What are the advantages and disadvantages of lasers?

Figure 17-2 presents the advantages and disadvantages of lasers.[2–4]

Advantages	Disadvantages
• Relatively bloodless • Minimal swelling and scarring • Coagulation • Minimal suturing • Less postsurgical pain	• Minimal evidence for use as a monotherapy • Not been shown to be better than scaling and root planing • May have delayed scar contraction (wound healing) • Expensive • There is potential for root surface damage (especially Er:YAG) • May reach the patient's eyes (need to prevent irradiation to eyes)

Fig 17-2 Advantages and disadvantages of lasers.

Different Types of Laser Therapies

Q: What is photodynamic therapy?

Photodynamic therapy unites low-level laser light with a photosensitizer (a nontoxic dye), which attaches to the target cells and destroys microorganisms.[1]

Q: What is the laser-assisted new attachment procedure (LANAP)?

LANAP (Millennium Dental Technologies) uses the Nd:YAG laser to remove the pocket epithelium and necrotic epithelium; however, the connective tissue is spared, allowing healing and regeneration to occur. The manufacturer claims decreased postoperative bleeding and recession compared with conventional osseous surgery.

Effectiveness

Q: Have lasers been found to be effective in treating chronic periodontitis?

Cobb's review[4] found that in terms of reducing pocket depth and subgingival bacterial populations, Nd:YAG and Er:YAG lasers have been shown to be as effective as scaling and root planing (SRP) in the treatment of chronic periodontitis. However, he described the evidence for laser therapy being superior to traditional nonsurgical periodontal therapy regarding gain in clinical attachment level (the "gold standard") as "minimal at best." Karlsson et al[5] did not find consistent evidence to support the effectiveness of adjunctive laser treatment in adults with chronic periodontitis.

Q: Are lasers more effective than traditional SRP?

A recent best evidence consensus by the American Academy of Periodontology (AAP) found that laser therapy as an adjunct to conventional therapy may provide less than 1 mm in clinical improvement in probing depth and clinical attachment level compared with traditional therapy treating chronic and aggressive forms of periodontitis. The authors also found evidence to suggest that adjunctive use of Nd:YAG and Er:YAG was superior to traditional therapy alone in pockets with probing depth 7 mm or greater. There is inadequate evidence to determine laser therapy alone is better or comparable to traditional periodontal therapy.[6]

A statement by the AAP[3] reported "minimal evidence" supporting the use of lasers as a monotherapy or adjunctively with SRP for subgingival debridement. It went on to state that although in vitro studies have shown the Er:YAG laser to remove calculus and to negate endotoxin, there is a risk of damage to the root surface during calculus removal due to the inability of the laser operator to see the area being lased by the hard tissue laser. It concluded that on the whole lasers have been shown to be "unpredictable and inconsistent in their ability to reduce subgingival microbial loads" to a greater degree than SRP alone.

Cobb[4] found limited proof that lasers used in an adjunctive capacity to SRP may offer some further benefit.

Eberhard et al[7] found that, although the efficacy of Er:YAG did not reach that achieved by hand instrumentation, it was capable of removing calculus from periodontally involved root surfaces. He also found that, opposed to →

scaling and root planing, the lack of cementum removal may qualify the laser as a different approach during supportive periodontal therapy.

In Slot et al's review[8] of initial treatment of periodontitis, they found that studies confirmed no beneficial effect for a pulsed Nd:YAG laser compared with conventional therapy.

Q: Is there evidence of reparative/regenerative responses following the treatment of periodontitis with lasers?

No, it has yet to be established.[6]

Q: Do lasers work better than SRP alone in patients with peri-implant mucositis or peri-implantitis?

There is no evidence supporting the use of laser treatment in peri-implant mucositis long term. There is limited evidence for benefits for adjunctive laser use and surgical treatment of peri-implantitis.[6]

Q: Can lasers be used for crown lengthening?

Presently, there are no controlled longitudinal or cohort studies demonstrating the use of lasers for clinical crown lengthening using the closed flap technique.[4]

Q: Is photodynamic therapy effective?

The best evidence consensus by the AAP found photodynamic therapy as an adjunct to conventional therapy may provide a modest improvement of less than 1 mm in clinical attachment level and probing depth when compared to conventional treatment.[6]

Braham et al[9] found that antimicrobial photodynamic therapy may enhance the outcomes of periodontal treatment through its bactericidal activity and ability to inactivate bacterial virulence factors and host cytokines that impede healing. Berakdar et al[1] demonstrated a slightly higher improvement of clinical parameters with photodynamic therapy in addition to SRP than with SRP alone.

Azarpazhooh et al[10] demonstrated in a meta-analysis that photodynamic therapy as an independent treatment or as an adjunct to SRP was not superior to SRP alone and as a result did not recommend photodynamic therapy

→

to routinely treat periodontitis. According to a statement by the AAP,[3] photo-dynamic therapy is arbitrary and variable.

Q: Is LANAP successful?

In a statement regarding the use of dental lasers for excisional new attachment procedures (ENAP), the AAP[11] states that there is a lack of evidence that "laser ENAP" or "laser curettage" provides clinical advantages in terms of treatment results compared with traditional periodontal therapy. They also point to evidence suggesting that such use of lasers could interfere with normal cell attachment and healing on root surfaces and adjacent alveolar bone.

Yukna et al[12] found that LANAP-treated teeth displayed superior probing depth reductions and clinical probing attachment level gains compared with control teeth. New cementum and new connective tissue attachment was observed on all teeth treated with LANAP.

Q: What case management advantages are there for laser therapy?

Laser therapy can be an alternative nonsurgical therapy for medically compromised patients. It can cause less patient bleeding and assist in disease site disinfection.[6]

Safety

Q: What are potential risks of laser therapy?

The use of lasers on healthy sites could cause harm rather than benefit.
Damage (eg, overheating) can occur to the teeth and/or implant if proper protocols are not followed.[6]

Q: Can lasers be used around dental implants?

Wilcox et al[13] studied the Nd:YAG laser and found that prudent use of the laser unit yields temperature profiles within clinical parameters in the presence of dental implants. $\rightarrow$

Galli et al[14] recommended operating Er:YAG lasers with care on titanium surfaces based on evidence that the laser may reduce the viability and the activity of osteoblastic cells.

Romanos et al[15] studied the CO_2 laser and observed osteoblast growth on titanium surfaces. The study concluded that osteoblast attachment and bone formation may be fostered by laser irradiation of titanium surfaces.

Q: Is there potential for root surface damage with the Er:YAG laser?

According to a statement by the AAP,[3] there is a risk of damage to the root surface during calculus removal by Er:YAG laser due to the inability of the operator to see the area being lased by the hard tissue laser.

References

1. Berakdar M, Callaway A, Eddin MF, Ross A, Willershausen B. Comparison between scaling-root-planing (SRP) and SRP/photodynamic therapy: Six-month study. Head Face Med 2012;8:12.
2. Pick RM, Colvard MD. Current status of lasers in soft tissue dental surgery. J Periodontol 1993;64:589–602.
3. American Academy of Periodontology statement on the efficacy of lasers in the non-surgical treatment of inflammatory periodontal disease. J Periodontol 2011;82:513–514.
4. Cobb CM. Lasers in periodontics: A review of the literature. J Periodontol 2006;77:545–564.
5. Karlsson MR, Diogo Löfgren CI, Jansson HM. The effect of laser therapy to nonsurgical periodontal treatment in subjects with chronic periodontitis: A systematic review. J Periodontol 2008;79:2021–2028.
6. Mills MP, Rosen PS, Chambrone L, et al. American Academy of Periodontology best evidence consensus statement on the efficacy of laser therapy used alone or as an adjunct to non-surgical and surgical treatment of periodontitis and peri-implant diseases. J Periodontol 2018;89:737–742.
7. Eberhard J, Ehlers H, Falk W, Açil Y, Albers HK, Jepsen S. Efficacy of subgingival calculus removal with Er:YAG laser compared to mechanical debridement: An in situ study. J Clin Periodontol 2003;30:511–518.
8. Slot DE, Kranendonk AA, Paraskevas S, Van der Weijden F. The effect of a pulsed Nd:YAG laser in nonsurgical periodontal therapy. J Periodontol 2009;80:1041–1056.
9. Braham P, Herron C, Street C, Darveau R. Antimicrobial photodynamic therapy may promote periodontal healing through multiple mechanisms. J Periodontol 2009;80:1790–1798.
10. Azarpazhooh A, Shah PS, Tenenbaum HC, Goldberg MB. The effect of photodynamic therapy for periodontitis: A systematic review and meta-analysis. J Periodontol 2010;81:4–14.
11. American Academy of Periodontology. Statement Regarding Use of Dental Lasers for Excisional New Attachment Procedure (ENAP). August 1999.
12. Yukna RA, Carr RL, Evans GH. Histologic evaluation of an Nd:YAG laser-assisted new attachment procedure in humans. Int J Periodontics Restorative Dent 2007;27:577–587.

13. Wilcox CW, Wilwerding TM, Watson P, Morris JT. Use of electrosurgery and lasers in the presence of dental implants. Int J Oral Maxillofac Implants 2001;16:578–582.
14. Galli C, Macaluso GM, Elezi E, et al. The effects of Er:YAG laser treatment on titanium surface profile and osteoblastic cell activity: An in vitro study. J Periodontol 2011;82:1169–1177.
15. Romanos G, Crespi R, Barone A, Covani U. Osteoblast attachment on titanium disks after laser irradiation. Int J Oral Maxillofac Implants 2006;21:232–236.

Medical Emergencies

Cardiopulmonary Resuscitation (CPR)

Q: What is hands-only CPR?[1]

1. Kneel beside the person who needs help.
2. Place the heel of one hand on the center of the chest.
3. Place the heel of the other hand on top of the first hand, then lace your fingers together.
4. Position your body so that your shoulders are directly over your hands and keep your arms straight.
5. Push hard, push fast. Use your body weight to help you administer compressions that are at least 2 inches deep and delivered at a rate of at least 100 compressions per minute. (Just be sure to let chest rise completely between compressions.)
6. Keep pushing. Continue hands-only CPR until you see obvious signs of life, like breathing; another trained responder or EMS professional can take over; you're too exhausted to continue; an automated external defibrillator (AED) becomes available; or the scene becomes unsafe.

Q: What are the first steps that must be taken when you see an unconscious person?

C: Check the scene for safety.
C: Check the patient for responsiveness.
C: Call for 911, get an AED.

Q: Explain the first three steps that must be done with an AED.

1. Turn on the AED.
2. Place the pads.
3. Connect the connector and follow the AED voice.

After the AED delivers a shock, the rescuer should immediately restart CPR, beginning with chest compressions.

Emergency Drugs

Q: What are some essential drugs to have in the emergency kit?

Figure 18-1 presents drugs that are essential to an emergency kit.

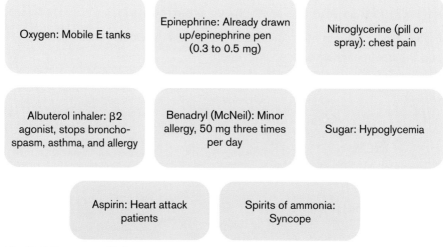

Oxygen: Mobile E tanks

Epinephrine: Already drawn up/epinephrine pen (0.3 to 0.5 mg)

Nitroglycerine (pill or spray): chest pain

Albuterol inhaler: β2 agonist, stops broncho-spasm, asthma, and allergy

Benadryl (McNeil): Minor allergy, 50 mg three times per day

Sugar: Hypoglycemia

Aspirin: Heart attack patients

Spirits of ammonia: Syncope

Fig 18-1 Emergency kit drugs.

Q: What are the secondary drugs that can be helpful in an emergency?

- Nitrous oxide: Pain control for heart attacks
- Glucagon: 1 mg for hypoglycemic patients
- Valium (Roche): Benzodiazepine for epilepsy
- Hydrocortisone: Allergy
- Reversal drugs: Intravenous (IV) sedation

Office Emergencies

Q: How can the diagnosis of an emergency condition be established?

Figure 18-2 presents the process of diagnosing a medical emergency.

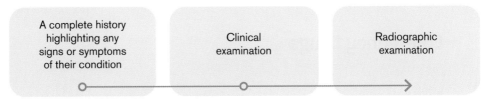

Fig 18-2 Diagnosis of a medical emergency.

Q: What are the common reasons a patient may lose consciousness and the associated treatments?

Figure 18-3 presents common reasons a patient may lose consciousness and the treatments associated with each.

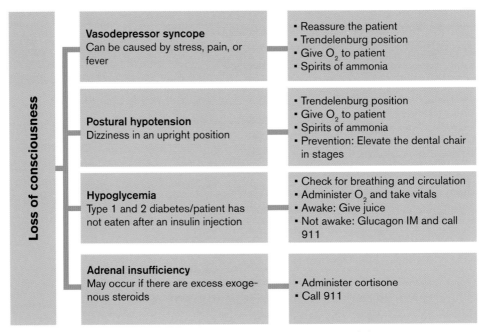

Fig 18-3 Causes and treatments of loss of consciousness. IM, intramuscularly.

Q: Describe a grand mal seizure.

Grand mal epilepsy is the most common form of seizure disorder. Causes include drug withdrawal, photic stimulation, menstruation, fatigue, alcohol, falling asleep, or awakening. The seizure could last 5 to 15 minutes.

Management of the patient includes protecting the airway (remove any objects from their mouth) and preventing the patient from injury. After being monitored, the patient can be discharged to an adult companion or friend.

Q: Describe prevention and symptoms of airway obstruction.

Prevention:

- Adequate protection of the oropharynx (rubber dam and throat screen)
- Ligatures around small dental objects

Possible symptoms:

- Coughing
- "Crowing" sounds
- Patient reaches for neck
- Inability to speak
- Cyanosis
- Loss of consciousness
- Death

Q: Describe the possible conditions that may result from respiratory distress and their management.

Management of the conditions that may result from respiratory distress is presented in Fig 18-4 (see next page).

Q: What are some reasons a patient may walk into the office confused?

Figure 18-5 presents possible causes for patient confusion (see next page).

Q: What are some reactions a patient may have to local anesthetic administration?

Possible patient reactions to local anesthetic administration include:

- Overdose: Watch patient and check vitals. $\rightarrow$

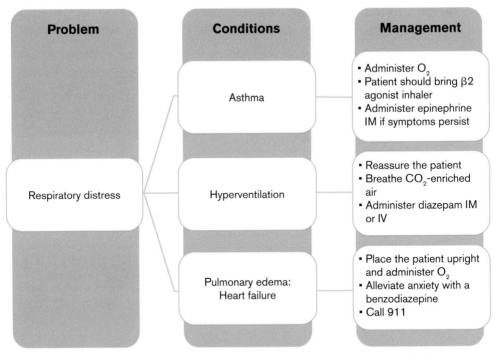

Fig 18-4 Management of conditions resulting from respiratory distress. IM, intramuscularly.

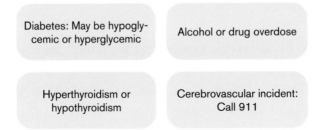

Fig 18-5 Causes of patient confusion.

- Allergy: Mild—50 mg Benadryl or a histamine blocker intramuscularly (IM); severe—epinephrine (0.3 to 0.5 mg) IM or IV and call 911.
- Hyperventilation: Reassure the patient and allow them to breathe CO_2-enriched air. It may be necessary to administer diazepam IM or IV.

Q: What are some reasons a patient walking into the practice may experience chest pain?

Figure 18-6 presents reasons for chest pain. For angina, a nitroglycerin tablet (0.3 to 0.5 mg) may be given. However, in potential cases of myocardial infarction, a call to 911 needs to be made as aspirin, nitrous oxide, and oxygen are administered.

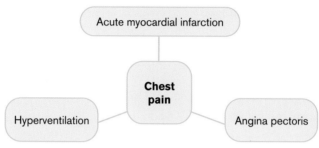

Fig 18-6 Causes of chest pain.

Q: What is the difference between angina and myocardial infarction?

The difference between angina and myocardial infarction is presented in Fig 18-7.

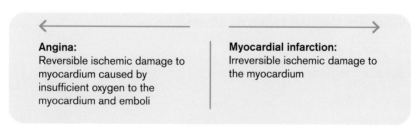

Fig 18-7 Difference between angina and myocardial infarction.

Q: Describe the symptoms and prevention techniques for a patient with congestive heart failure.[2]

A patient's whose heart does not pump properly may suffer from congestive heart disease. Possible causes include myocardial infarction or valvular heart disease. →

Recognition:

1. Shortness of breath
2. Rales heard with auscultation
3. Tachypnea
4. Agitation
5. Cyanosis
6. Pink frothy sputum

Prevention:

1. Confirm patient took cardiac medications
2. Treat in a more upright position
3. Reduce stress
4. Supplemental oxygen while monitoring heart rate
5. Limit volume and salt intake of IV fluids

Q: What are signs that a patient is having a stroke?[3]

- Sudden numbness or weakness in the face, arm, or leg, especially on one side of the body
- Sudden confusion, trouble speaking, or difficulty understanding speech
- Sudden trouble seeing in one or both eyes
- Sudden trouble walking, dizziness, loss of balance, or lack of coordination
- Sudden severe headache with no known cause

Q: What are the two types of stroke?

Hemorrhagic stroke:

- Risk factor: Hypertension

Occlusive stroke:

- 85% of strokes
- Most result from atherosclerotic disease and cardiac abnormalities
- Risk factors: Hypertension, diabetes, smoking, abnormal valves, atrial fibrillation, and prior transient ischemic attack

Q: How would you treat the patient?[3]

If you think someone may be having a stroke, act F.A.S.T. and do the following simple test:

- F—Face: Ask the person to smile. Does one side of the face droop? →

- A—Arms: Ask the person to raise both arms. Does one arm drift downward?
- S—Speech: Ask the person to repeat a simple phrase. Is the speech slurred or strange?
- T—Time: If you see any of these signs, call 911 right away.

The stroke treatments that work best are available only if the stroke is recognized and diagnosed within 3 hours of the first symptoms.

Management in the chair till help arrives[4] (after calling 911):

1. Sit the patient upright (if conscious). If the patient is unconscious, he/she should be supine. (If blood pressure is elevated, the head and chest should be elevated slightly.)
2. Assess the patient's breathing and circulation.
3. Monitor the vital signs. (The heartbeat should be recorded every 5 minutes.)
4. O_2 can be administered.

References

1. The American Red Cross website. How to perform hands-only CPR. redcross.org/take-a-class/cpr/performing-cpr/hands-only-cpr. Accessed 4 December 2019.
2. Camargo P, Freymiller EG. Medical emergencies in the dental office. Webinar. Fall 2019.
3. Centers for Disease Control and Prevention. Stroke signs and symptoms. https://www.cdc.gov/stroke/signs_symptoms.htm. Accessed 5 November 2019.
4. Malamed S. Medical Emergencies in the Dental Office, ed 5. St Lous: Mosby, 2000:299.

Treatment Planning **19**

Read the case presentations, then answer the questions that follow. Teeth are numbered according to the two-digit FDI notation.

Case 1

Patient identification

- Age: 36 years
- Ethnicity: White

History of present illness

Chief complaint: "My dentist told me to come see a periodontist. I was told that I need gum surgery."

Medical history

- Significant past illnesses: None
- Medications: None
- Allergies: None

Current medical history

General health: Good

- Head/eyes/ears/nose/throat: None
- Neuromuscular: None
- Respiratory: None
- Cardiovascular: None $\rightarrow$

- Gastrointestinal: None
- Genitourinary: None
- Hematologic/immune: None

Family history

- Diabetes: None
- Cardiovascular disease: None
- Bleeding disorders: None
- Tuberculosis: None
- Mental/emotional disorders: None
- Periodontal disease: None

Social history

- Diet: Healthy
- Smoking: Past marijuana smoker (12 years)
- Exercise: Seldom
- Alcohol: 1 to 2 drinks/week

Dental history

- Restorative experience: Minimal
- Orthodontics: None reported
- Frequency of prior care: Infrequent
- Oral hygiene: Fair
    - Brushing: Once a day
    - Flossing: Twice a day

Clinical examination

Dental examination:

- Missing: 18 and 28 (Fig 19-1a)
- Restorations:
    - 26 distal/occlusal/buccal/lingual: silver
    - 36 distal/occlusal and buccal pit: silver (Fig 19-1b)
    - 46 occlusal: silver
- Open contacts: None (Fig 19-1c)
- Wear facets/attrition: Generalized moderate occlusal and incisal wear
- Abrasion: None
- Abfraction: None
- Parafunctional activity: Suspected clenching/grinding →

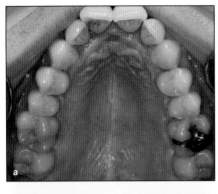
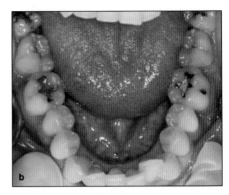
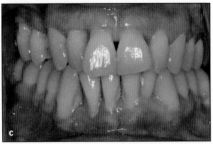
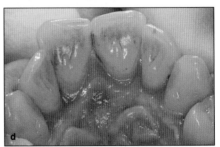
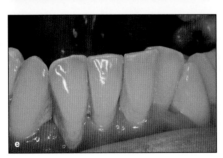

Fig 19-1 *(a)* Maxillary occlusal view. *(b)* Mandibular occlusal view. *(c)* Frontal view. *(d)* Lingual view of the maxillary anterior teeth. *(e)* Facial view of the mandibular anterior teeth.

- Marginal ridge discrepancies: 37 and 38; 47 and 48
- Staining: Moderate generalized staining (Figs 19-1d and 19-1e)

Occlusal examination:

- Angle classification: Dental molar Class I
- Canine relationship: Class I on the left; edge to edge on the right
- Centric relation: Repeatable
- Left lateral guidance: Lateral anterior guidance
- Right lateral guidance: Lateral anterior guidance
- Protrusive guidance: 11, 21, 31, 32, 41, and 42
- Incisal relationship:
  - Horizontal overlap: 2 mm
  - Vertical overlap: 2 mm →

- Fremitus: 12
- Crossbite: None

Periodontal examination (Fig 19-2):

- Plaque/calculus: Generalized plaque accumulation with moderate to heavy supragingival and subgingival calculus
- Oral hygiene: Poor
- Plaque free: 34% (initial)
- Marginal bleeding: 14% (initial)
- Periodontal tissues:
    - Color: Pink with localized areas of erythematous tissue and blunted papillae
    - Texture: Generalized smooth appearance
    - Tone: Generally fibrous and edematous at the gingival margin; interdental papillae are spongy
- Probing depths: Generalized 2 to 7 mm
- Bleeding on probing (BOP): Localized
- Suppuration: 14
- Recession (Miller):
    - Class 1: 11, 12, 21 to 23, 26, 31, 32, 41 to 44, 47
    - Class 2: 14B
- Mucogingival problems: 14, no keratinized attached tissue
- Vestibular depth: Good vestibular depth except for 38 and 48
- Mobility (Miller):
    - Class I: 11, 12, 21, 22, 31, 32, 41, 42
    - Class II: 14
- Furcation (Glickman):
    - Grade I: 27B, 38B, 37B, 47B, and 48B
    - Grade II: 17B, 17DL, 16B, 16ML, 16DL, 26B, 26DL, 36BL, and 46B
    - Grade III: 14BMD
- Anatomical considerations: Thin periodontal biotype, short root trunk, and the sinus is proximal to the maxillary molar roots

Radiographic examination (Fig 19-3):

- Bone loss: Generalized moderate to advanced horizontal bone loss, with localized vertical defects
- Radiographic bone loss:
    - Mesial bone loss: 16, 47
    - Distal bone loss: 17, 48
    - Mesial and distal bone loss: 11, 12, 14, 21, 22, 26, 27, 31, 35 to 38, 41, 42, 46 →

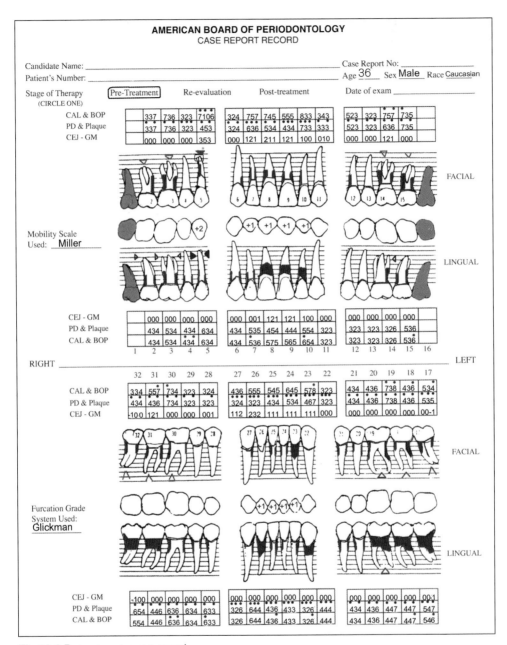

Fig 19-2 Pretreatment report record.

- Periapical radiolucencies: 14
- Root form: Long and tapering
- Furcation radiolucencies: 14, 16, 17, 26, 27, 36, 46 →

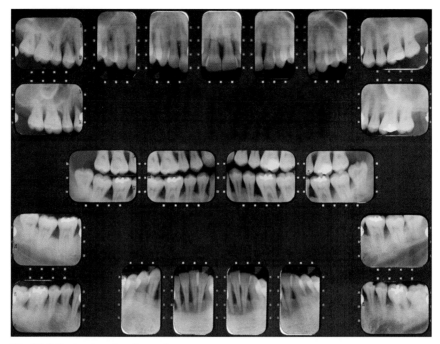

Fig 19-3 Pretreatment radiographs.

- Restorations:
    - 26 distal/occlusal/buccal/lingual: silver
    - 36 occlusal and buccal pit: silver
    - 46 occlusal: silver
- Calculus: Generalized moderate to heavy (11D, M12, 25D, 31M, 32M, 41M, 42D, and 46M)

Q: What is your diagnosis of the patient?

Note: Always include a medical diagnosis when answering this question.

- Medical: American Society of Anesthesiologists (ASA) 1, healthy, past marijuana smoker (12 years)
- Periodontal: Generalized severe chronic periodontitis; American Academy of Periodontology (AAP) Type IV
- New classification: Stage III Grade C
- Dental
    - Parafunctional activity: Bruxism (sleeping)
    - Temporomandibular joint (TMJ)/musculature: No clicking or popping

Q: What etiology do you suspect to have caused this condition?

- Primary etiologic agent: Microbial plaque secondary to poor oral hygiene
- Distribution of plaque and calculus: Patient has generalized supra- and subgingival calculus
- Possible risk factors:
  - Genetics: No known occurrences of periodontal disease among family members
  - Poor oral hygiene
  - Smoking: Smoked marijuana two times per week for 12 years
  - Stress (coping)
  - Systemic factors: None

Q: What bacteria would you expect if you were to perform sensitivity testing?

Based on the diagnosis, one would expect *Prevotella intermedia*, *Tannerella forsythia*, and *Fusobacterium nucleatum*. The sensitivity testing confirmed this (Table 19-1; see next page). Clindamycin was prescribed based on the sensitivity testing.

Q: What is the prognosis of the teeth in both the short and long term?

- Overall: Fair (McGuire and Nunn classification[1])—The prognosis is highly dependent upon the strategic removal of the most compromised teeth, improved oral hygiene, and consistent preventive maintenance care.
- Individual short term (< 5 years):
  - Hopeless: 14
  - Poor: 11, 12, 16, 17, 21, 22, 31, 32, 38, 41, 42, 48
  - Fair: 26, 27, 34 to 36, 46
  - Good: 13, 15, 23 to 25, 33, 37, 43 to 45, 47
- Individual long term (> 5 years):
  - Hopeless: 14, 38, 48
  - Poor: 11, 12, 16, 17, 21, 22, 31, 32, 41, 42
  - Fair: 24 to 27, 34 to 36, 44 to 46
  - Good: 13, 15, 23, 33, 37, 43, 47

Table 19-1 Sensitivity testing results: Presumptive identification of periodontal pathogens*

Culture	Microbiota (%)	Inhibition (%)				
		Clindamycin	Amoxicillin	Metronida-zole	Ciprofloxacin	Azithromycin
Aggregatibacter actinomycetemcomitans	0					
Porphyromonas gingivalis	0					
Prevotella intermedia	6.1	100	0	100	0	86
Tannerella forsythia	4.3	100	100	100	87	100
Campylobacter species	5.2	100	100	100	100	100
Eubacterium species	0					
Fusobacterium species	7.0	100	0	100	0	82
Peptostreptococcus micros	0					
Enteric gram-negative rods	0					
Beta hemolytic streptococci	0					
Yeast	0					
Eikenella corrodens	0					
Staphylococcus species	0					
Dialister pneumosintes	4.3	100	100	100	100	100

*Paper points placed on the mesial of 26 and 36.

Q: What are your goals when strategizing the treatment plan for the patient?

- Eradicate and change etiologic factors for periodontal disease
- Educate the patient on the causes and prevention of periodontal disease
- Improve oral hygiene and plaque control
- Reduce plaque and calculus to below disease threshold
- Establish and maintain the health of the periodontium
- Extract periodontally compromised teeth (14, 38, 48)
- Surgically reduce the deep periodontal pockets (more cleansable environment)
- Schedule regular periodontal maintenance recalls for monitoring and preventive care

Q: What is your treatment plan for this patient?

- Systemic: Encourage patient to maintain healthy lifestyle
- Diagnostic phase:
  - Emergency treatment: None
  - Examination
  - Diagnostic evaluation, study casts
  - Treatment plan/options presentation
  - Restorative consultation
- Preparatory phase:
  - Patient education/oral hygiene instructions (OHI)
  - Explanation of the disease etiology
  - Current diagnosis and periodontal condition
  - Explanation of risk factors: Poor oral hygiene
  - Options: Nonsurgical vs surgical treatment vs extraction vs no treatment
  - OHI: Modified Bass technique/interproximal brushes, rubber tip, and floss
- Phase I periodontal therapy (nonsurgical therapy):
  - Microbiologic sensitivity testing
  - Maxillary and mandibular left scaling and root planing (SRP)
  - Maxillary and mandibular right SRP
  - Periodontal reevaluation
- Surgical phase (periodontal surgery):
  - Extraction of 14 with socket preservation
  - Pocket reduction for 23 to 27
  - Pocket reduction for 34 to 37 and extraction of 38 →

- Pocket reduction for 15 to 17
- Pocket reduction for 43 to 47 and extraction of 48
- Maintenance phase:
  - Supportive periodontal therapy with 3-month recall and monitoring

Results at reevaluation (Fig 19-4; see next page):

- Phase I therapy has been effective in this patient. Improvements in oral hygiene, reduction in pocket depths, a decrease in marginal bleeding, and an increase in the percentage of teeth that are plaque free have all been observed.
- Oral hygiene improved, as noted by the increase in plaque-free areas (34% to 76%) and decrease in marginal bleeding index.
- A significant number of sites with pocket depth of 4 to 6 mm remained.

Q: What is your rationale for surgical pocket reduction therapy?

- Surgical pocket reduction therapy was indicated because of the high number of remaining deep periodontal pockets and for further removal of calculus and its associated subgingival microflora. This may provide improvements in clinical attachment level, minimize further inflammation, and achieve reduction and stability in probing depths for supportive periodontal therapy.
- Goals of surgical therapy:
  - Provide access to the roots for effective plaque and calculus removal
  - Decrease remaining pocket depths through soft tissue reduction and osseous recontouring
  - Allow for oral hygiene access for the patient and periodontist
- Stambaugh et al[2] showed that trained hygienists who scaled teeth under local anesthesia achieved a "curet efficiency" of 3.73 mm. The instrument limit where evidence of instrumentation could be seen was 6.21 mm.
- Caffesse et al[3] noted that while scaling only and scaling with a flap increased the percentage of root surface without calculus, scaling following the reflection of a flap aided calculus removal in pockets 4 mm and deeper. Percentages of tooth surfaces completely free of calculus following scaling only versus scaling with a flap, respectively, at various pocket depths were 86% for both techniques for 1- to 3-mm pockets, 43% versus 76% for 4- to 6-mm pockets, and 32% versus 50% for pockets deeper than 6 mm.

371

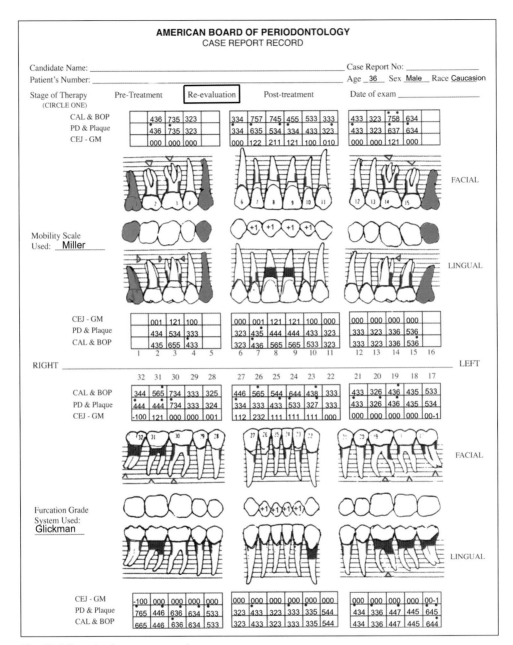

AMERICAN BOARD OF PERIODONTOLOGY
CASE REPORT RECORD

Candidate Name: _____ Case Report No: _____
Patient's Number: _____ Age _36_ Sex _Male_ Race _Caucasion_

Stage of Therapy   Pre-Treatment   [Re-evaluation]   Post-treatment   Date of exam _____
(CIRCLE ONE)

Mobility Scale Used: _Miller_

FACIAL

LINGUAL

RIGHT _____ LEFT

Furcation Grade System Used: _Glickman_

FACIAL

LINGUAL

Fig 19-4 Reevaluation report record.

Q: Please show and describe how you would extract tooth 14 and graft the site.

Figure 19-5 shows the radiographic appearance of tooth 14 before extraction. The surgical procedure was performed as follows: →

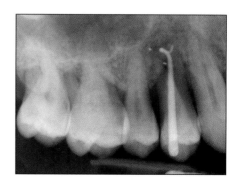

Fig 19-5 Radiograph of tooth 14 showing gutta-percha extending to the apex.

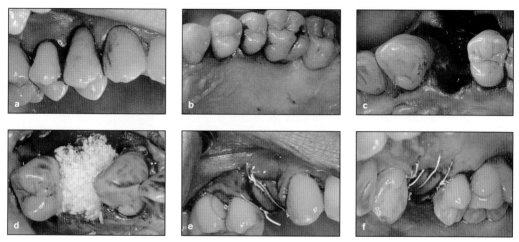

Fig 19-6 Bone graft at site 14. *(a)* Initial buccal incisions. *(b)* Initial palatal incisions. *(c)* Extraction of the tooth. *(d)* Placement of bone graft and membrane. *(e)* Buccal view of sutures. *(f)* Lingual view of sutures.

- Buccal: A sulcular incision was made from the facial of tooth 16 to the mesial aspect of tooth 13 (Fig 19-6a).
- Palatal: A sulcular incision was made from the palatal of tooth 16 to the mesial aspect of tooth 13 (Fig 19-6b).
- The tooth was extracted. No buccal plate was evident (Fig 19-6c).
- Soft tissue and granulation removal were performed, followed by thorough SRP with hand instruments. Freeze-dried bone allograft (FDBA) was placed into the defect with two layers of Bio-Gide membrane (Geistlich) because of the lack of a buccal plate (Fig 19-6d).
- Interrupted sutures (Gore-Tex, W. L. Gore) were placed from the mesial aspect of tooth 15 to the distal aspect of tooth 13 (Figs 19-6e and 19-6f).

$\rightarrow$

▪ The patient was given one tablet of ibuprofen (800 mg) and an ice pack. He was also prescribed 500 mg amoxicillin three times per day for 1 week.

Q: Provide the rationale for the choice of graft and barrier.

Graft

▪ Mellonig[4] demonstrated complete or greater than 50% bone fill in 67% of sites treated with FDBA alone and in 78% of sites treated with FDBA and autogenous bone.
▪ A 2005 AAP position paper[5] found bone fill ranging from 1.3 to 2.6 mm when FDBA was used to treat defects. Human trials using demineralized FDBA (DFDBA) have demonstrated bone fill similar to that achieved with FDBA, ranging from 1.7 to 2.9 mm.
▪ Comparisons between bone allografts and alloplasts suggest that they produce similar clinical results.[5]
▪ A meta-analysis by Vignoletti et al[6] found that socket preservation therapies resulted in significantly less vertical and horizontal contraction of the alveolar bone crest.

Barrier

▪ The membrane will prevent apical migration of the epithelium and protect the wound.
▪ Resorbable membrane: Laurell et al[7] reviewed studies presented during the last 20 years on the surgical treatment of intrabony defects, analyzing treatment results of open flap debridement, bone replacement grafts, and guided tissue regeneration. No difference was found between resorbable and nonresorbable membranes.

Q: Discuss implant placement in site 14.

▪ Study casts and photographs are important for planning treatment when the patient is not present.
▪ Cone beam computed tomography (CBCT) scans are necessary to determine the height of available bone in three dimensions and therefore to select the appropriate implant. They also may be needed to determine the location of anatomical structures (eg, nerves, vessels, and the sinus).
▪ Written informed consent is discussed between the surgeon and the patient.
▪ Figure 19-7 presents the implant placement procedures. →

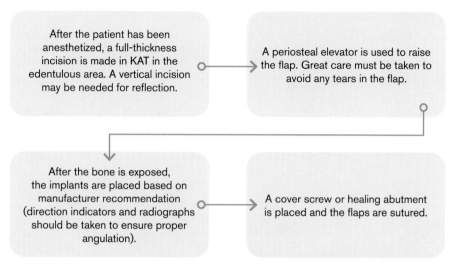

After the patient has been anesthetized, a full-thickness incision is made in KAT in the edentulous area. A vertical incision may be needed for reflection.

A periosteal elevator is used to raise the flap. Great care must be taken to avoid any tears in the flap.

After the bone is exposed, the implants are placed based on manufacturer recommendation (direction indicators and radiographs should be taken to ensure proper angulation).

A cover screw or healing abutment is placed and the flaps are sutured.

Fig 19-7 Implant placement procedures. KAT, keratinized attached tissue.

Q: Describe your technique for performing osseous resective surgery on the maxillary left quadrant.

The procedures for resective osseous surgery in the maxillary left quadrant are presented in Fig 19-8 and outlined below:

1. Buccal: A sulcular incision is made from the facial of tooth 23 to the disto-facial aspect of tooth 27 (see Fig 19-8c).
2. Palatal: A sulcular incision is made from the mesial aspect of tooth 23 to the distal aspect of tooth 27 (see Fig 19-8d). (A distal wedge incision is made on the distal aspect of tooth 27.)
3. Full-thickness reflection is performed, followed by degranulation and SRP using Cavitron (Dentsply) and hand instruments (see Figs 19-8e and 19-8f).
4. Osteoplasty and ostectomy are done with a handpiece and hand instruments to maintain positive architecture (see Figs 19-8g and 19-8h).
5. The buccal and lingual flaps are sutured with interrupted (chromic gut) sutures (see Figs 19-8i and 19-8j).
6. Coe-Pak (GC America) is placed, and the patient is prescribed ibuprofen 800 mg (1 tablet every 6 hours) as an anti-inflammatory and for pain management. Adequate postoperative healing is noted at the follow-up appointment. →

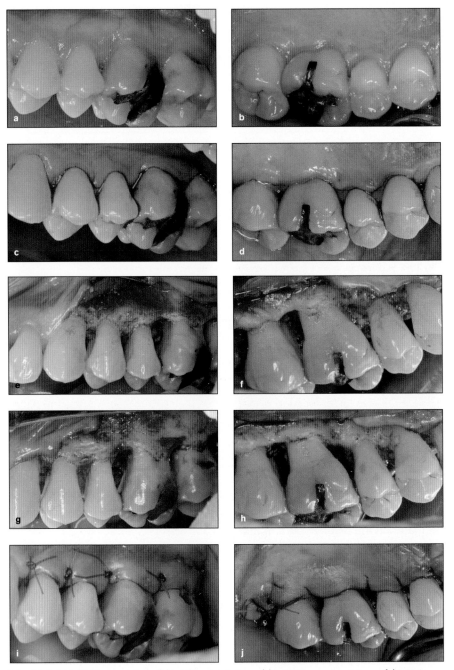

Fig 19-8 *(a)* Initial buccal view. *(b)* Initial palatal view. *(c)* Initial buccal incisions. *(d)* Initial palatal incisions. *(e)* Buccal view before osseous resective surgery. *(f)* Palatal view before osseous resective surgery. *(g)* Buccal view following osseous resective surgery. *(h)* Palatal view following osseous resective surgery. *(i)* Buccal sutures. *(j)* Palatal sutures.

Q: Discuss the reasoning behind using a dressing, and then explain why a surgeon may decide not to use a dressing.

Figure 19-9 presents the rationale for placing or not placing a dressing.[8]

Placing	Not placing
• Protects the wound. • Increases patient comfort. • Stabilizes the flap. • Retains the graft material.	• Increases postoperative pain. • Irritates. • Increases plaque retention (increased bacteria): Powell et al[8] found that the use of a postsurgical dressing demonstrated a slightly higher rate of infection (8 infections in 300 procedures, 2.67%) than nonuse of a dressing (14 infections in 753 procedures, 1.86%).

Fig 19-9 Rationale for placing or not placing a dressing.

Q: Describe the specific technique for the treatment of teeth 43 to 48.

Procedures for resective osseous surgery in the mandibular right quadrant and extraction of tooth 48 are presented in Fig 19-10 and described below:

1. Buccal: A sulcular incision is made from the facial of tooth 43 to the distal aspect of tooth 48 (see Fig 19-10c).
2. Lingual: A sulcular incision is made from the lingual of tooth 43 to the mesial aspect of tooth 48 (see Fig 19-10d).
3. Full-thickness reflection is performed, followed by degranulation and SRP using Cavitron and hand instruments (see Figs 19-10e and 19-10f).
4. Tooth 48 is extracted, and ostectomy is performed with a handpiece and hand instruments between teeth 46 and 47 and between teeth 45 and 46.
5. The buccal and lingual flaps are sutured with interrupted (silk) sutures (see Figs 19-10g and 19-10h).
6. Coe-Pak is placed, and the patient is prescribed ibuprofen 800 mg (1 tablet every 6 hours) as an anti-inflammatory and for pain management. Adequate postoperative healing is noted at the follow-up appointment. →

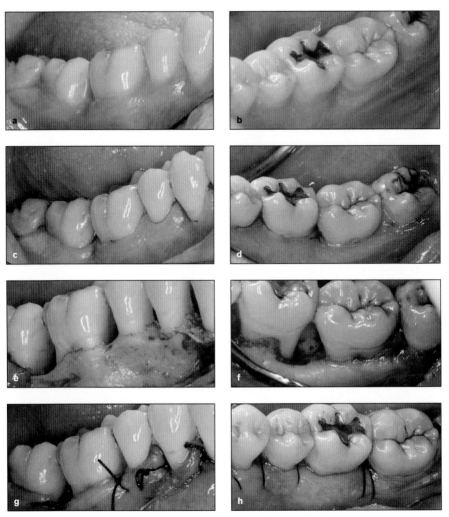

Fig 19-10 *(a)* Initial buccal view. *(b)* Initial lingual view. *(c)* Initial buccal incisions. *(d)* Initial lingual incisions. *(e)* Buccal view before osseous resective surgery. *(f)* Lingual view before osseous resective surgery. *(g)* Buccal sutures. *(h)* Lingual sutures.

Q: What instructions should be provided to the patient after surgery?

Figure 19-11 presents instructions that should be provided to the patient after surgery. $\rightarrow$

Care of your mouth: Immediately after surgery, keep ice cold water or other cold foods such as ice cream or frozen yogurt in your mouth for 6 to 8 hours. Do not brush your teeth in the areas that have dressing or sutures. Do all normal cleaning of teeth that did not undergo surgery.	Activity: Reduce your activity following surgery. No running, weight lifting, or any strenuous aerobic activity or contact sports for 48 hours.	Discomfort: Following all types of surgery, you can expect some discomfort. Take pain medication as prescribed; do not drink alcoholic beverages in combination with pain medication.
Swelling: In some cases swelling may be expected, but it will go away in 3 to 4 days.	Eating: Eat only cold, soft foods on the day of surgery. After the first day, stay on a soft but balanced diet. Do not eat hard, crunchy, or spicy foods.	Smoking: Do not smoke following surgery. Tobacco smoke is an irritant and delays healing of the tissue. Refrain from smoking for as long as possible.

Fig 19-11 Postoperative instructions.

Q: What factors would you consider when evaluating the results of therapy?

1. Examination:
   - Periodontal tissues
     - Color: Pink fibrotic tissue
     - Texture: Generalized firm tissue
     - Tone: Gingival tissues are generally fibrotic
   - Probing depths: Generalized 2- to 5-mm pockets with localized 6-mm pockets (Table 19-2 and Fig 19-12)

Table 19-2	Results of therapy		
Parameter	Initial	Reevalutaion	Postsurgery
Marginal bleeding	14%	6%	5%
Plaque-free areas	34%	76%	87%
Pockets > 3 mm with BOP	17%	12%	11%
Pockets < 3 mm	78 (43%)	92 (54%)	126 (78%)
Pockets 4 to 6 mm	91 (51%)	74 (43%)	34 (21%)
Pockets > 6 mm	10 (6%)	6 (3%)	2 (1%)

→

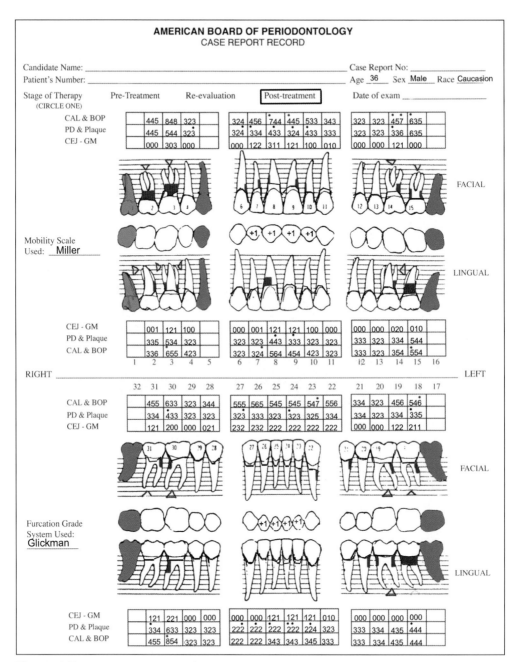

AMERICAN BOARD OF PERIODONTOLOGY
CASE REPORT RECORD

Candidate Name: _____   Case Report No: _____

Patient's Number: _____   Age _36_ Sex _Male_ Race _Caucasion_

Stage of Therapy   Pre-Treatment   Re-evaluation   [Post-treatment]   Date of exam _____
(CIRCLE ONE)

Maxillary Facial:

CAL & BOP	445	848	323		324	456	744	445	533	343	
PD & Plaque	445	544	323		324	334	433	324	433	333	
CEJ - GM	000	303	000		000	122	311	121	100	010	

323	323	457	635
323	323	336	635
000	000	121	000

FACIAL

Mobility Scale
Used: _Miller_

Maxillary teeth: +1 +1 +1 +1

LINGUAL

Maxillary Lingual:

CEJ - GM	001	121	100		000	001	121	121	100	000	
PD & Plaque	335	534	323		323	323	443	333	323	323	
CAL & BOP	336	655	423		323	324	564	454	423	323	

000	000	020	010
333	323	334	544
333	323	354	554

Tooth numbers: 1 2 3 4 5 | 6 7 8 9 10 11 | 12 13 14 15 16

RIGHT _____ LEFT

Tooth numbers: 32 31 30 29 28 | 27 26 25 24 23 22 | 21 20 19 18 17

CAL & BOP	455	633	323	344	555	565	545	545	547	556	
PD & Plaque	334	433	323	323	323	333	323	323	325	334	
CEJ - GM	121	200	000	021	232	232	222	222	222	222	

334	323	456	546
334	323	334	335
000	000	122	211

FACIAL

Furcation Grade
System Used:
Glickman

Mandibular teeth: +1 +1 +1 +1

LINGUAL

Mandibular Lingual:

CEJ - GM	121	221	000	000	000	000	121	121	121	010	
PD & Plaque	334	633	323	323	222	222	222	222	224	323	
CAL & BOP	455	854	323	323	222	222	343	343	345	333	

000	000	000	000
333	334	435	444
333	334	435	444

Fig 19-12 Posttreatment report record.

- Recession: Generalized moderate recession on 11, 12, 21 to 23, 26, 31, 32, 41 to 44, and 47 (Fig 19-13)
- Mobility: Miller Class I: 11, 12, 21, 22, 31, 32, 41, and 42 →

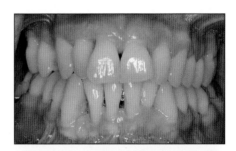

Fig 19-13 Intraoral frontal view following periodontal therapy.

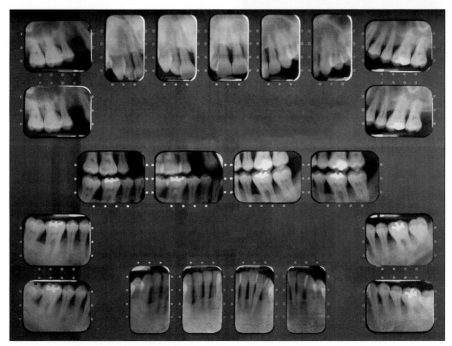

Fig 19-14 Posttreatment radiographs.

- Furcation (Glickman):
  - Grade I: 27B, 37B, and 47B
  - Grade II: 16B, 16ML, 16DL, 17B, 17DL, 26B, 26DL, 36BL, and 46B
  - Grade III: None
2. Sensitivity testing:
  - The antibiotic regimen (clindamycin) in conjunction with the periodontal therapy was successful in reducing the periodontal pathogens in the mouth. No more microbiota were found in the final sensitivity testing.
3. Radiographs:
  - Although the radiographs show bone loss, it has improved, and no calculus is shown (Fig 19-14). $\rightarrow$

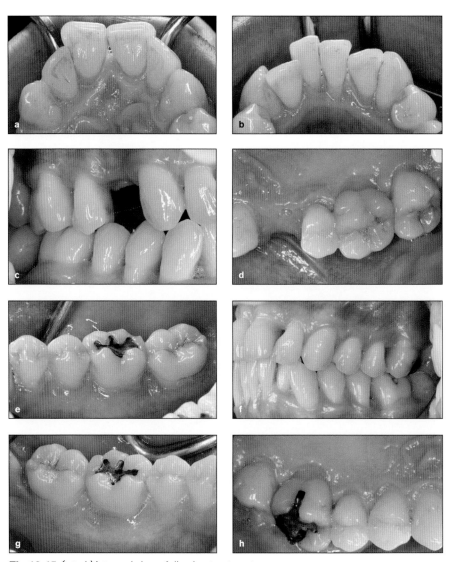

Fig 19-15 *(a to h)* Intraoral views following treatment.

4. Photographs:
   ▪ The photographs show pink, healthy tissues with no plaque or calculus present (Fig 19-15).
5. All three goals of surgical therapy (see question on page 372) have been met:
   ▪ Provide access to the roots for effective plaque and calculus removal

$\rightarrow$

- Decrease remaining pocket depths through soft tissue reduction and osseous recontouring
- Allow for oral hygiene access for the patient and periodontist

Q: What factors would you consider in developing an optimal maintenance schedule for this patient?

Following are the factors to be considered in developing an optimal maintenance schedule[9]:

- BOP greater than 25% (patient has 11%)
- Pocket depth (patient has localized areas with greater than 4-mm probing depth)
- Tooth loss (patient is missing four teeth)
- Age in relation to loss of periodontal support (patient is young)
- Systemic and genetic factors (none reported)
- Environment (history of smoking)
- Oral hygiene (poor)
- Compliance (patient is much more compliant)

Studies have reported that patients who have had a history of periodontal disease need to be recalled at least four times per year.[10]

Q: If the mandibular right quadrant started to show further bone loss in 10 years, would you re-treat it?

Note: There is no wrong answer, but the answer will need to be supported by logical thinking.

Yes. There was a study done that found that nearly half of the patients who were originally treated for periodontal disease and consistently kept their follow-up appointments needed retreatment at least once during a 13-year period. Comprehensive maintenance care and surgical retreatments appeared to limit additional tooth loss for patients at risk because of indeterminate or poor preliminary prognosis, erratic or poor compliance, and a family history of periodontal disease.[11]

Case 2

Patient identification

- Age: 43 years
- Sex: Male
- Ethnicity: Indian
- No history of smoking

History of present illness

Chief complaint: Maxillary anterior teeth "are getting more loose every day" (Fig 19-16).

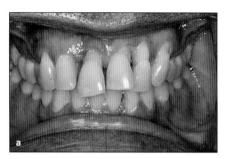 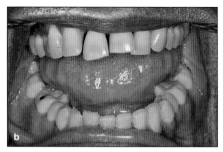

Fig 19-16 Frontal view with the jaws closed (a) and with the jaws open (b).

Medical history

- General health: Good
- Medications: None
- Allergies: None

Family history

- Diabetes: None
- Cardiovascular disease: None
- Bleeding disorders: None
- Tuberculosis: None
- Mental/emotional disorders: None
- Periodontal disease: None

Dental history

- Restorative experience: Minimal (see Fig 19-16b)
- Orthodontics: None reported →

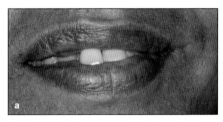 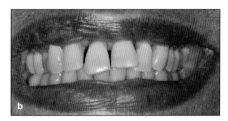

Fig 19-17 Patient at rest *(a)* and smiling *(b)*.

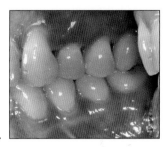

Fig 19-18 Posterior occlusion.

- Frequency of prior care: Infrequent
- Oral hygiene: Fair
  - Brushing: Twice a day
  - Flossing: Twice a day

Clinical examination

Dental examination:

- Missing: 18, 28, and 38
- Wear facets/attrition: Generalized moderate occlusal and incisal wear
- Abrasion: None
- Abfraction: None
- Parafunctional activity: Suspected clenching/grinding
- Staining: Moderate generalized staining
- Display at rest: Maxillary teeth 1 to 2 mm (Fig 19-17a)
- Display during smiling: Maxillary teeth to first molar, 1 to 2 mm of gingival tissue and mandibular teeth (Fig 19-17b)

Occlusal examination:

- Angle classification: Dental molar Class I (Fig 19-18)
- Canine relationship: Class I on both sides
- Centric relation: Repeatable →

- Left lateral guidance: Group
- Right lateral guidance: Group
- Incisal relationship:
  - Horizontal overlap: 5 to 6 mm (because of the mobility of tooth 11)
  - Vertical overlap: 3 mm (tooth 11 supererupted)

Periodontal examination:

- Plaque/calculus: Generalized heavy plaque with heavy supragingival and subgingival calculus
- Oral hygiene: Poor
- Plaque free: 65% (initial)
- Marginal bleeding: 25% (initial)
- Periodontal tissues: Generalized areas of compromised tissue with localized moderate to severe cyanotic areas and blunted papillae
- Probing depths: Generalized 3 to 9 mm
- BOP: Localized
- Recession (Miller):
  - Class 2: 13, 23
  - Class 3: 11, 12, 21, 22
- Mobility (Miller):
  - Class II: 12, 22
  - Class III: 11, 21

Radiographic examination:

- Bone loss: Generalized moderate horizontal bone loss with localized vertical defects (Fig 19-19; see next page)
- Radiolucencies: 11
- Calculus: Generalized moderate to heavy deposits

Q: What is your diagnosis of the patient?

- Medical: ASA 1, healthy
- Periodontal: Generalized moderate chronic periodontitis and localized severe chronic periodontitis with BOP (patient may have had aggressive periodontitis when he was younger); AAP Type III.
- New classification: Stage III Grade B
- Mucogingival deformities and conditions around teeth: Facial and/or lingual recession and interproximal recession type 2 under developmental or acquired deformities and conditions.

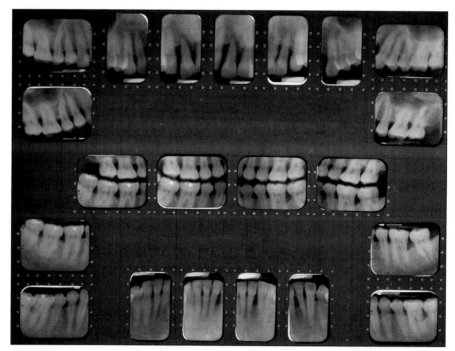

Fig 19-19 Pretreatment radiographs.

Q: What is the etiology of the bone loss?

- Primary etiologic agent: Microbial plaque secondary to poor oral hygiene
- Distribution of plaque and calculus: Generalized supra- and subgingival calculus (Fig 19-20)
- Possible risk factors:
  - Genetics: No known occurrences of periodontal disease among family members
  - Poor oral hygiene
  - Stress (coping)
  - Systemic factors: None

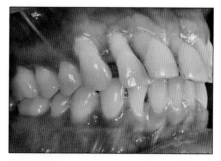

Fig 19-20 Intraoral lateral view of teeth in occlusion.

Q: What is the prognosis for the maxillary incisors?

Based on the classification by Kwok and Caton,[12] the prognosis is unfavorable. There are many local factors that indicate an unfavorable prognosis for these teeth:

- Deep probing depths and attachment loss
- Anatomical plaque-related factors (open contacts)
- Class II and III mobility

Q: What are the treatment options for the maxillary incisors?

Figure 19-21 presents the treatment options for the maxillary incisors.

Option 1: No further treatment

Option 2: Implants
1. Preoperative assessment/diagnostic information
   - Wax-up
   - Fabrication of surgical stent
   - CT scan
2. Bone graft/soft tissue augmentation
3. Implant-supported fixed partial denture (11, 12, 21, 22)

Option 3: Fixed partial denture (canine to canine)

Option 4: Maxillary removable partial denture

Fig 19-21 Treatment options for the maxillary incisors.

Q: You indicated that a bone graft would most likely be needed before implant placement. What are the options for a horizontal bone graft?

- Socket grafting: Placing a bone graft into the socket may allow for preservation of the ridge in the esthetic zone.
- Bone and membrane guided bone regeneration using FDBA or DFDBA.
- Autogenous block graft (eg, tuberosity, chin, and lateral ramus).
- Ridge splitting: May reduce treatment time and morbidity.
- Distraction osteogenesis: No graft requirement and concurrent enlargement of soft tissue.
- Block allograft: Not living bone, must be hydrated, and air bubbles must be removed.

Q: Which option did you choose and why?

Note: There is no wrong answer to this question as long as it is well supported.

FDBA and a resorbable membrane were used to horizontally augment the ridge in preparation for implants. The CBCT scan shows that the buccal plate is not thick enough in the esthetic area to allow proper implant placement (Fig 19-22). According to Beitlitum et al,[13] good clinical results can be achieved by placing FDBA and barrier membranes to treat large vertical and/or horizontal ridge deficiencies. Geurs et al[14] found that lateral alveolar ridge augmentation resulting from the use of a synthetic long-term resorbable membrane and an allograft was comparable to that obtained using other materials while avoiding the need to harvest a graft or perform a second surgery to remove the membrane.

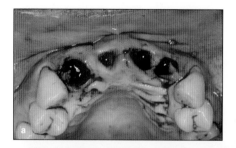
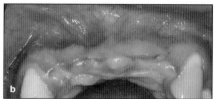
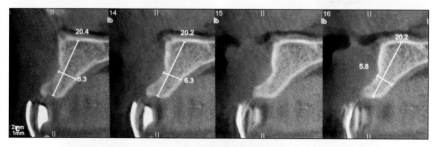
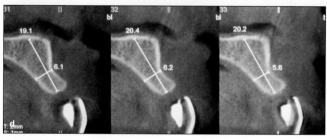

Fig 19-22 *(a)* Extraction of the maxillary incisors. *(b)* Clinical view of the ridge before bone graft placement, 7 months after extraction. *(c)* CBCT scans of implant position for site 12. *(d)* CBCT scans of implant position for site 22.

Q: Describe your technique for grafting the anterior maxilla.

Incisions were made in keratinized tissue, and a flap was reflected. The Bio-Gide membrane was cut to fit the site, and FDBA was placed under the membrane. The anterior maxilla was then sutured with silk and Gore-Tex sutures using the horizontal mattress and interrupted suture technique (Fig 19-23).

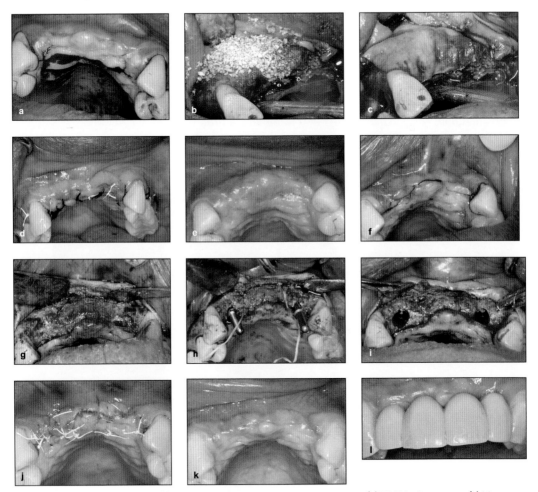

Fig 19-23 Bone graft surgery. (a) Initial incisions for bone graft placement. (b) FDBA placement. (c) Membrane positioning. (d) Suture placement. (e) One month postoperative. (f) Initial incisions for implant placement. (g) Bone morphology before implant placement. (h) Direction indicators placed before implant placement. (i) Implants placed. (j) Sutures (Gore-Tex) positioned. (k) Three months after implant placement. (l) One year after implant placement.

Q: What should be evaluated when placing the anterior implants?

The following should be included in the evaluation prior to placing anterior implants[15]:

- Mesiodistal dimension of the edentulous area
- 3D imaging of the site
- Neighboring teeth (tooth dimensions, form, position, and orientation; periodontal/endodontic status; length of roots; crown-to-root ratio)
- Interarch relationships (vertical dimension of occlusion, interocclusal space)
- Esthetic parameters (height of upper smile line, lower lip line, occlusal plane orientation, dental and facial symmetry)
- Patient expectations
- Oral hygiene
- Primary stability of the implants

Q: Discuss implant placement in the esthetic area.

- Low trauma
- Precise 3D positioning
- Slightly palatal positioning to preserve keratinized tissue on the labial aspect
- Use of a screw-retained implant to prevent subgingival cement placement
- Deeper placement of the implants in sites 12 and 22 to allow the superstructure to be hidden and a gradual emergence profile

Q: How will you evaluate the success of the implants at maintenance visits?

The following parameters are used to evaluate the success of implants[16,17]:

- The implants should be immobile (less than 1 mm in any direction) and functioning.
- Radiographs show no radiolucency.
- Vertical bone loss is less than 0.2 mm annually following the implant's first year of service.
- Implant has no persistent and/or irreversible signs.
- Patient and clinician are satisfied.
- The hard and soft tissues are healthy.

Case 3 (by Dr Sejal Thacker and Dr Khadijeh Al-Abedalla)

Please note the tooth numbers are universal, not in FDI notation like the rest of the chapter.

Patient identification

- Age: 76 years
- Sex: Male
- Ethnicity: Asian

Medical history

- Hypercholesterolemia
- Medications: Simvastatin

Dental history

- Maintained by general dentist and hygienist, scaling and prophylaxis every 6 months
- Smoking history: Nonsmoker

Extraoral examination

- Within normal limits.

Clinical examination limited to mandibular right quadrant (Figs 19-24 to 19-26)

- Missing tooth 28
- Mesial migration of tooth 29
- Supraeruption of 30
- Teeth 30 and 31 cementoenamel projection on buccal
- Recessions on teeth 29, 30, and 31
- Hamp F2 furcation involvement on buccal of tooth 30 and F1 furcation on lingual of tooth 30
- F1 furcation involvement on buccal of tooth 31
- Oral hygiene is good
- Plaque Index: 20%
- Bleeding Index: 5%
- Probing depths and recessions as charted →

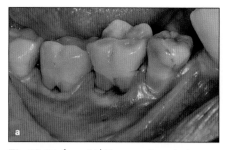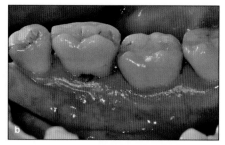

Fig 19-24 *(a and b)* Preoperative photos.

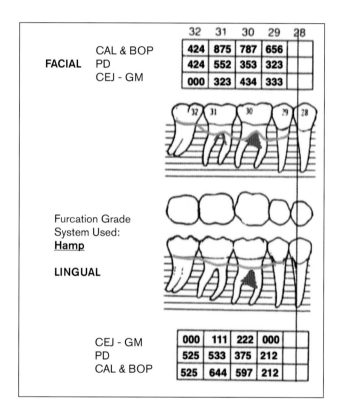

Fig 19-25 Preoperative chart.

		32	31	30	29	28
FACIAL	CAL & BOP	424	875	787	656	
	PD	424	552	353	323	
	CEJ - GM	000	323	434	333	

Furcation Grade System Used: **Hamp**

LINGUAL

	32	31	30	29	28
CEJ - GM	000	111	222	000	
PD	525	533	375	212	
CAL & BOP	525	644	597	212	

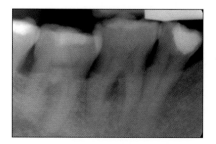

Fig 19-26 Preoperative radiograph.

Q: What is your diagnosis in this case (based on the new AAP classification)?

- Medical: ASA 2
- According to the new AAP classification this case can be classified as: Localized Stage III, Grade B periodontitis

The patient has root proximity ⟶ localized tooth-related factors, which is a subcategory of developmental or acquired deformities and conditions.

Justification

- The clinical attachment level in this case is ≥ 5 mm, bone loss is at the middle to the apical third of the tooth, tooth loss in this patient is ≤ 4, and probing depth is ≥ 6 mm with F1 and F3 furcation involvement.
- Localized because the extent is <30% of teeth.
- Though we do not have previous radiographs to provide information about the history of his periodontal disease, percentage bone loss by age is < 1, and the patient is a nonsmoker and nondiabetic.

Q: What are the primary etiologic factors and risk factors associated with periodontal disease in this patient? Please elaborate on the risk factors in this case scenario.

Primary etiology

- Microbial plaque

Risk factors

- Local risk factors: Malposition of teeth, cervical enamel projections (CEPs)[18,19]
- Individual risk indicators: Age, sex

Risk factors justification/elaboration

- Tooth malposition: Supraeruption (as seen in this case) can result in attachment loss.[20] There is also root proximity between teeth 29 and 30, which could hinder maintenance and accelerate periodontal breakdown.[21]
- CEPs: This patient presents with Grade III CEPs in both teeth 30 and 31 according to the Masters and Hoskins classification.[22] These projections are an anatomical anomaly that prevents connective tissue attachment. →

They are frequently seen in mandibular first molars and when present are associated with furcation involvement in almost 80% of molars.[23]

- Age: Aging has been shown to be weakly related to prevalence of periodontal disease. This relationship may be due to age-related cumulative periodontal breakdown, nutritional deficiencies, concurrent medical diseases and complications, and behavioral incapability to perform oral hygiene measures.[24]

- Sex: Sex exhibits a significant association with prevalence, with males having almost 9% higher prevalence of periodontal disease than females. This difference is attributable to lifestyle, hormonal disparity leading to dimorphism in immune response, and host susceptibility.[25,26]

Q: **What are your treatment options for this patient? What is your preferred option? Why?**

The various treatment options for this patient in the mandibular right quadrant include the following:

- Open flap debridement
- Osseous surgery with tunneling
- Extraction of tooth 30 followed by rehabilitation with implant placement
- Do nothing

Preferred treatment for this patient

- Osseous surgery with tunneling in tooth 30

Justification of preferred treatment option

Patient has good overall oral hygiene, is compliant, root trunk length of tooth 30 is average, root length is long, and there is absence of baseline mobility.

Q: **Describe in brief the surgical procedure and flap management for this procedure.**

The surgical procedure should be done only after ascertaining low caries risk, OHI, and reevaluating patient compliance toward a maintenance regimen.

The surgery would involve the following steps geared toward achieving a positive architecture and apically positioning the flap to provide adequate space for home care measures in the tooth 30 furcation (Fig 19-27):

- Subsulcular incision with full-thickness flap elevation from teeth 29 to 32
- Degranulation and debridement →

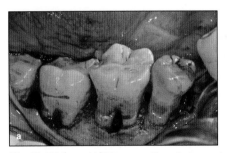 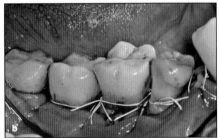

Fig 19-27 *(a and b)* Intraoperative photographs after odontoplasty, ostectomy, osteoplasty, and suturing.

- Odontoplasty to remove CEPs on teeth 30 and 31 and also to eliminate furcation involvement in tooth 31
- Osteoplasty and ostectomy to create positive or flat architecture and adequate biologic width apical to the furcation of 30 to keep furcation patent for hygiene measures
- Sutures to facilitate apical positioning of the flap: external mattress or continuous sling sutures

Q: Elaborate on postoperative instructions and care for this patient.

- Ice packs, anti-inflammatory medications, and minimal disturbance to the surgical site.
- Soft brushing and chlorhexidine rinse from the day after, refrain from interdental aids until sutures are removed.
- Suture removal in 10 days, reinforce OHI.
- Three month maintenance; reevaluate probing depths in 6 weeks.
- If patient is at a moderate risk for caries, prescribe fluoride toothpaste.

Q: How and when will you evaluate the patient and assess the outcome of the surgery?

Patient will be evaluated for outcome 6 weeks after the surgery.[27,28] Probing depths, attachment loss, furcation involvement, BOP, and plaque will be noted (Fig 19-28). Patient's ability to access and clean the tunneled site will be evaluated based on these parameters. $\rightarrow$

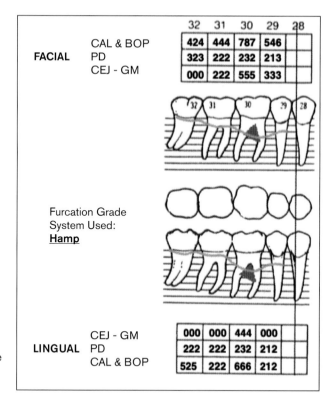

		32	31	30	29	28
FACIAL	CAL & BOP	424	444	787	546	
	PD	323	222	232	213	
	CEJ - GM	000	222	555	333	

Furcation Grade
System Used:
Hamp

		32	31	30	29	28
LINGUAL	CEJ - GM	000	000	444	000	
	PD	222	222	232	212	
	CAL & BOP	525	222	666	212	

Fig 19-28 Postoperative chart.

Q: What are the short- and long-term prognoses of a patient treated with tunneling to manage furcation involvement?

The short- and long-term studies by multiple groups[29-31] have shown that the prognosis of this procedure is good provided the compliance to supportive periodontal therapy is good (Figs 19-29 and 19-30). The most common cause of failure of these procedures is root caries that can develop in exposed furcation areas.[32,33]

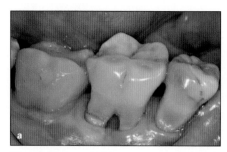
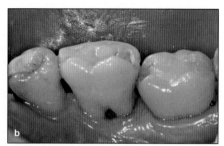

Fig 19-29 *(a and b)* 1-year postoperative photographs.

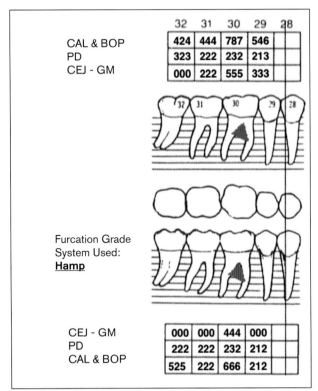

	32	31	30	29	28
CAL & BOP	424	444	787	546	
PD	323	222	232	213	
CEJ - GM	000	222	555	333	

Furcation Grade
System Used:
Hamp

CEJ - GM	000	000	444	000	
PD	222	222	232	212	
CAL & BOP	525	222	666	212	

Fig 19-30 1-year postoperative chart.

Case 4 (By Dr Sejal Thacker)

Patient identification

- Age: 35 years
- Sex: Female
- Ethnicity: Caucasian

Chief complaint

"Sensitivity in maxillary left quadrant, and my dentist says the gums are receding."

Medical history

Noncontributory

Dental history

Orthodontic treatment as a teenager, first premolars were extracted, compliant, and goes for maintenance to general dentist every 6 months. →

Extraoral examination

- Within normal limits

Intraoral examination

Clinical and radiographic findings were as follows:

- Probing depths and bone levels in radiographs within normal limits.
- Oral hygiene is good, and BOP is 15% with plaque index of 20%.
- Teeth 13 and 14 present with recession of 5 to 6 mm with 3 mm keratinized tissue, adequate vestibular depth, and no frenal pull.
- Palatal vault is average in depth.

Q: What is the etiology of recession?

The primary etiology of recession is mechanical trauma from toothbrushing or plaque-induced inflammation[34,35] (Fig 19-31). Other contributing/predisposing factors include the following:

- Buccal position of the tooth
- Orthodontic treatment
- Subgingival restorations
- Smoking and lip piercing
- Thin gingival tissue[36]
- Frenal and muscle attachment pull
- Genetics

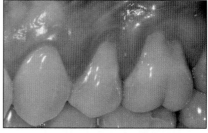

Fig 19-31 Baseline recession 4 to 5 mm.

Q: What is the diagnosis?

- ASA I
- Gingival recession Miller Class I or Cairo RT1[37,38] ⟶ Mucogingival deformities and conditions around teeth, which is a subcategory of developmental or acquired deformities and conditions.

Q: How can this be managed surgically? What will be your technique of choice? Why?

There are multiple techniques to manage this recession defect surgically. Broadly these can be divided into the following:

- Autogenous gingival grafts
- Free soft tissue grafts →

- Pedicle grafts (lateral or coronally advanced)
- Bilaminar techniques (combination of free grafts and pedicle grafts)
- Guided tissue regeneration
- Allografts (eg, AlloDerm, BioHorizons)

Though all of these techniques are effective and have been validated, the surgical technique of choice will be a bilaminar technique—a coronally advanced flap (CAF) with a subepithelial connective tissue graft (SCTG). The surgical procedure will be aimed at thickening the tissue biotype, gaining root coverage, and reducing sensitivity.

The treatment plan will include the following:

- Phase I: OHI (show proper brushing technique), prophylaxis, and reevaluation
- Phase II: CAF + SCTG harvested from the palate
- Phase III: Maintenance, reinforce OHI, and reevaluate patient symptoms

The rationale for CAF + SCTG:

There is strong evidence in the literature for CAF + SCTG being the gold standard in terms of root coverage, cost effectiveness, and long-term stability of the results achieved.[39-41]

Q: Elaborate on your preferred surgical procedure to manage the recession.

The surgical technique for CAF + SCTG (as described by Zucchelli et al[42]) involves the following steps (Fig 19-32):

- Adequate anesthesia.
- Supragingival scaling.
- Include one tooth distal and mesial while creating an envelope flap, dissecting the papilla.
- All surgical papillae are dissected split thickness, and the soft tissue apical to the exposed roots is elevated full thickness to expose 3 mm of bone. This is followed by a split-thickness elevation to release the tension and facilitate coronal advancement.
- A single-incision technique is used to harvest a subepithelial connective tissue graft from the palate.[43,44] The graft is harvested from premolar/canine sites.[45] The palate is sutured and hemostasis achieved. →

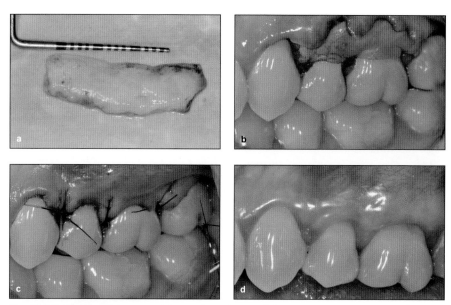

Fig 19-32 *(a)* CT graft harvested from palate. *(b and c)* Coronally advanced flap with suturing. *(d)* Six months postoperative.

- The graft will be stabilized in the envelope created in the recipient site. The envelope will be coronally advanced and sutured with nonresorbable sutures such as polypropylene or nylon with a sling technique.

Q: What are the postoperative instructions to the patient?

- Postoperative pain management with anti-inflammatory medication such as ibuprofen
- Intermittent ice compresses for 6 to 8 hours postsurgery
- Avoid trauma to the surgical site
- Avoid foods that can disturb healing
- Resume careful mechanical tooth cleaning 3 to 4 weeks postsurgery
- Suture removal in 10 to 15 days
- Professional scaling 1, 2, 4, and 8 weeks postsurgery

Q: When can you evaluate the outcome of the procedure?

Soft tissue healing will be complete in 4 to 6 weeks,[46] although creeping attachment and remodeling of the site can be expected for 1 year postsurgery.[47] The following outcome variables can be evaluated at 6 weeks:

- Root coverage
- Probing depth, attachment level, BOP, and Plaque Index →

- Amount of remnant root coverage
- Esthetics and color match
- Papillary height pre- and postsurgery

Q: What are the short- and long-term prognoses of this surgical procedure?

A good outcome can be anticipated considering the fact that the recession is Miller Class I, indicating that 97% to 98% root coverage can be obtained and maintained over the long term, provided brushing technique is changed and other risk factors are controlled. The results obtained by the CAF + CTG approach has been shown to be maintained in 5- to 10-year follow-up studies.[41,48]

Case 5

The patient is a 65-year-old white man complaining of oral malodor. His dentist referred him to you to access the mandibular right second molar because of swelling, pus, and soreness. When he sits in your chair, he seems disoriented and irritable. When you look in his mouth, you find generalized inflammation of the gingiva and an abscess on the buccal aspect of the mandibular right second molar with suppuration (Fig 19-33). Charting demonstrates an 8-mm facial pocket and 6-mm palatal and interproximal pockets.

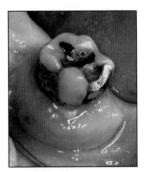

Fig 19-33 Abscess on the buccal aspect of the mandibular right second molar.

Q: What is your diagnosis of the patient?

Medical

There are a number of reasons for the patient to appear dazed and irritable:

- Hypoglycemia or hyperglycemia
- Alcohol or drug overdose
- Hyperthyroidism or hypothyroidism
- Cerebrovascular incident →

Dental

▪ The patient may have diabetes mellitus, which falls under the heading of other systemic disorders that influence the pathogenesis of periodontal disease, which is a subcategory of systemic diseases associated with loss of periodontal supporting tissues.
▪ The patient has a periodontal abscess (as opposed to a non-periodontitis abscess), which is a subclassification of periodontal abscess.

Q: What could have led to the abscess formation?

▪ Diabetes: According to Bjelland et al,[49] multiple periodontal abscesses may result from uncontrolled hyperglycemia. Rees[50] listed multiple or recurrent periodontal abscesses among the possible indications of undiagnosed or poorly controlled diabetes mellitus.
▪ The abscess may also be caused by a preexisting periodontal pocket in association with bacteria at the depth of the pocket.
▪ A foreign body can also cause a periodontal abscess.

Q: How will you treat the periodontal abscess?

▪ Ask the patient if he has seen his physician recently and whether he knows his hemoglobin A1c levels to determine if the abscess may be associated with diabetes (only his medical doctor can make that diagnosis).
▪ An incision at a 90-degree angle to the long axis of the tooth will drain the exudate. Without removal of the cause (foreign body, bacteria, or calculus), the abscess will recur. If this is not possible, extraction might be necessary.[51]
▪ Antibiotics and analgesics should be prescribed. A follow-up with a dentist is also needed.[52]

Case 6

An 80-year-old patient presents to the office with a chief complaint of a continuous burning feeling on his palate (Fig 19-34). Upon examination you find that the patient is extremely sensitive. When you finish your examination, the patient complains of sudden chest pain. He starts to sweat and has labored breathing. →

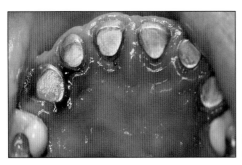

Fig 19-34 Clinical view of the patient's palate.

Q: What is your diagnosis of the patient?

- Medical: There are a number of possibilities for the patient to have chest pain and labored breathing. The patient might be experiencing an acute myocardial infarction, hyperventilation, or angina pectoris.
- Dental: The patient has a *Candida* species infection, which is a gingival disease of fungal origin. It is a subcategory of gingival diseases—non-dental biofilm-induced. It is also known as *atrophic (erythematous) candidiasis.*

Q: How will you manage the patient if he is having a myocardial infarction?

1. Stop the dental procedure.
2. Administer oxygen to the patient at 4 to 6 liters per minute.
3. Call 911.
4. Administer nitroglycerin from the emergency kit (if pain continues, most likely not angina).
5. Administer aspirin (fibrinolytic properties).
6. Monitor vital signs.
7. Manage the patient's pain with opioids (morphine) or nitrous oxide.

Q: What is your approach to treating the dental condition of this patient?

First treat the condition with a topical antifungal (eg, nystatin or clotrimazole troches) applied to the tissue side of the denture four to six times a day for 2 to 3 weeks. If the fungal infection persists, treat the patient with 100 mg fluconazole daily.

References

1. McGuire MK. Prognosis versus actual outcome: A long-term survey of 100 treated periodontal patients under maintenance care. J Periodontol 1991;62:51–58.
2. Stambaugh RV, Dragoo M, Smith DM, Carasali L. The limits of subgingival scaling. Int J Periodontics Restorative Dent 1981;1(5):30–41.
3. Caffesse RG, Sweeney PL, Smith BA. Scaling and root planing with and without periodontal flap surgery. J Clin Periodontol 1986;13:205–210.
4. Mellonig JT. Freeze-dried bone allografts in periodontal reconstructive surgery. Dent Clin North Am 1991;35:505–520.
5. Wang HL, Greenwell H, Fiorellini W; Research, Schience and Therapy Committee of the American Academy of Periodontolgy. Position paper: Periodontal regeneration. J Periodontol 2005;76:1601–1622.
6. Vignoletti F, Matesanz P, Rodrigo D, Figuero E, Martin C, Sanz M. Surgical protocols for ridge preservation after tooth extraction. A systematic review. Clin Oral Implants Res 2012;23(suppl 5):22–38.
7. Laurell L, Gottlow J, Zybutz M, Persson R. Treatment of intrabony defects by different surgical procedures. A literature review. J Periodontol 1998;69:303–313.
8. Powell CA, Mealey BL, Deas DE, McDonnell HT, Moritz AJ. Post-surgical infections: Prevalence associated with various periodontal surgical procedures. J Periodontol 2005;76:329–333.
9. Lang NP, Brägger U, Salvi GE, Tonetti MS. Supportive periodontal therapy (SPT). In: Lindhe J, Lang NP, Karring T. Clinical Periodontology and Implant Dentistry, ed 5. Oxford, UK: Blackwell Munksgaard 2008:1303.
10. Cohen RE; Research, Science and Therapy Committee of the American Academy of Periodontology. Position paper: Periodontal maintenance. J Periodontol 2003;74:1395–1401.
11. Fardal O, Linden GJ. Re-treatment profiles during long-term maintenance therapy in a periodontal practice in Norway. J Clin Periodontol 2005;32:744–749.
12. Kwok V, Caton JG. Commentary: Prognosis revisited: A system for assigning periodontal prognosis. J Periodontol 2007;78:2063–2071.
13. Beitlitum I, Artzi Z, Nemcovsky CE. Clinical evaluation of particulate allogeneic with and without autogenous bone grafts and resorbable collagen membranes for bone augmentation of atrophic alveolar ridges. Clin Oral Implants Res 2010;21:1242–1250.
14. Geurs NC, Korostoff JM, Vassilopoulos PJ, et al. Clinical and histologic assessment of lateral alveolar ridge augmentation using a synthetic long-term bioabsorbable membrane and an allograft. J Periodontol 2008;79:1133–1140.
15. Cortellini P, Tonetti MS. Regenerative periodontal therapy. In: Lindhe J, Lang NP, Karring T. Clinical Periodontology and Implant Dentistry, ed 5. Oxford, UK: Blackwell Munksgaard 2008:918.
16. Zarb GA, Albrektsson T. Criteria for determining clinical success with osseointegrated dental implants [in French]. Cah Prothese 1990;(71):19–26.
17. Cochran DL. A comparison of endosseous dental implant surfaces. J Periodontol 1999;70:1523–1539.
18. Grossi SG, Zambon JJ, Ho AW, et al. Assessment of risk for periodontal disease. I. Risk indicators for attachment loss. J Periodontol 2010;65:260–267.
19. Nunn ME. Understanding the etiology of periodontitis: An overview of periodontal risk factors. Periodontol 2000 2003;32:11–23.
20. Craddock HL, Youngson CC, Manogue M, Blance A. Occlusal changes following posterior tooth loss in adults. Part 1: A study of clinical parameters associated with the extent and type of supraeruption in unopposed posterior teeth: Clinical research. J Prosthodont 2007;16:485–494.
21. Heins PJ, Wieder SM. A histologic study of the width and nature of inter-radicular spaces in human adult pre-molars and molars. J Dent Res 1986;65:948–951.
22. Masters DH, Hoskins SW. Projection of cervical enamel into molar furcations. J Periodontol 2015;35:49–53.

23. Hou GL, Tsai CC. Relationship between periodontal furcation involvement and molar cervical enamel projections. J Periodontol 1987;58:715–721.
24. Eke PI, Dye BA, Wei L, et al. Update on prevalence of periodontitis in adults in the United States: NHANES 2009 to 2012. J Periodontol 2015;86:611–622.
25. Shiau HJ, Reynolds MA. Sex differences in destructive periodontal disease: Exploring the biologic basis. J Periodontol 2010;81:1505–1517.
26. Shiau HJ, Reynolds MA. Sex differences in destructive periodontal disease: A systematic review. J Periodontol 2010;81:1379–1389.
27. Engler WO, Ramfjord SP, Hiniker JJ. Healing following simple gingivectomy. A tritiated thymidine radioautographic study. I. Epithelialization. J Periodontol 1966;37:298–308.
28. Ramfjord SP, Engler WO, Hiniker JJ. A radioautographic study of healing following simple gingivectomy. II The connective tissue. J Periodontol 1966;37:179–189.
29. Fugazzotto PA. A comparison of the success of root resected molars and molar position implants in function in a private practice: Results of up to 15-plus years. J Periodontol 2005;72:1113–1123.
30. Lindhe J, Nyman S. Long-term maintenance of patients treated for advanced periodontal disease. J Clin Periodontol 1984;11:504–514.
31. Kaldahl WB, Kalkwarf KL, Patil KD, Dyer JK, Bates RE Jr. Evaluation of four modalities of periodontal therapy: Mean probing depth, probing attachment level and recession changes. J Periodontol 1988;59:783–793.
32. Huynh-Ba G, Kuonen P, Hofer D, Schmid J, Lang NP, Salvi GE. The effect of periodontal therapy on the survival rate and incidence of complications of multirooted teeth with furcation involvement after an observation period of at least 5 years: A systematic review. J Clin Periodontol 2009;36:164–176.
33. Hamp SE, Nyman S, Lindhe J. Periodontal treatment of multi rooted teeth. Results after 5 years. J Clin Periodontol 1975;2:126–135.
34. Baker DL, Seymour GJ. The possible pathogenesis of gingival recession: A histological study of induced recession in the rat. J Clin Periodontol 1976;3:208–219.
35. Löe H, Anerud A, Boysen H, Morrison E. Natural history of periodontal disease in man: Rapid, moderate and no loss of attachment in Sri Lankan laborers 14 to 46 years of age. J Clin Periodontol 1986;13:431–435.
36. Merijohn GK. Management and prevention of gingival recession. Periodontol 2000 2016;7:228–242.
37. Cairo F, Nieri M, Cincinelli S, Mervelt J, Pagliaro U. The interproximal clinical attachment level to classify gingival recessions and predict root coverage outcomes: An explorative and reliability study. J Clin Periodontol 2011;38:661–666.
38. Cortellini P, Bissada NF. Mucogingival conditions in the natural dentition: Narrative review, case definitions, and diagnostic considerations. J Clin Periodontol 2018;89(suppl 1):S204–S213.
39. Chambrone L, Salinas Ortega MA, Sukekava F, et al. Root coverage procedures for treating localised and multiple recession-type defects. Cochrane Database Syst Rev 2018;10:CD007161.
40. Roccuzzo M, Bunino M, Needleman I, Sanz M. Periodontal plastic surgery for treatment of localized gingival recessions: A systematic review. J Clin Periodontol. 2002;29(suppl 3):178–194.
41. Chambrone L, Tatakis DN. Periodontal soft tissue root coverage procedures: A systematic review from the AAP Regeneration Workshop. J Periodontol 2015;86(2 suppl):S8–S51.
42. Zucchelli G, Mele M, Mazzotti C, Marzadori M, Montebugnoli L, De Sanctis M. Coronally advanced flap with and without vertical releasing incisions for the treatment of multiple gingival recessions: A comparative controlled randomized clinical trial. J Periodontol 2009;80:1083–1094.
43. Fickl S, Fischer KR, Jockel-Schneider Y, Stappert CFJ, Schlagenhauf U, Kebschull M. Early wound healing and patient morbidity after single-incision vs. trap-door graft harvesting from the palate—A clinical study. Clin Oral Investig 2014;18:2213–2219.
44. Hürzeler MB, Weng D. A single-incision technique to harvest subepithelial connective tissue grafts from the palate. Int J Periodontics Restorative Dent 1999;19:279–287.

45. Studer SP, Allen EP, Rees TC, Kouba A. The thickness of masticatory mucosa in the human hard palate and tuberosity as potential donor sites for ridge augmentation procedures. J Periodontol 1997;68:145–151.

46. Engler WO, Ramfjord SP, Hiniker JJ. Healing following simple gingivectomy. A tritiated thymidine radioautographic study. I. Epithelialization. J Periodontol 2015;37:298–308.

47. Harris RJ. Creeping attachment associated with the connective tissue with partial-thickness double pedicle graft. J Periodontol 2012;68:890–899.

48. Dai A, Huang JP, Ding PH, Chen LL. Long-term stability of root coverage procedures for single gingival recessions: A systematic review and meta-analysis. J Clin Periodontol 2019;46:572–585.

49. Bjelland S, Bray P, Gupta N, Hirscht R. Dentists, diabetes and periodontitis. Aust Dent J 2002;47:202–207.

50. Rees TD. Periodontal management of the patient with diabetes mellitus. Periodontol 2000 2000;23:63–72.

51. Sivapathasundharam B. Diseases of the periodontium. In: Rajendran R, Sivapathasundharam B (eds). Shafer's Textbook of Oral Pathology, ed 6. New Delhi: Elsevier, 2009:404.

52. DeFlitch CJ. Throat and oropharynx. In: Aghababian R (ed). Essentials of Emergency Medicine. Sudbury, MA: Jones and Bartlett, 2006:238.

Appendix

Classification of Periodontal and Peri-implant Diseases and Conditions

I. Periodontal health, gingival diseases/conditions
    A. Periodontal health and gingival health
        1. Clinical gingival health on an intact periodontium (bleeing on probing [BOP] < 10% without attachment loss, erythema, edema, and radiographic bone loss, no probing depths of 4 mm or greater that bleed on probing)
        2. Clinical gingival health on a reduced periodontium
            a. Stable periodontitis patient (no BOP, erythema, and edema in the presence of reduced bone and clinical attachment levels, no probing depths of 4 mm or greater with BOP)
            b. Non-periodontitis patient
    B. Gingivitis, dental biofilm-induced
        1. Associated with dental biofilm alone
            a. Plaque-induced gingivitis on an intact periodontium
                1) Localized: BOP $\geq$ 10% and $\leq$ 30% without attachment loss and radiographic bone loss
                2) Generalized: BOP score > 30% without attachment loss and radiographic bone loss
            b. Plaque-induced gingivitis on a reduced periodontium (criteria: without a history of periodontitis, possible radiographic bone loss, all probing depths $\leq$ 3 mm)[6]
                1) Non-periodontitis patient (eg, recession, crown lengthening)
                    a) Localized: BOP $\geq$ 10% and $\leq$ 30%
                    b) Generalized: BOP > 30%
                2) Successfully treated periodontitis patient

a) Localized: BOP ≥ 10% and ≤ 30%
b) Generalized: BOP > 30%
2. Mediated by systemic or local risk factors
   a. Systemic risk factors (modifying factors)
      1) Smoking
      2) Hyperglycemia
      3) Nutritional factors
      4) Pharmacologic agents
      5) Sex steroid hormones
         a) Puberty (inflammation in presence of small amounts of plaque during adolescence)
         b) Menstrual cycle
         c) Pregnancy (inflammation in presence of small amounts of plaque during pregnancy)
         d) Oral contraceptives
      6) Hematologic conditions
   b. Oral factors enhancing plaque accumulation
      1) Prominent subgingival restoration margins
      2) Hyposalivation
3. Drug-influenced gingival enlargement
C. Gingival diseases, non–dental biofilm–induced[7] (not caused by plaque and do not resolve following plaque removal)
   1. Genetic/developmental disorders
      a. Hereditary gingival fibromatosis
   2. Specific infections
      a. Bacterial origin
         1) Necrotizing periodontal disease (*Treponema* spp, *Selenomonas* spp, *Fusobacterium* spp, *Prevotella intermedia*, and others)
         2) *Neisseria gonorrhoeae* (gonorrhea)
         3) *Treponema pallidum* (syphilis)
         4) *Myobacterium tuberculosis* (tuberculosis)
         5) *Streptococcal gingivitis* (strains of streptococcus)
      b. Viral origin
         1) Coxsackie virus (hand-foot-and-mouth disease)
         2) Herpes simplex 1/2 (primary or recurrent)
         3) Varicella-zoster virus (chicken pox or shingles affecting V nerve)
         4) Molluscum contagiosum virus
         5) Human papilloma virus (squamous cell papilloma, condyloma acuminatum, verrucca vulgaris, and focal epithelial hyperplasia)
      c. Fungal
         1) Candidosis
         2) Other mycoses (eg, histoplasmosis, aspergillosis)
   3. Inflammatory and immune conditions

      a. Hypersensitivity reactions
         1) Contact allergy
         2) Plasma cell gingivitis
         3) Erythema multiforme
      b. Autoimmune diseases of skin and mucous membranes (see chapter 16 for more detail)
         1) Pemphigus vulgaris
         2) Pemphigoid
         3) Lichen planus
         4) Lupus erythematosus
            a) Systemic lupus erythematosus
            b) Discoid lupus erythematosus
      c. Granulomatous inflammatory condition (orofacial granulomatosis)
         1) Crohn disease
         2) Sarcoidosis
   4. Reactive processes
      a. Epulides
         1) Fibrous epulis
         2) Calcifying fibroblastic granuloma
         3) Pyogenic granuloma (vascular epulis)
         4) Peripheral giant cell granuloma (or central)
   5. Neoplasms
      a. Premalignant
         1) Leukoplakia
         2) Erythroplakia
      b. Malignant
         1) Squamous cell carcinoma
         2) Leukemia
         3) Lymphoma
            a) Hodgkin
            b) Non-Hodgkin
   6. Endocrine, nutritional, and metabolic diseases
      a. Vitamin deficiencies
         1) Vitamin C deficiency (scurvy)
   7. Traumatic lesions
      a. Physical/mechanical insults
         1) Frictional keratosis
         2) Mechanically (toothbrushing) induced gingival ulceration
         3) Factitious injury (self-harm)
      b. Chemical (toxic) insults
         1) Etching
         2) Chlorhexidine
         3) Acetylsalicyclic acid

   4) Cocaine

   5) Hydrogen peroxide

   6) Dentifrice detergents

   7) Paraformaldehyde or calcium hydroxide

  c. Thermal insults

   1) Burns of mucosa

 8. Gingival pigmentation

  a. Gingival pigmentation/melanoplakia

  b. Smoker's melanosis

  c. Drug-induced pigmentation (antimalarials; minocycline)

  d. Amalgam tattoo

II. Periodontitis

 A. Staging based on severity, complexity, extent, and distribution

  1. Stage 1: Slight

- Interdental CAL 1 to 2 mm at site of greatest loss
- Radiographic bone loss < 15% in coronal third of the root, mostly horizontal
- Probing depths 3 to 4 mm

  2. Stage 2: Moderate

- Interdental CAL 3 to 4 mm at site of greatest loss
- Radiographic bone loss 15% to 33% in coronal third of root, mostly horizontal
- Probing depths 4 to 5 mm

  3. Stage 3: Severe

- Interdental CAL $\geq$ 5 mm
- Radiographic bone loss extending to middle third of root.
- Vertical defects $\geq$ 3 mm
- Probing depths $\geq$ 6 mm
- Furcation involvement grade II and III
- Masticatory function is preserved
- Moderate ridge defect
- Periodontal tooth loss $\leq$ 4 teeth

  4. Stage 4: Very severe

- Interdental CAL $\geq$ 5 mm
- Radiographic bone loss extending to middle third of root and beyond
- Probing depths $\geq$ 6 mm
- Furcation involvement grade II and III
- Masticatory dysfunction—need for complex rehabilitation
- Secondary occlusal trauma, mobility $\geq$ 2
- Bite collapse
- Less than 20 remaining teeth

- Severe ridge defect
- Periodontal tooth loss ≥ 5 teeth

B. Grading based on past progression, risk of future progression, anticipated treatment outcome, and general health status
  1. Grade A: Slow rate of progression
  2. Grade B: Moderate rate of progression
  3. Grade C: Rapid rate of progression

III. Systemic diseases associated with loss of periodontal supporting tissues
  A. Systemic disorders that have a major impact on the loss of periodontal supporting tissues by influencing periodontal inflammation
    1. Genetic disorders
      a. Diseases associated with immunologic disorders
        1) Down syndrome
        2) Leukocyte adhesion deficiency syndromes
        3) Papillon-Lefèvre syndrome
        4) Haim-Munk syndrome
        5) Chediak-Higashi syndrome
        6) Congenital neutropenia (Kostmann syndrome)
        7) Primary immunodeficiency diseases
          a) Chronic granulomatous disease
          b) Hyperimmunoglobulin E syndromes
        8) Cohen syndrome
      b. Diseases affecting the oral mucosa and gingival tissue
        1) Epidermolysis bullosa
          a) Dystrophic epidermolysis bullosa
          b) Kindler syndrome
        2) Plasminogen deficiency
      c. Diseases affecting the connective tissues
        1) Ehlers-Danlos syndromes (types IV, VIII)
        2) Angioedema (C1-inhibitor deficiency)
        3) Systemic lupus erythematosus
      d. Metabolic and endocrine disorders
        1) Glycogen storage disease
        2) Gaucher disease
        3) Hypophosphatasia
        4) Hypophosphatemic rickets
        5) Hajdu-Cheney syndrome
    2. Acquired immunodeficiency diseases
      a. Acquired neutropenia
      b. Human immunodeficiency virus infection
    3. Inflammatory immune diseases
      a. Epidermolysis bullosa acquisita
      b. Inflammatory bowel disease

B. Other systemic disorders that influence the pathogenesis of periodontal diseases
  1. Diabetes mellitus
  2. Obesity
  3. Osteoporosis
  4. Arthritis
      a. Rheumatoid arthritis
      b. Osteoarthritis
  5. Emotional stress and depression
  6. Smoking (nicotine dependence)
  7. Medications
C. Systemic disorders that can result in loss of periodontal tissues independent of periodontitis
  1. Neoplasms
      a. Primary neoplastic diseases of the periodontal tissues
          1) Squamous cell carcinoma
          2) Odontogenic tumors
          3) Other primary neoplasms
      b. Secondary metastatic neoplasms of the periodontal tissues
  2. Other disorders that may affect the periodontium
      a. Granulomatosis with polyangiitis
      b. Langerhans cell histiocytosis
      c. Giant cell granulomas
      d. Hyperparathyroidism
      e. Systemic sclerosis (scleroderma)
      f. Gorham-Stout disease (vanishing bone disease)
IV. Necrotizing periodontal diseases
  A. In severely compromised patients (eg, HIV+/AIDS, with CD4 counts < 200 and detectable viral load in adults, malnutrition and viral infections in kids)
    1. Necrotizing gingivitis (presence of necrosis/ulcer of the interdental papillae, gingival bleeding, and pain)
    2. Necrotizing periodontitis (presence of necrosis/ulcer of the interdental papillae, gingival bleeding, halitosis, pain, and rapid bone loss)
    3. Necrotizing stomatitis (severe inflammatory condition with soft tissue necrosis extending beyond the gingiva and bone denudation with formation of bone sequestrum)
    4. Noma (cancrum oris)
  B. In moderately/temporarily compromised patients (eg, uncontrolled factors, stress, nutrition, smoking)
    1. Necrotizing gingivitis
    2. Necrotizing periodontitis

V.   Periodontal abscesses
   A. In periodontitis patients (in a preexisting periodontal pocket)
      1. Acute exacerbation
         a. Untreated periodontitis
         b. Non-responsive to therapy
         c. Supportive periodontal therapy
      2. After treatment
         a. Post-scaling
         b. Postsurgery (eg, foreign body sutures or membranes)
         c. Post-medication (eg, systemic antimicrobials)
   B. In non-periodontitis patients (not mandatory to have a preexisting pocket)
      1. Impaction (eg, dental floss, rubber dam)
      2. Harmful habits (eg, nail biting)
      3. Orthodontic factors (eg, crossbite)
      4. Gingival overgrowth
      5. Alteration of the root surface
         a. Severe anatomical alterations (eg, invaginated tooth)
         b. Minor anatomical alterations (eg, cemental tears, enamel pearls)
         c. Iatrogenic conditions (eg, perforations)
         d. Severe root damage (eg, fissure or fracture)
         e. External root resorption
VI. Periodontitis associated with endodontic lesions
   A. Endodontic-periodontal lesion (pathologic communication between the pulpal and periodontal tissues at a given tooth)
      1. With root damage (pain)
         a. Root fracture/cracking
         b. Root canal or pulp chamber perforation
         c. External root resorption
      2. Without root damage
         a. In periodontitis site (slow and chronic without evident symptoms)
            1) Grade 1: Narrow deep periodontal pocket in one tooth surface
            2) Grade 2: Wide deep periodontal pocket in one tooth surface
            3) Grade 3: Deep periodontal pockets in more than one tooth surface
         b. In non-periodontitis site
            1) Grade 1: Narrow deep periodontal pocket in one tooth surface
            2) Grade 2: Wide deep periodontal pocket in one tooth surface
            3) Grade 3: Deep periodontal pockets in more than one tooth surface
VII. Developmental or acquired deformities and conditions
   A. Prostheses and tooth-related factors that modify or predispose to plaque-induced gingival diseases/periodontitis

1. Localized tooth-related factors
    a. Tooth anatomical factors
    b. Root fractures
    c. Cervical root resorption, cemental tears
    d. Root proximity
    e. Altered passive eruption
2. Localized dental prostheses–related factors
    a. Restoration margins placed within the supracrestal attached tissues
    b. Loss of periodontal supporting tissues caused by fabrication of indirect restoration
    c. Hypersensitivity/toxicity reactions to dental materials
B. Mucogingival deformities and conditions around teeth
    1. Gingival phenotype
        a. Thin scalloped (Fig 6-2)
        b. Thick scalloped (Fig 6-3)
        c. Thick flat
    2. Gingival/soft tissue recession
        a. Facial or lingual surfaces
        b. Interproximal (papillary)
        c. Severity of recession[8] (Fig 6-4)
            1) Recession type 1 (RT1): Gingival recession with no loss of interproximal attachment. Interproximal CEJ is clinically not detectable at both mesial and distal aspects of the tooth.
            2) Recession type 2 (RT2): Gingival recession associated with loss of interproximal attachment. The amount of interproximal attachment loss (measured from the interproximal CEJ to the depth of the interproximal sulcus/pocket) is less than or equal to the buccal attachment loss (measured from the buccal CEJ to the apical end of the buccal sulcus/pocket).
            3) Recession type 3 (RT3): Gingival recession associated with loss of interproximal attachment. The amount of interproximal attachment loss (measured from the interproximal CEJ to the apical end of the sulcus/pocket) is greater than the buccal attachment loss (measured from the buccal CEJ to the apical end of the buccal sulcus/pocket).
        d. Gingival thickness
        e. Gingival width
        f. Presence of noncarious cervical lesions (NCCL)/cervical caries
        g. Patient esthetic concern (smile esthetic index)
        h. Presence of hypersensitivity
    3. Lack of keratinized gingiva
    4. Decreased vestibular depth

5. Aberrant frenum/muscle position
6. Gingival excess
   a. Pseudopocket
   b. Inconsistent gingival margin
   c. Excessive gingival display
   d. Gingival enlargement
7. Abnormal color
8. Root surface condition
C. Traumatic occlusal forces
  1. Primary occlusal trauma
  2. Secondary occlusal trauma
  3. Orthodontic forces
VIII. Peri-implant diseases and conditions
  A. Peri-implant health
    1. Normal bone height
    2. Reduced bone height
  B. Peri-implant mucositis
  C. Peri-implantitis
  D. Peri-implant soft and hard tissue deficiencies
    1. Soft tissue deficiencies
      a. Thin peri-implant mucosa
      b. Lack of keratinized peri-implant mucosa
      c. Reduced papilla height
      d. Peri-implant frenum attachments
    2. Hard tissue deficiencies
      a. Horizontal ridge deficiency
      b. Vertical ridge deficiency
      c. Pneumatization of maxillary sinus
      d. Thin/absent buccal and lingual bone plates

Index

Page numbers followed by "t" denote tables; those followed by "f" denote figures

resorbable, 230f, 230–231, 389

tacks used to stabilize, 234

titanium-reinforced, 231

Meniscal derangement, 14

Mental nerve, 265

Meperidine, 69

Mepivacaine, 66t

Merkel cells, 10

Meta-analyses, 3f

Metabolic disorders, 305–306

Metastases, 330

Metronidazole, 55t–56t, 56, 157, 338

Micro-macroporous biphasic calcium phosphate, 228

Microsurgery
  advantages of, 175
  macrosurgery versus, for graft placement, 197

Midazolam, 68–69

Miller classification
  of gingival recession-type defects, 209f
  of mobility, 126–127
  of soft tissue resection, 192f

Minimally invasive surgery, 170–173

Minimally invasive surgical technique, 171

Minocycline, 55t, 56, 59t

MIS. See Minimally invasive surgery.

Misch bone density scale, 223

MIST. See Minimally invasive surgical technique.

M-MIST. See Modified minimally invasive surgical technique.

Mobile implant, 279

Mobility, 126–128

Moderate periodontitis, 105

Modified Gingival Index, 35

Modified minimally invasive surgical technique, 172, 227

Modified Widman flap, 167–168

Moi-Stir moistening solution, 75

Molars
  with accessory canals, 25
  implant therapy versus root resection in, 122–123

loss of, tooth-related factors for, 114–115

restorations, furcation lesions in, 28

root coverage of, 216

root debridement in, 141

uprighting of, using orthodontics, 136

Mouth breathing, 40

Mouthrinses, 76

MTA pulp capping, 121t

Mucocele, 336, 337t

Mucoepidermoid carcinoma, 345

Mucogingival defects, Sullivan and Atkins classification of, 192, 192f

Mucogingival deformities, 102–104

Mucogingival junction, 7f

Mucogingival surgery, smoking effects on, 202

Mucogingival therapy
  anatomy for, 203–204
  definition of, 186
  enamel matrix derivative for, 207
  endpoints of, 187
  side effects of, 188

Mucositis, peri-implant
  adjunctive therapy for, 281
  causes of, 277–278
  chlorhexidine for, 281
  definition of, 273
  description of, 104–105
  diabetes and, 279
  gingivitis versus, 258t
  illustration of, 280f
  incidence of, 280
  laser treatment for, 350
  peri-implantitis and, 257, 274t–275t, 280
  prevalence of, 280

Mucous membrane pemphigoid, 333f, 337t

Mucus retention cyst, 336, 337t

Mycelex troches, 77

Mylohyoid muscle, 16

Myocardial infarction, 316, 359, 404

N

Nabers probe, 17

Naloxone, 70

NCCLs. See Noncarious cervical lesions.

Nd:YAG laser, 347f, 351

Neck lumps, 342

Necrotizing gingivitis, 119

Necrotizing periodontal diseases, 47, 47f, 97–98

Necrotizing ulcerative periodontitis
  features of, 338, 338f
  prognosis of, 119
  treatment of, 338

Neurofibroma, 339

Neutropenia, 311

New attachment, 221

Nikolsky test, 333

Nitrous oxide, 68, 355

Noncarious cervical lesions, 125

Non–cross-linked membranes, 233

Nonfunctional contacts, 132

Nonresorbable membranes, 230f, 230–231

Nonspecific plaque hypothesis, 43

Nonspecific ulcer, 340

Nonsteroidal anti-inflammatory drugs, 60t

Nonsurgical root canal therapy, 121t

Nonsurgical therapy
  irrigation, 156–158
  scaling and root planing. See Scaling and root planing.
  surgical therapy versus, 154t, 177
  types of, 139

Nystatin, 77

O

Obesity
  inflammation and, 305–306
  osteoarthritis risks, 307
  periodontitis risks, 33

Occlusal adjustment, 133f, 133–134

Occlusal contacts, 131–132

Occlusal discrepancies, 131–132

Occlusal forces, 131, 134–135

Occlusal overload, 129

Occlusal trauma
  definition of, 125